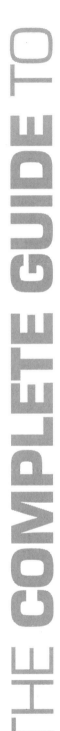

THE **COMPLETE GUIDE TO**

SPORTS
NUTRITION

Other Titles in THE **COMPLETE GUIDE** SERIES

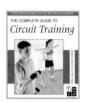
The Complete Guide to
Circuit Training
by Debbie Lawrence, Bob Hope

The Complete Guide to
Postnatal Fitness 2nd edition
by Judy DiFiore

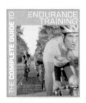
The Complete Guide to
Endurance Training
by Jon Ackland

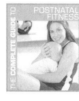
The Complete Guide to
Strength Training
by Anita Bean

The Complete Guide to
Exercise in Water
by Debbie Lawrence

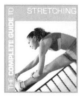
The Complete Guide to
Stretching
by Christopher Norris

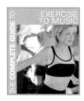
The Complete Guide to
Exercise to Music 2nd edition
by Debbie Lawrence

The Complete Guide to
Sports Massage
by Tim Paine

THE **COMPLETE GUIDE TO**

Anita Bean

SPORTS
NUTRITION

4th edition

A & C Black • London

Note

Whilst every effort has been made to ensure that the content of this book is as technically accurate and as sound as possible, neither the author nor the publishers can accept responsibility for any injury or loss sustained as a result of the use of this material

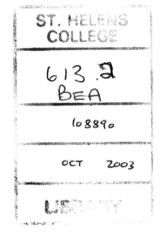
Published by A & C Black Publishers Ltd
37 Soho Square, London W1D 3QZ
www.acblack.com

Fourth edition 2003
Third edition 2000; reprinted 2001
Second edition 1996; reprinted 1997 (twice), 1998, 1999, 2000
First edition 1993; reprinted 1994, 1995

ISBN 0 7136 6741 9

A CIP catalogue record for this book is available from the British Library.

Cover photograph courtesy of Empics

Illustration on page vi © Tina Howe

All other illustrations © Clive Goodyer

Author photograph © Grant Pritchard

A & C Black uses paper produced with elemental chlorine-free pulp, harvested from managed sustainable forests.

Typeset in 10½ on 12pt Baskerville BE Regular.

Printed and bound in Great Britain by
Biddles Ltd, Guildford and Kings Lynn.

CONTENTS

APPENDICES

ACKNOWLEDGEMENTS

Thanks to my ever-patient husband for keeping me calm when the going gets tough. You always manage to stay optimistic and cheerful, giving me loads of encouragement to write the best book I can. Huge thanks to my two lovely daughters who are a constant source of inspiration for everything I do. You make it all worthwhile.

Over the last four editions I have had the privilege to work with excellent editors – Jane, Jonathan, Penny, Cheryl, Sally, Charlotte and Hannah – and am very grateful for their expert guidance and advice.

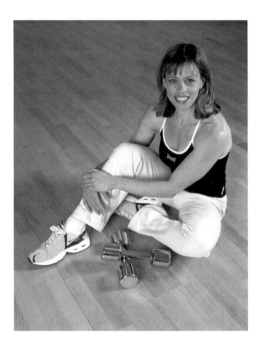

FOREWORD

In many ways, there are close similarities between the human body and a high performance car. No matter how good the chassis, engine or driver, if you put in poor quality fuel, the car won't produce its optimum performance. Our bodies are exactly the same. Even those blessed with world-class talent, or dedicated to the hardest training programmes, will not achieve their full potential if they don't eat the right foods. This is why the fourth edition of *The Complete Guide to Sports Nutrition* is such a valuable aid to anyone involved with sport and exercise, whether as a coach, teacher or athlete, or as someone simply wishing to keep fit and healthy.

All of the information in the book is based on sound, scientific theories – something that is so crucial at a time when unfounded fads and trends are all too easily adopted by athletes looking for a short cut to success. The underlying science behind correct sports nutrition is explained clearly and simply with a combination of text and diagrams, and this is used as the basis for the practical advice and information that is the essential ingredient of this text.

Over the years I have conducted research into sports nutrition, and also worked with many elite sportsmen and women. I have known Anita Bean for many years and I know from first-hand experience that the advice and help provided in this book will undoubtedly help improve and sustain optimal sports performance. I would therefore thoroughly recommend it to anyone with an interest in sport and exercise, and congratulate Anita on the fourth edition of an excellent book that has already found its way to the 'top table' of sports nutrition texts!

Jim Brewer
Director,
Lilleshall Sports Injury & Human
Performance Centre

PREFACE TO THE FOURTH EDITION

I wrote this book for everyone who takes their training seriously. It contains 18 years of my professional experience of helping athletes achieve their sporting potential through improved nutrition. The intention is to cut through the hype and confusion about what athletes should eat and drink as well as providing clear, concise and practical nutritional information.

I wanted to write a book for sportspeople that evolved from science, not heresay, and that dealt with key nutrition issues, such as what, when and how much to eat and drink. Most important of all, I want the book to be easy to understand without confusing scientific jargon or long-winded, unnecessary anecdotes: hence its question and answer style throughout, and light-hearted illustrations.

This fourth edition has been updated to include the latest scientific findings on, and recent trends in, sports nutrition. In particular, I have revised the chapters on eating before, during and after exercise, and sports supplements. New studies, reports and consensuses constantly improve our understanding and I endeavour to include the findings in each new edition of *The Complete Guide to Sports Nutrition*. I have further referenced this fourth edition to support all of the new information presented and to give you the opportunity to seek further information, should you require it.

I, too, love fitness and sport. As a former competitive athlete (British Natural Body-building Champion in 1991), I know how difficult it is to eat the right diet while maintaining a heavy training programme, full-time work and a family life. I also have first-hand experience of preparing for competition, making weight, pre-contest nerves and travelling abroad to compete. Though I no longer compete, I continue to train regularly, including weight-training, running, pilates and dance fitness in my exercise schedule. I seem to be writing more and more prolifically nowadays, as well as being a full-time mum to my two beautiful daughters, Chloe and Lucy.

Hopefully, this book will inspire you to eat healthily in order to get more out of your training programme. Remember, it's important to enjoy your food even when you are training hard or extremely busy!

Enjoy!

Anita Bean
March 2003

THE FITNESS FOOD PYRAMID

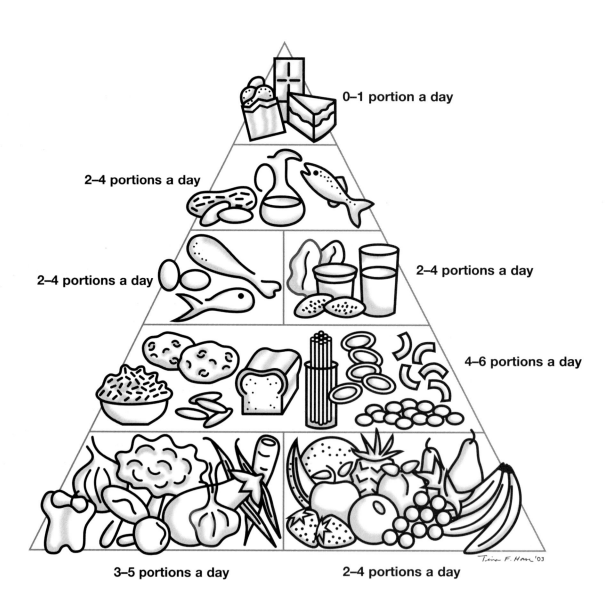

0–1 portion a day

2–4 portions a day

2–4 portions a day

2–4 portions a day

4–6 portions a day

3–5 portions a day

2–4 portions a day

The Fitness Food Pyramid is designed to meet the nutritional needs of regular exercisers and athletes. Use it as a base for developing your daily training diet.

The pyramid divides food into seven categories: fruit; vegetables; carbohydrate-rich foods; calcium-rich foods; protein-rich foods; healthy fats and junk foods. The foods in the lower layers of the pyramid should form the main part of your diet while those at the top should be eaten in smaller quantities.

- Include foods from each group in the pyramid each day
- Make sure you include a variety of foods within each group
- Aim to include the suggested number of portions from each food group each day

Fruit and vegetables
3–5 portions of vegetables a day
2–4 portions of fruit a day

Fruit and vegetables contain vitamins, minerals, fibre, antioxidants and other phytonutrients (see pages 47–57) which are vital for health, immunity and optimum performance.

Healthy carbohydrates
4–6 portions a day

A diet rich in wholegrain foods – wholewheat bread, breakfast cereas, rice, pasta, porridge oats, – beans, lentils and potatoes, maintains high glycogen (stored carbohydrate) levels, needed to fuel hard training (see p. 15).

Calcium-rich foods
2–4 portions a day

Including dairy products, nuts, pulses and tinned fish in your daily diet is the easiest way to get calcium, which is needed for strong bones (see p 62).

Protein-rich foods
2–4 portions a day

Regular exercisers need more protein than inactive people (see pages 37–8), so include lean meat, poultry, fish, eggs, soya or quorn in your daily diet. Beans, lentils, dairy foods and protein supplements can also be counted towards your daily target.

Healthy fats
2–4 portions a day

The oils found in nuts, seeds, rapeseed oil, olive oil, flax seed oil, sunflower oil, and oily fish may improve endurance, recovery as well as protect against heart disease (see pages 108–10).

Junk foods
0–1 portion a day

Biscuits, cakes, puddings, soft drinks, confectionery and crisps should be eaten only in moderation because they supply very few essential nutrients yet lots of calories, processed fats and sugars.

What counts as one portion?	
Food group	Portion size
Fruit	85–125 g (about the size of a tennis ball): 1 medium fruit, e.g. apple, 2 small fruit, e.g. kiwi fruit, 1 cupful of berries, e.g. strawberries, 1 large slice of large fruit, e.g. melon
Vegetables	85–125 g (about the size of your palm): 1 bowl of salad; 2 tbsp cooked vegetables, e.g. broccoli
Carbohydrate-rich foods	Cooked pasta, rice, grains, cereal, pulses (size of your palm); 1 baked potato (size of your fist); 2 slices bread; 1 roll or bagel
Calcium-rich foods	1 cup milk; 1 carton yoghurt; 40 g cheese (size of 4 dice)
Protein-rich foods	Meat, poultry, fish, quorn, tofu (size of a deck of cards); pulses (size of your palm); 2 eggs
Healthy fats	2 tsp oil; ½ Avocado; 2 tbsp nuts or seeds; oily fish (size of a deck of cards)

ENERGY FOR PERFORMANCE

When you exercise, your body must start producing energy much faster than it does when it is at rest. The muscles start to contract more strenuously, the heart beats faster to pump blood around the body more rapidly, and the lungs work harder. All these processes require extra energy. Where does it come from, and how can you make sure you have enough to last through a training session?

Before we can fully answer such questions, it is important to understand how the body produces energy, and what happens to it. This chapter looks at what takes place in the body when you exercise, where extra energy comes from, and how the fuel mixture used differs according to the type of exercise. It explains why fatigue occurs, how it can be delayed, and how you can get more out of training by changing your diet.

What is energy?

Although we cannot actually see energy, we can see and feel its effects in terms of heat and physical work. But what exactly is it?

Energy is produced by the splitting of a chemical bond in a substance called adenosine triphosphate (ATP). This is often referred to as the body's 'energy currency'. It is produced in every cell of the body from the breakdown of carbohydrate, fat, protein and alcohol – four fuels that are transported and transformed by various biochemical processes into the same end product.

What is ATP?

ATP is a small molecule consisting of an adenosine 'backbone' with three phosphate groups attached.

Energy is released when one of the phosphate groups splits off. When ATP loses one of its phosphate groups it becomes adenosine diphosphate, or ADP. Some energy is used to carry out work (such as muscle contractions), but most (around three-quarters) is given off as heat. This is why you feel warmer when you exercise. Once this has happened, ADP is converted back into ATP. A continual cycle takes place, in which ATP forms ADP and then becomes ATP again.

Figure 1.1 ATP

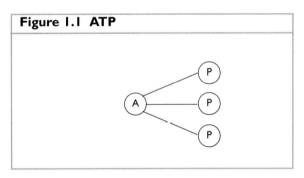

The inter-conversion of ATP and ADP

The body stores only very small amounts of ATP at any one time. There is just enough to keep up basic energy requirements while you are at rest – sufficient to keep the body ticking over. When you start exercising, energy demand suddenly increases, and the supply of ATP is used up within a few seconds. As more ATP must be produced to continue exercising, more fuel must be broken down.

Figure 1.2 The relationship between ATP and ADP

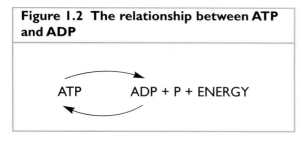

$$ATP \rightleftharpoons ADP + P + ENERGY$$

Where does energy come from?

There are four components in food and drink that are capable of producing energy:

- carbohydrate
- protein
- fat
- alcohol.

When you eat a meal or have a drink, these components are broken down in the digestive system into their various constituents or building blocks. Then they are absorbed into the bloodstream. Carbohydrates are broken down into small, single sugar units: glucose (the most common unit), fructose and galactose. Fats are broken down into fatty acids, and proteins into amino acids. Alcohol is mostly absorbed directly into the blood.

The ultimate fate of all of these components is energy production, although carbohydrates, proteins and fats also have other important functions.

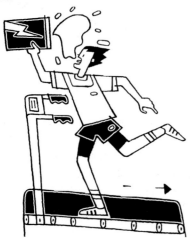

Carbohydrates and alcohol are used mainly for energy in the short term, while fats are used as a long-term energy store. Proteins can be used to produce energy either in 'emergencies' (for instance, when carbohydrates are in short supply) or when they have reached the end of their useful life. Sooner or later, all food and drink components are broken down to release energy.

How is energy measured?

Energy is ultimately given off from the body as heat. It is measured in units of heat, called joules. In scientific terms, 1 joule (J) is the energy used to move a weight of 1 kilogram (kg) over 1 metre (m) by a force of 1 newton (N). However, imperial units of energy, calories, are still used more commonly than joules. One calorie (cal) is defined as the amount of heat required to increase the temperature of 1 gram (g) of water by 1 degree centigrade (°C).

As the calorie and the joule represent very small amounts of energy, kilocalories (kcal or Cal) and kilojoules (kJ) are more often used. As their names suggest, a kilocalorie is 1000 calories and a kilojoule 1000 joules. You have probably seen these units on food labels. When we mention calories in the everyday sense, we are really talking about Calories with a capital C, or kilocalories (Cal or kcal).

To convert kilocalories into kilojoules, simply multiply by 4.2. For example:

1 kcal = 4.2 kJ
10 kcal = 42 kJ

To convert kilojoules into kilocalories, divide by 4.2. For example, if 100 g of food provides 400 kJ, and you wish to know how many kilocalories that is, divide 400 by 4.2 to find the equivalent number of kilocalories:

400 kJ ÷ 4.2 = 95 kcal

Metabolism

Metabolism is the sum of all the biochemical processes that occur in the body. There are two directions: *anabolism* is the formation of larger molecules; *catabolism* is the breakdown of larger molecules into smaller molecules. *Aerobic metabolism* includes oxygen in the processes; *anaerobic metabolism* takes place without oxygen. A *metabolite* is a product of metabolism. That means that anything made in the body is a metabolite.

The body's rate of energy expenditure is called the *metabolic rate*. Your *basal metabolic rate (BMR)* is the number of calories expended to maintain essential processes such as breathing and organ function during sleep. However, most methods measure the *resting metabolic rate (RMR)*, which is the number of calories burned over 24 hours while lying down but not sleeping.

Why do different foods provide different amounts of energy?

Foods are made of different amounts of carbohydrates, fats, proteins and alcohol. Each of these nutrients provides a certain quantity of energy when it is broken down in the body. For instance, 1 g of carbohydrate or protein releases about 4 kcal of energy, while 1 g of fat releases 9 kcal, and 1 g of alcohol releases 7 kcal.

The energy value of different food components

1 g provides:
- carbohydrate 4 kcal (17 kJ)
- fat 9 kcal (38 kJ)
- protein 4 kcal (17 kJ)
- alcohol 7 kcal (29 kJ).

Fat is the most concentrated form of energy, providing the body with more than twice as much energy as carbohydrate or protein, and also more than alcohol. However, it is not necessarily the 'best' form of energy for exercise.

All foods contain a mixture of nutrients, and the energy value of a particular food depends on the amount of carbohydrate, fat and protein it contains. For example, one slice of wholemeal bread provides roughly the same amount of energy as one pat (7 g) of butter. However, their composition is very different. In bread, most energy (75%) comes from carbohydrate, while in butter, virtually all (99.7%) comes from fat.

How does my body store carbohydrate?

Carbohydrate is stored as *glycogen* in the muscles and liver, along with about three times its own weight of water. Altogether there is about three times more glycogen stored in the muscles than in the liver. Glycogen is a large molecule, similar to starch, made up of many glucose units joined together. However, the body can store only a relatively small amount of glycogen – there is no endless supply! Like the petrol tank in a car, the body can only hold a certain amount.

The total store of glycogen in the average body amounts to about 500 g; with approximately 400 g in the muscles and 100 g in the liver. This store is equivalent to 1600–2000 kcal – enough to last one day if you were to eat nothing. This is why a low-carbohydrate diet tends to make people lose quite a lot of weight in the first few days. The weight loss is almost entirely due to loss of glycogen and water. Endurance athletes have higher muscle glycogen concentrations compared with sedentary people. Increasing your muscle mass will also increase your storage capacity for glygocen.

The purpose of liver glycogen is to maintain blood glucose levels at rest and during prolonged exercise.

Small amounts of glucose are present in the blood (approximately 15 g, which is equivalent to 60 kcal) and in the brain (about 2 g or 8 kcal) and their concentrations are kept within a very narrow range, both at rest and during exercise. This allows normal body functions to continue.

How does my body store fat?

Fat is stored as *adipose* (fat) tissue in almost every region of the body. A small amount of fat, about 300–400 g, is stored in muscles – this is called intramuscular fat – but the majority is stored around the organs and beneath the skin. The amount stored in different parts of the body depends on genetic make-up and individual hormone balance. The average 70 kg person stores 10–15 kg fat. Interestingly, people who store fat mostly around their abdomen (the classic pot-belly shape) have a higher risk of heart disease than those who store fat mostly around their hips and thighs (the classic pear shape).

Unfortunately, there is little you can do to change the way that your body distributes fat. But you can definitely change the *amount* of fat that is stored, as you will see in Chapter 7.

You will probably find that your basic shape is similar to that of one or both of your parents. Males usually take after their father, and females after their mother. Female hormones tend to favour fat storage around the hips and thighs, while male hormones encourage fat storage around the middle. This is why, in general, women are 'pear shaped' and men are 'apple shaped'.

How does my body store protein?

Protein is not stored in the same way as carbohydrate and fat. It forms muscle and organ tissue, so it is mainly used as a building material rather than an energy store. However, proteins *can* be broken down to release energy if need be, so muscles and organs represent a large source of potential energy.

Which fuels are most important for exercise?

Carbohydrates, fats and proteins are all capable of providing energy for exercise; they can all be transported to, and broken down in, muscle cells. Alcohol, however, cannot be used directly by muscles for energy during exercise, no matter how strenuously they may be working. Only the liver has the specific enzymes needed to break down alcohol. You cannot break down alcohol faster by exercising harder either – the liver carries out its job at a fixed speed. Do not think you can work off a few drinks by going for a jog, or by drinking a cup of black coffee!

Proteins do not make a substantial contribution to the fuel mixture. It is only during very prolonged or very intense bouts of exercise that proteins play a more important role in giving the body energy.

The production of ATP during most forms of exercise comes mainly from broken down carbohydrates and fats.

Table 1.1 illustrates the potential energy available from the different types of fuel that are stored in the body.

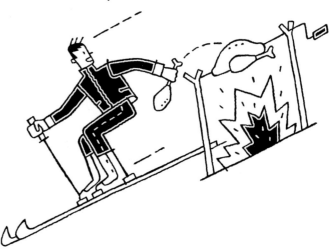

Table 1.1	Fuel reserves in a person weighing 70 kg		
Fuel stores	Potential energy available (kcal)		
	Glycogen	Fat	Protein
Liver	400	450	400
Adipose tissue (fat)	0	135,000	0
Muscle	1200	350	24,000

Source: Cahill, 1976.

When is protein used for energy?

Protein is not usually a major source of energy, but it may play a more important role during the latter stages of very strenuous or prolonged exercise as glycogen stores become depleted. For example, during the last stages of a marathon or a long distance cycle race, when glycogen stores are exhausted, the proteins in muscles (and organs) may make up around 10% of the body's fuel mixture.

During a period of semi-starvation, or if a person follows a low-carbohydrate diet, glycogen would be in short supply, so more proteins would be broken down to provide the body with fuel. Up to half of the weight lost by someone following a low-calorie or low-carbohydrate diet comes from protein (muscle) loss. Some people think that if they deplete their glycogen stores by following a low-carbohydrate diet, they will force their body to break down more fat and lose weight. This is not the case: you risk losing muscle as well as fat, and there are many other disadvantages, too. These are discussed in Chapter 8.

HOW IS ENERGY PRODUCED?

The body has three main energy systems it can use for different types of physical activity. These are called:

1 the ATP–PC (phosphagen) system

2 the anaerobic glycolytic, or lactic acid, system
3 the aerobic system – comprising of the glycolytic (carbohydrate) and lipolytic (fat) systems.

At rest, muscle cells contain only a very small amount of ATP, enough to maintain basic energy needs and allow you to exercise at maximal intensity for about 1 second. To continue exercising, ATP must be regenerated from one of the three energy systems, each of which has a very different biochemical pathway and rate at which it produces ATP.

How does the ATP–PC system work?

This system uses ATP and phosphocreatine (PC) that is stored within the muscle cells, to generate energy for maximal bursts of strength and speed that last for up to 6 seconds. The ATP–PC system would be used, for example, during a 20-metre sprint, a near-maximal lift in the gym, or a single jump. Phosphocreatine is a high-energy compound formed when the protein, creatine, is linked to a phosphate molecule (see box 'What is creatine?'). The PC system can be thought of as a back-up to ATP. The job of PC is to regenerate ATP rapidly (see Fig. 1.3). PC breaks down into creatine and phosphate, and the free phosphate bond transfers to a molecule of ADP forming a new ATP molecule. The ATP–PC system can

Figure 1.3 PC splits to release energy to regenerate ATP rapidly

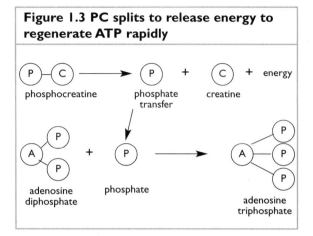

release energy very quickly, but, unfortunately, it is in very limited supply and can only provide 3–4 kcal. After this the amount of energy produced by the ATP–PC system falls dramatically, and ATP must be produced from other fuels, such as glycogen or fat. When this happens, other systems take over.

What is creatine?

Creatine is a compound that's made naturally in our bodies to supply energy. It is mainly produced in the liver from the amino acids glycine, arginine and methionine. From the liver it is transported in the blood to the muscle cells where it is combined with phosphate to make *phosphocreatine* (PC).

The muscle cells turnover about 2–3 g of creatine a day. Once PC is broken down into ATP (energy), it can be recycled into PC or converted into another substance called creatinine, which is then removed via the kidneys in the urine.

Creatine can be obtained in the diet from fish (tuna, salmon, cod), beef and pork (approx. 3–5 g creatine/kg uncooked fish or meat). That means vegetarians have no dietary sources. However, to have a performance-boosting effect, creatine has to be taken in large doses. This is higher than you could reasonably expect to get from food. You would need to eat at least 2 kg of raw steak a day to load your muscles with creatine.

The average-sized person stores about 120 g creatine, almost all in skeletal muscles (higher levels in fast-twitch muscle fibres, see p. 8). Of this amount, 60–70% is stored as PC, 30–40% as free creatine.

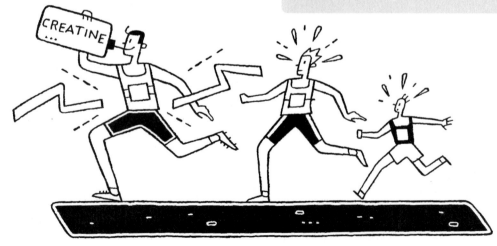

How does the anaerobic glycolytic system work?

This system is activated as soon as you begin high-intensity activity. It dominates in events lasting up to 90 seconds, such as a weight training set in the gym or a 400–800 m sprint. In order to meet sudden, large demands for energy, glucose bypasses the energy producing pathways that would normally use oxygen, and follows a different route that does not use oxygen. This saves a good deal of time. After 30 seconds of high-intensity exercise this system contributes up to 60% of your energy output; after 2 minutes its contribution falls to only 35%.

The anaerobic glycolytic system uses carbohydrate in the form of muscle glycogen or glucose as fuel. Glycogen is broken down to glucose, which rapidly breaks down in the absence of oxygen to form ATP and lactic acid (*see* Fig. 1.4). Each glucose molecule produces only two ATP molecules under anaerobic conditions, making it a very inefficient system. The body's glycogen stores dwindle quickly, proving that the benefits of a fast delivery service come at a price. The gradual build-up of lactic

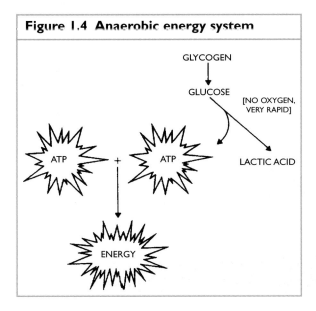

Figure 1.4 Anaerobic energy system

What happens to the lactic acid?

Lactic acid produced by the muscles is not a wasted by-product. It constitutes a valuable fuel. When the exercise intensity is reduced or you stop exercising, lactic acid has two possible fates. Some may be converted into another substance called *pyruvic acid*, which can then be broken down in the presence of oxygen into ATP. In other words, lactic acid produces ATP and constitutes a valuable fuel for aerobic exercise. Alternatively, lactic acid may be carried away from the muscle in the bloodstream to the liver where it can be converted back into glucose, released back into the bloodstream or stored as glycogen in the liver (a process called *gluconeogenesis). This mechanism for removing* lactic acid from the muscles is called the lactic acid shuttle.

This explains why the muscle soreness and stiffness experienced after hard training is not due to lactic acid accumulation. In fact, the lactic acid is usually cleared within 15 minutes of exercise.

acid will eventually cause fatigue and prevent further muscle contractions. (Contrary to popular belief, it is not lactic acid, but the build up of hydrogen ions and acidity that causes the 'burning' feeling during or immediately after maximal exercise – see p. 12.)

How does the aerobic system work?

The aerobic system can generate ATP from the breakdown of carbohydrates (by glycolysis) and fat (by lipolysis) in the presence of oxygen (*see* Fig. 1.5). Although the aerobic system cannot produce ATP as rapidly as can the other two anaerobic systems, it can produce larger amounts. When you start to exercise, you initially use the ATP–PC and anaerobic

Figure 1.5 Aerobic energy system

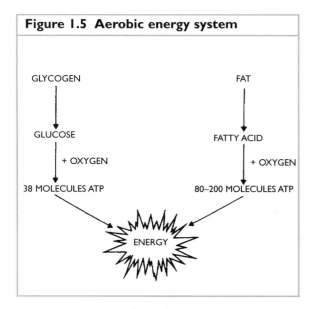

GLYCOGEN

GLUCOSE

+ OXYGEN

38 MOLECULES ATP

FAT

FATTY ACID

+ OXYGEN

80–200 MOLECULES ATP

ENERGY

glycolytic systems, but after a few minutes your energy supply gradually switches to the aerobic system.

Most of the carbohydrate which fuels aerobic glycolysis comes from muscle glycogen. Additional glucose from the bloodstream becomes more important as exercise continues for longer than 1 hour and muscle glycogen concentration dwindles. Typically, after 2 hours of high-intensity exercise (greater than 70% VO_2max), almost all of your muscle glycogen will be depleted. Glucose delivered from the bloodstream is then used to fuel your muscles, along with increasing amounts of fat (lipolytic glycolysis). Glucose from the bloodstream may be derived from the breakdown of liver glycogen or from carbohydrate consumed during exercise.

In aerobic exercise, the demand for energy is slower and smaller than in an anaerobic activity, so there is more time to transport sufficient oxygen from the lungs to the muscles and for glucose to generate ATP with the help of the oxygen. Under these circumstances, one molecule of glucose can create up to 38 molecules of ATP. Thus, aerobic energy production is about 20 times more efficient than anaerobic energy production.

Anaerobic exercise uses only glycogen, whereas aerobic exercise uses both glycogen and fat, so it can be kept up for longer. The disadvantage, though, is that it produces energy more slowly.

Fats can also be used to produce energy in the aerobic system. One fatty acid can produce between 80 and 200 ATP molecules, depending on its type (*see* Fig. 1.5). Fats are therefore an even more efficient energy source than carbohydrates. However, they can only be broken down into ATP under aerobic conditions when energy demands are relatively low, and so energy production is slower.

Muscle fibre types and energy production

The body has several different muscle fibre types, which can be broadly classified into fast-twitch (FT) or type II, and slow-twitch (ST) or type I (endurance) fibres. Both muscle fibre types use all three energy systems to produce ATP but the FT fibres use mainly the ATP–PC and anaerobic glycolytic systems, while the ST fibres use mainly the aerobic system.

Everyone is born with a specific distribution of muscle fibre types; the proportion of FT fibres to ST fibres can vary quite considerably between individuals. The proportions of each muscle fibre type you have has implications for sport. For example, top sprinters have a greater proportion of FT fibres than average and thus can generate explosive power and speed. Distance runners, on the other hand, have proportionally more ST fibres and are better able to develop aerobic power and endurance.

How do my muscles decide whether to use fat or carbo-hydrate during aerobic exercise?

During aerobic exercise the use of carbohydrate relative to fat varies according to a number of factors. The most important are:

1 the intensity of exercise
2 the duration of exercise
3 your fitness level
4 your pre-exercise diet.

Intensity

The higher the intensity of your exercise, the greater the reliance on muscle glycogen (*see* Fig. 1.6). During anaerobic exercise, energy is produced by the ATP–PC and anaerobic glycolytic systems. So, for example, during sprints, heavy weight training and intermittent maximal bursts during sports like football and rugby, muscle glycogen, rather than fat, is the major fuel.

During aerobic exercise you will use a mixture of muscle glycogen and fat for energy. Exercise at a low intensity (less than 50% of VO$_2$max) is fuelled mainly by fat. As you increase your exercise intensity, for example, as you increase your running speed, you will use a higher proportion of glycogen than fat. During

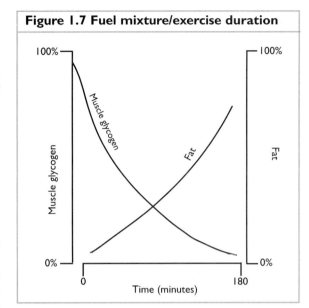

Figure 1.7 Fuel mixture/exercise duration

moderate-intensity exercise (50–70% VO$_2$max), muscle glycogen supplies around half your energy needs; the rest comes from fat. When your exercise intensity exceeds 70% VO$_2$max, fat cannot be broken down and transported fast enough to meet energy demands so muscle glycogen provides at least 75% of your energy needs.

Duration

Muscle glycogen is unable to provide energy indefinitely as it is stored in relatively small quantities. As you continue exercising, your muscle glycogen stores become progressively lower (*see* Fig. 1.7). Thus, as muscle glycogen concentration drops, the contribution that blood glucose makes to your energy needs increases. The proportion of fat used for energy also increases but it can never be burned without the presence of carbohydrate.

On average, you have enough muscle glycogen to fuel 90–180 minutes of endurance activity; the higher the intensity, the faster your muscle glycogen stores will be depleted. During

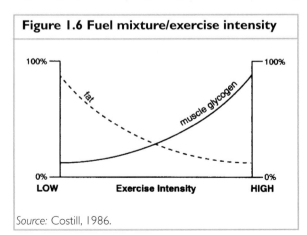

Figure 1.6 Fuel mixture/exercise intensity

Source: Costill, 1986.

interval training, i.e. a mixture of endurance and anaerobic activity, muscle glycogen stores will become depleted after 45–90 minutes. During mainly anaerobic activities, muscle glycogen will deplete within 30–45 minutes.

Once muscle glycogen stores are depleted, protein makes an increasing contribution to energy needs. Muscle proteins break down to provide amino acids for energy production and to maintain normal blood glucose levels.

Fitness level

As a result of aerobic training, your muscles make a number of adaptations to improve your performance, and your body's ability to use fat as a fuel improves. Aerobic training increases the numbers of key fat-oxidising enzymes, such as hormone-sensitive lipase, which means your body becomes more efficient in breaking down fat into fatty acids. The number of blood capillaries serving the muscle increases so you can transport the fatty acids to the muscle cells. The number of mitochondria (the sites of fatty acid oxidation) also increases which means you have a greater capacity to burn fatty acids in each muscle cell. Thus, improved aerobic fitness enables you to break down fat at a faster rate at any given intensity, thus allowing you to spare glycogen (*see* Fig. 1.8). This is important because glycogen is in much shorter supply than fat. By using proportionally more fat, you will be able to exercise for longer before muscle glycogen is depleted and fatigue sets in.

Figure 1.8 Trained people use less glycogen and more fat

Glycogen utilisation (Low to High) vs Exercise intensity (Low to High), showing "untrained" and "trained" curves.

Pre-exercise diet

A low-carbohydrate diet will result in low muscle and liver glycogen stores. Many studies have shown that initial muscle glycogen concentration is critical to your performance and that low muscle glycogen can reduce your ability to sustain exercise at 70% VO_2max for longer than 1 hour (Bergstrom et al., 1967). It also affects your ability to perform during shorter periods of maximal power output.

When your muscle glycogen stores are low, your body will rely heavily on fat and protein. However, this is not a recommended strategy for fat loss, as you will lose lean tissue. (See Chapter 8 for appropriate ways of reducing body fat.)

WHICH ENERGY SYSTEMS DO I USE IN MY SPORT?

Virtually every activity uses all three energy systems to a greater or lesser extent. No single energy system is used exclusively and at any given time energy is being derived from each of the three systems (*see* Fig. 1.9). In every activity,

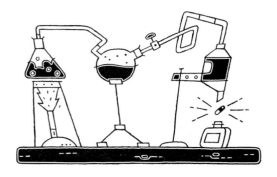

ATP is always used and is replaced by PC. Anaerobic glycolysis and aerobic energy production depend on exercise intensity.

For example, during explosive strength and power activities lasting up to 5 seconds, such as a sprint start, the existing store of ATP is the primary energy source. For activities involving high power and speed lasting 5–30 seconds, such as 100–200 m sprints, the ATP–PC system is the primary energy source, together with some muscle glycogen broken down through anaerobic glycolysis. During power endurance activities such as 400–800 m events, muscle glycogen is the primary energy source and produces ATP via both anaerobic and aerobic glycolysis. In aerobic power activities, such as running 5–10 km, muscle glycogen is the primary energy source producing ATP via

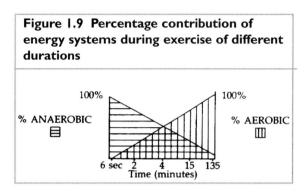

Figure 1.9 Percentage contribution of energy systems during exercise of different durations

aerobic glycolysis. During aerobic events lasting 2 hours or more, such as half- and full marathons, muscle glycogen, liver glycogen, intra-muscular fat and fat from adipose tissue are the main fuels used. The energy systems and fuels used for various types of activities are summarised in Table 1.2.

Table 1.2	The main energy systems used during different types of exercise	
Type of exercise	Main energy system	Major storage fuels used
Maximal short bursts lasting less than 6 sec	ATP–PC (phosphagen)	ATP and PC
High intensity lasting up to 30 sec	ATP–PC Anaerobic glycolytic	ATP and PC Muscle glycogen
High intensity lasting up to 15 min	Anaerobic glycolytic Aerobic	Muscle glycogen
Moderate–high intensity lasting 15–60 min	Aerobic	Muscle glycogen Adipose tissue
Moderate–high intensity lasting 60–90 min	Aerobic	Muscle glycogen Liver glycogen Blood glucose Intra-muscular fat Adipose tissue
Moderate intensity lasting longer than 90 min	Aerobic	Muscle glycogen Liver glycogen Blood glucose Intra-muscular fat Adipose tissue

What happens in my body when I start exercising?

When you begin to exercise, energy is produced without oxygen for at least the first few seconds, before your breathing rate and heart can catch up with energy demands. Therefore, a build-up of lactic acid takes place. As the heart and lungs work harder, getting more oxygen into your body, carbohydrates and fats can be broken down aerobically. If you are exercising fairly gently (i.e. your oxygen supply keeps up with your energy demands), any lactic acid that accumulated earlier can be removed easily since there is now enough oxygen around.

If you continue to exercise aerobically, more oxygen is delivered around the body and more fat starts to be broken down into fatty acids. They are taken to muscle cells via the bloodstream and then broken down with oxygen to produce energy.

In effect, the anaerobic system 'buys time' in the first few minutes of an exercise, before the body's slower aerobic system can start to function.

For the first 5–15 minutes of exercise (depending on your aerobic fitness level) the main fuel is carbohydrate (glycogen). As time goes on, however, more oxygen is delivered to the muscles, and you will use proportionally less carbohydrate and more fat.

On the other hand, if you begin exercising very strenuously (e.g. by running fast), lactic acid quickly builds up in the muscles. The delivery of oxygen cannot keep pace with the huge energy demand, so lactic acid continues to accumulate and very soon you will feel fatigue. You must then either slow down and run more slowly, or stop. Nobody can maintain a fast run for very long.

If you start a distance race or training run too fast, you will suffer from fatigue early on and be forced to reduce your pace considerably. A head start will not necessarily give any benefit at all. Warm up *before* the start of a race (by walking, slow jogging, or performing gentle mobility exercises), so that the heart and lungs can start to work a little harder, and oxygen delivery to the muscles can increase. Start the race at a moderate pace, gradually building up to an optimal speed. This will prevent a large 'oxygen debt' and avoid an early depletion of glycogen. In this way, your optimal pace can be sustained for longer.

The anaerobic system can also 'cut in' to help energy production, for instance when the demand for energy temporarily exceeds the body's oxygen supply. If you run uphill at the same pace as on the flat, your energy demand increases. The body will generate extra energy by breaking down glycogen/glucose anaerobically. However, this can only be kept up for a short period of time, because there will be a gradual build-up of lactic acid. The lactic acid can be removed aerobically afterwards, by running back down the hill, for example.

The same principle applies during fast bursts of activity in interval training, when energy is produced anaerobically. Lactic acid accumulates and is then removed during the rest interval.

WHAT IS FATIGUE?

In scientific terms, fatigue is an inability to sustain a given power output or speed. It is a mismatch between the demand for energy by the exercising muscles and the supply of energy in the form of ATP. Runners experience fatigue when they are no longer able to maintain their speed; footballers are slower to sprint for the ball and their technical ability falters; in the gym, you can no longer lift the weight; in an aerobics class, you will be unable to maintain the pace and intensity. Subjectively, you will find that exercise feels much harder to perform, your legs may feel hollow and it becomes increasingly hard to push yourself.

Why does fatigue develop during anaerobic exercise?

During explosive activities involving maximal power output, fatigue develops due to ATP and PC depletion. In other words, the demand for ATP exceeds the readily available supply.

During activities lasting between 30 seconds and 30 minutes, fatigue is caused by a different mechanism. The rate of lactic acid removal in the bloodstream cannot keep pace with the rate of lactic acid production. So during high-intensity exercise lasting up to half an hour there is a gradual increase in muscle acidity, which reduces the ability of the muscles to maintain intense contractions. It is not possible to continue high-intensity exercise indefinitely because the acute acid environment in your muscles would inhibit further contractions and cause cell death. The burning feeling you experience when a high concentration of lactic acid develops is a kind of safety mechanism, preventing the muscle cells from destruction.

Reducing your exercise intensity will lower the rate of lactic acid production, reduce the build-up, and enable the muscles to switch to the aerobic energy system, thus enabling you to continue exercising.

Why does fatigue develop during aerobic exercise?

Fatigue during moderate and high-intensity aerobic exercise lasting longer than 1 hour occurs when muscle glycogen stores are depleted. It's like running out of petrol in your car. Muscle glycogen is in short supply compared with the body's fat stores. Liver glycogen can help maintain blood glucose levels and a supply of carbohydrate to the exercising

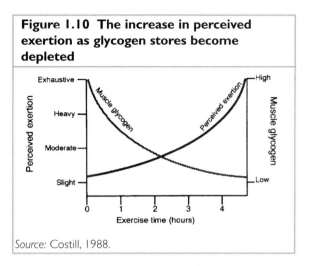

Figure 1.10 The increase in perceived exertion as glycogen stores become depleted

Source: Costill, 1988.

muscles, however stores are also very limited and eventually fatigue will develop as a result of both muscle and liver glycogen depletion and hypoglycaemia (*see* Fig. 1.10).

During low–moderate-intensity exercise lasting more than three hours, fatigue is caused by additional factors. Once glycogen stores have been exhausted, the body switches to the aerobic lipolytic system where fat is able to supply most (not all) of the fuel for low-intensity exercise. However, despite having relatively large fat reserves, you will not be able to continue

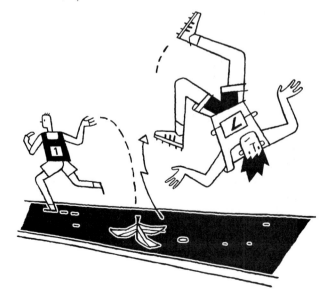

exercise indefinitely as fat cannot be converted to energy fast enough to keep up with the demand by exercising muscles. Even if you slowed your pace to enable the energy supplied by fat to meet the energy demand, other factors will cause you to fatigue. These include a rise in the concentration of the brain chemical serotonin, which results in an overall feeling of tiredness, acute muscle damage, and fatigue due to lack of sleep.

How can I delay fatigue?

Glycogen is used during virtually every type of activity. Therefore the amount of glycogen stored in your muscles and, in certain events, your liver, before you begin exercise will have a direct affect on your performance. The greater your pre-exercise muscle glycogen store the longer you will be able to maintain your exercise intensity, and delay the onset of fatigue. Conversely, sub-optimal muscle glycogen stores can cause earlier fatigue, reduce your endurance, reduce your intensity level and result in smaller training gains.

You may also delay fatigue by reducing the rate at which you use up muscle glycogen. You can do this by pacing yourself, gradually building up to your optimal intensity.

SUMMARY OF KEY POINTS

- The body uses three energy systems: (1) the ATP–PC, or phosphagen, system; (2) the anaerobic glycolytic, or lactic acid, system; (3) the aerobic system, which comprises both glycolytic (carbohydrate) and lipolytic (fat) systems.
- The ATP–PC system fuels maximal bursts of activity lasting up to 6 seconds.

- Anaerobic glycolysis provides energy for short-duration high-intensity exercise lasting from 30 seconds to several minutes. Muscle glycogen is the main fuel.
- The lactic acid produced during anaerobic glycolysis is a valuable fuel for further energy production when exercise intensity is reduced.
- The aerobic system provides energy from the breakdown of carbohydrate and fat for sub-maximal intensity, prolonged exercise.
- Factors that influence the type of energy system and fuel usage are exercise intensity and duration, your fitness level and your pre-exercise diet.
- The proportion of muscle glycogen used for energy increases with exercise intensity and decreases with exercise duration.
- For most activities lasting longer than 30 seconds, all three energy systems are used to a greater or lesser extent; however, one system usually dominates.
- The main cause of fatigue during anaerobic activities lasting less than 6 seconds is ATP and PC depletion; during activities lasting between 30 seconds and 30 minutes it is lactic acid accumulation and muscle cell acidity.
- Fatigue during moderate and high-intensity exercise lasting longer than 1 hour is usually due to muscle glycogen depletion. For events lasting longer than 2 hours fatigue is associated with low liver glycogen and low blood sugar levels.
- For most activities, performance is limited by the amount of glycogen in the muscles. Low pre-exercise glycogen stores lead to early fatigue, reduced exercise intensity and reduced training gains.

BEFORE, DURING AND AFTER EXERCISE 2

Carbohydrate is needed to fuel almost every type of activity and the amount of glycogen stored in your muscles and liver has a direct effect on your exercise performance. A high muscle-glycogen concentration will allow you to train at your optimal intensity and achieve a greater training effect. A low muscle-glycogen concentration, on the other hand, will lead to early fatigue, reduced training intensity and sub-optimal performance.

Clearly, then, glycogen is the most important and most valuable fuel for any type of exercise. This chapter explains what happens if you fail to eat enough carbohydrate and glycogen levels become depleted. It shows you how to calculate your precise carbohydrate requirements and considers the latest research on the timing of carbohydrate intake in relation to training.

Each different carbohydrate produces a different response in the body, so this chapter gives advice on which types of carbohydrate foods to eat. It presents comprehensive information on the glycaemic index (GI), a key part of every athlete's nutritional tool box. Finally, it considers the current thinking on carbohydrate loading before a competition.

The relationship between muscle glycogen and performance

The importance of carbohydrates in relation to exercise performance was first demonstrated in 1939. Christensen and Hansen, found that a high-carbohydrate diet significantly increased endurance. However, it wasn't until the 1970s that scientists discovered that the capacity for endurance exercise is related to pre-exercise glycogen stores and that a high-carbohydrate diet increases glycogen stores.

In a pioneering study, three groups of athletes were given a low-carbohydrate diet, a high-carbohydrate diet or moderate-carbohydrate diet (Bergstrom et al., 1967). Researchers measured the concentration of glycogen in their leg muscles and found that those athletes eating the high-carbohydrate diet stored twice as much glycogen as those on the moderate-carbohydrate diet and 7 times as much as those eating the low-carbohydrate diet. Afterwards, the athletes were instructed to cycle to exhaustion on a stationary bicycle at 75% of VO_2max. Those on the high-carbohydrate diet managed to cycle for 170 minutes, considerably longer than those on the moderate-carbohydrate diet (115 minutes) or the low-carbohydrate diet (60 minutes) (*see* Fig 2.1).

Figure 2.1 The effect of carbohydrate intake on performance

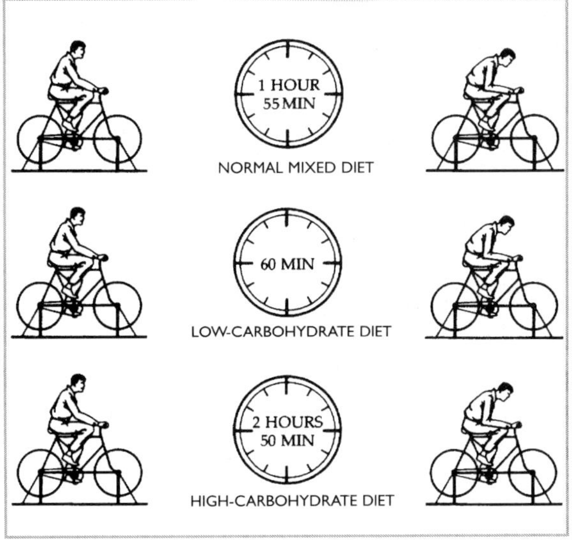

1 HOUR 55 MIN

NORMAL MIXED DIET

60 MIN

LOW-CARBOHYDRATE DIET

2 HOURS 50 MIN

HIGH-CARBOHYDRATE DIET

HOW MUCH CARBOHYDRATE SHOULD I EAT PER DAY?

Sports nutritionists and exercise physiologists consistently recommend that regular exercisers consume a diet containing a relatively high percentage of energy from carbohydrate and a relatively low percentage of energy from fat (American Dietetic Association, 1993). There is plentiful evidence that such a diet enhances endurance and performance during training.

This recommendation is based on the fact that carbohydrate is very important for endurance exercise since carbohydrate stores – as muscle and liver glycogen – are limited. Depletion of these stores results in fatigue and reduced performance. This can easily happen if your pre-exercise glycogen stores are low. In order to get the most out of your training session, you should ensure your pre-exercise glycogen stores are high. This will help to improve your endurance, delay exhaustion and help you exercise longer and harder (Coyle, 1988; Costill & Hargreaves, 1992).

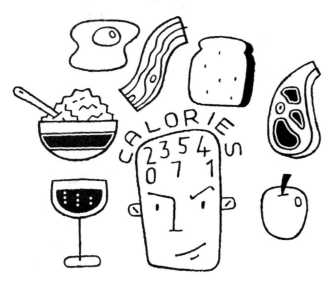

You can estimate your optimum carbohydrate intake in one of two ways:

From your energy intake

The International Conference on Foods, Nutrition & Performance in 1991, recommended a diet containing *60–70% energy from carbohydrate* (Williams & Devlin, 1992). You can estimate your usual energy (calorie) intake by keeping a weighed food diary over several consecutive days then looking up the calorie values of each food using food tables or a calorie counter (e.g. Chan, W., 2003).

Alternatively, you can use the formulae based on RMR (*see* Chapter 8, steps 1–4, p. 118) to estimate your energy needs. Multiply this value by 60% (or 0.6) then divide by 4 (because 1 g carbohydrate yields 4 kcal) to get your ideal daily carbohydrate intake in grams.

Example:

Energy intake = 3000
Calories from Carbohydrate = 3000 × 60%
$$= 1800$$
g Carbohydrate = 1800 ÷ 4 = 450 g

However, this method can be misleading in terms of providing optimum nutrition. For those with high energy requirements – say, 4000–5000 calories daily – even a diet providing 50% of energy from carbohydrate would contain 500–600 g of carbohydrate, which is more than enough to maintain muscle glycogen stores (Coyle, 1995). Conversely, for those with low energy requirements – say, less than 2000 calories daily – even a diet providing 60% energy from carbohydrate would not contain enough carbohydrate to maintain muscle glycogen stores.

From your body weight and activity level

This method, based on individuals' body weight and training volumes, is more popular among sports nutritionists and sports scientists who consider it to be more accurate. It is more flexible as it takes account of different training requirements and can be calculated independent of calorie intake (Schokman, 1999). Table 2.1 indicates the amount of carbohydrate per kg of body weight needed per day according to your activity level.

Example based on a male athlete who exercises for one hour a day:

Body weight = 70 kg
Carbohydrate need = 6 g/kg of body weight
Daily carbohydrate need = 70 × 6 = 420 g

WHICH CARBOHYDRATES ARE BEST?

Carbohydrates are traditionally classified according to their chemical structure. The most simplistic method divides them into two categories: *simple* (sugars) and *complex* (starches and fibres). These terms simply refer to the number of sugar units in the molecule.

Simple carbohydrates are very small molecules consisting of one or two sugar units.

Is a high carbohydrate diet practical?

In practice, eating a high carbohydrate diet can be difficult, particularly for those athletes with high energy needs. Many complex carbohydrate foods, such as bread, potatoes and pasta are quite bulky and the diet quickly becomes very filling, particularly if whole grain and high fibre foods make up most of your carbohydrate intake. Several surveys have found that endurance athletes often fail to consume the recommended carbohydrate levels (Frentsos, 1999; Jacobs & Sherman, 1999). Most get between 45 and 65% of their calories from carbohydrate. This may be partly due to the large number of calories needed and therefore the bulk of their diet, and partly due to lack of awareness of the benefits of a higher carbohydrate intake. It is interesting that most of the studies upon which the carbohydrate recommendations were made, used liquid carbohydrates (i.e. drinks) to supplement meals. Tour de France cyclists and triathletes consume up to one third of their carbohydrate in liquid form. If you are finding a high carbohydrate diet impractical, try eating smaller more frequent meals and supplementing your food with liquid forms of carbohydrate such as meal replacement shakes (see p. 67) and glucose polymer drinks (see p. 91).

Table 2.1	How much carbohydrate?
Activity level*	g carbohydrate/kg body weight/day
3–5 hours/week	4–5
5–7 hours/week	5–6
1–2 hours/day	6–7
2–4 hours/day	7–8
More than 4 hours/day	8–10

*Number of hours of moderate intensity exercise or sport

They comprise the *monosaccharides* (1-sugar units): glucose (dextrose), fructose (fruit sugar) and galactose; and the *disaccharides* (2-sugar units): sucrose (table sugar, which comprises a glucose and fructose molecule joined together) and lactose (milk sugar, which comprises a glucose and galactose molecule joined together).

Complex carbohydrates are much larger molecules, consisting of between 10- and several thousand-sugar units (mostly glucose) joined together. They include the starches, amylose and amylopectin, and the non-starch polysaccharides (dietary fibre), such as cellulose, pectin and hemicellulose.

In between simple and complex carbohydrates are glucose polymers and maltodextrin, which comprise between 3- and 10-sugar units. They are made from the partial breakdown of corn starch in food processing, and are widely used as bulking and thickening agents in processed foods, such as sauces, dairy desserts, baby food, puddings and soft drinks. They are popular ingredients in sports drinks and engineered meal-replacement products, owing to their low sweetness and high energy density relative to sucrose.

In practice, many foods contain a mixture of both simple and complex carbohydrates, making the traditional classification of foods into 'simple' and 'complex' very confusing. For example, biscuits and cakes contain flour (complex) and sugar (simple), and bananas contain a mixture of sugars and starches depending on their degree of ripeness.

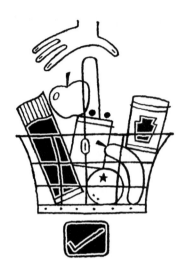

Not all carbohydrates are equal

It's tempting to think that simple carbohydrates, due to their smaller molecular size, are absorbed more quickly than complex carbohydrates, and produce a large and rapid rise in blood sugar. Unfortunately, it's not that straightforward. For example, apples (containing simple carbo-hydrates) produce a small and prolonged rise in blood sugar, despite being high in simple carbohydrates. Many starchy foods (complex carbohydrates), such as potatoes and bread, are digested and absorbed very quickly and give a rapid rise in blood sugar. So the old notion about simple carbohydrates giving fast-released energy and complex carbohydrates giving slow-released energy is incorrect and misleading.

What is more important as far as sports performance is concerned is how rapidly the carbohydrate is absorbed from the small intestine into your bloodstream. The faster this transfer, the more rapidly the carbohydrate can be taken up by muscle cells (or other cells of the body) and make a difference to your training and recovery.

THE GLYCAEMIC INDEX

To describe more accurately the effect different foods have on your blood sugar levels, scientists developed the glycaemic index (GI). It is a ranking of foods from 0 to 100 based on their immediate effect on blood sugar levels, a measure of the speed at which you digest food and convert it into glucose. The faster the rise in blood glucose the higher the rating on the index. To make a fair comparison, all foods are compared with a reference food, such as glucose, and are tested in equivalent carbohydrate amounts. The GI of foods is very useful to know because it tells you how the body responds to them. If you need to get carbohydrates into your bloodstream and muscle cells rapidly, for example immediately after exercise to kick-start glycogen replenishment, you would choose high GI foods.

How is the GI worked out?

An amount of food containing 50 g carbohydrate is consumed. For example, to test baked potatoes, you would eat 250 g potatoes, which contain 50 g of carbohydrate. Over the next two hours, a sample of blood is taken every 15 minutes and the blood sugar level measured. The blood sugar level is plotted on a graph and the area under the curve calculated using a computer programme (*see* Fig. 2.2). Your response to the test food (e.g. potato) is compared with your blood sugar response to 50 g glucose (the reference food). The GI is given as a percentage which is calculated by dividing the area under the curve after you've eaten potatoes by the area under the curve after you've eaten the glucose. So, the GI of baked potatoes is 85, which means that eating baked potato produces a rise in blood sugar which is 85% as great as that produced after eating an equivalent amount of glucose.

The GI of more than 600 foods is known. Most values lie somewhere between 20 and 100 and many sports nutritionists find it useful to classify foods as *high GI* (60–100), *medium GI* (40–59) and *low GI* (less than 40). This simply makes it easier to select the appropriate food before, during and after exercise. In a nutshell, the higher the GI, the higher the blood sugar levels after eating that food. In general, refined starchy foods, including potatoes, white rice and white bread, as well as sugary foods, such as soft drinks and biscuits are high on the glycaemic index. For example, baked potatoes (GI 85) and white rice (GI 87) produce a rise in blood sugar almost the same as eating pure glucose (yes, you read correctly!). Less refined starchy foods – porridge, beans, lentils, muesli – as well as fruit and dairy products are lower on the glycaemic index. They produce a much smaller rise in blood sugar compared with glucose. The GI of various foods is listed in Appendix 1.

What makes one food have a high GI and another food a low GI?

Factors that influence the GI of a food include the size of the food particle, the biochemical make-up of the carbohydrate (the ratio of amylose to amylopectin), the degree of cooking (which affects starch gelatinisation), and the presence of fat, sugar, protein and fibre. How these factors influence the GI of a food is summarised in Table 2.2.

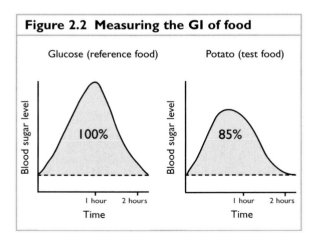

Figure 2.2 Measuring the GI of food

Glucose (reference food)   Potato (test food)

Blood sugar level   100%   Blood sugar level   85%

1 hour 2 hours   1 hour 2 hours

Time   Time

Table 2.2	Factors that influence the GI of a food	
Factor	How it works	Examples of foods
Particle size	Processing reduces particle size and makes it easier for digestive enzymes to access the starch. The smaller the particle size (i.e. the more processed the food), the higher the GI.	Most breakfast cereals, e.g. cornflakes and rice crispies have a higher GI than muesli or porridge.
Degree of starch gelatinisation	The more gelatinised (swollen with water) the starch, the greater the surface area for enzymes to attack, the faster the digestion and rise in blood sugar, i.e. higher GI.	Cooked potatoes (high GI); biscuits (lower GI).
Amylose to amylopectin ratio	There are two types of starch: amylose (long straight molecule, difficult access by enzymes) and amylopectin (branched molecule, easier access by enzymes). The more amylose a food contains the slower it is digested, i.e. lower GI.	Beans, lentils, peas and basmati rice have high amylose content, i.e. low GI; wheat flour and products containing it have high amylopectin content, i.e. high GI.
Fat	Fat slows down rate of stomach emptying, slowing down digestion and lowering GI.	Potato crisps have a lower GI than plain boiled potatoes; adding butter or cheese to bread lowers GI.
Sugar (sucrose)	Sucrose is broken down into 1 molecule of fructose and 1 molecule of glucose. Fructose is converted into glucose in the liver slowly, giving smaller rise in blood sugar.	Sweet biscuits, cakes, sweet breakfast cereals, honey.
Soluble fibre	Soluble fibre increases viscosity of food in digestive tract and slows digestion, producing lower blood sugar rise, i.e. lowers GI.	Beans, lentils, peas, oats, porridge, barley, fruit.
Protein	Protein slows stomach emptying and therefore carbohydrate digestion, producing a smaller blood sugar rise, i.e. lowers GI.	Beans, lentils, peas, pasta (all contain protein as well as carbohydrate). Eating chicken with rice lowers the GI.

Table 2.3	How to calculate the GI of a meal			
Food	Carbohydrate (g)	% total carbohydrate	GI	Contribution to meal GI
Orange juice (150 ml)	12.5	26	46	26% × 46 = 12
Weetabix (30 g)	21	43	69	43% × 69 = 30
Milk (150 ml)	7	15	27	15% × 27 = 4
1 slice toast	13	27	70	27% × 70 = 19
Total	48	100		Meal GI = 65

Source: Leeds et al., 2000.

How can you calculate the GI of a meal?

To date, only the GIs of single foods have been directly measured. In reality, it is more useful to know the GI of a meal, as we are more likely to eat combinations of foods. It is possible to *estimate* the GI of a meal by working out its total carbohydrate content, and then the contribution of each food to the total carbohydrate content. Table 2.3 shows how to calculate the overall GI of a typical breakfast.

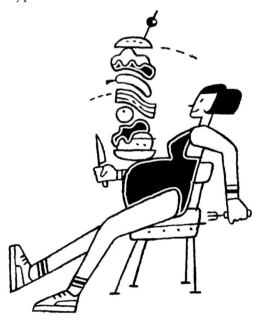

For a quick estimate of a simple meal, such as beans on toast, you may assume that half the carbohydrate is coming from the bread and half from the beans. So you can add the GI values of the two foods together and divide by 2: (70 + 48) ÷ 2 = 59.

If you have uneven proportions of two foods, for example 75% milk: 25% muesli, then 75% of the GI of milk can be added to 25% of the GI of muesli.

How can the GI help your performance?

While the GI concept was originally developed to help diabetics control their blood sugar levels, it can benefit everyone else too. In particular, it can be used to help people manage their weight and regular exercisers improve performance.

The key to efficient glycogen refuelling – and minimal fat storage – is to maintain steady levels of blood glucose and insulin. When glucose levels are high (for example, after consuming high GI foods), large amounts of insulin are produced, which shunts the excess glucose into fat cells. But it is the combined effect of a large amount of carbohydrate as well a food's GI value that really matters. This is called the glycaemic load. A high glycaemic load can result from eating large quantities of any carbohydrate or moderate amounts of high GI foods. This produces a large surge in blood glucose and insulin.

Conversely, eating smaller amounts of any carbohydrate or low GI foods produces a low glycaemic 'load'. This results in a small yet sustained rise in blood glucose.

So, to optimise glycogen storage and minimise fat storage, aim to achieve a small or moderate glycaemic load – eat little and often, avoid overloading on carbohydrates, and stick to balanced combinations of carbohydrate, protein and healthy fat.

There's no need to cut out high glycaemic foods. The key is to eat them with protein and/or a little healthy fat. Combining your carbs with protein (and healthy fat) results in steadier insulin levels and less fat storage. For example, have a baked potato (high GI food) with a little cheese or tuna (both low GI foods). Both protein and fat put a brake on the digestive process, slowing down the release of glucose.

Scientists say that high GI foods have a smaller effect on blood glucose and insulin in regular exercisers compared with non-exercisers. That's because exercise modifies the glycaemic response. Studies at the University of Sydney in Australia have found that when athletes are fed high GI foods, they produce much less insulin than would be predicted from GI tables. In other

How much fibre?

Aim to get the majority of your carbohydrate from unrefined and unprocessed foods – whole grain bread, oats, rice, pasta, potatoes, fruit – which not only have a higher content of vitamins and minerals but also contain more fibre. The Department of Health recommends between 18 g and 24 g a day. The average intake in the UK is a mere 13 g a day, though. Fibre helps your digestive system work properly and modifies the glycaemic effect of a meal. The soluble kind slows the digestion of carbohydrate, producing a slower blood glucose rise. The richest sources are beans, lentils, oats, rye, fruit and vegetables. Insoluble fibre – found mainly in whole grain cereals such as whole wheat bread, Weetabix and whole wheat pasta, brown rice and vegetables – helps speed the passage of food through the gut, and prevent constipation and bowel problems.

words, they don't show the same peaks and troughs in insulin as sedentary people do. Regard the GI index as a rough guide to how various foods are likely to behave in your body.

BEFORE EXERCISE

What, when and how much you eat before exercise will effect your performance, strength and endurance.

When is the best time to eat before exercise?

Ideally, you should eat between 2 and 4 hours before training, leaving enough time for your stomach to settle so that you feel comfortable – not too full and not too hungry. Clearly, the exact timing of your pre-exercise meal will

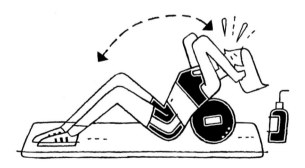

depend on your daily schedule and the time of day you plan to train.

Researchers at the University of North Carolina found that performance during moderate to high intensity exercise lasting 35–40 minutes was improved after eating a moderately high carbohydrate, low fat meal 3 hours before exercise (Maffucci & McMurray, 2000). In this study, the volunteers were able to run significantly longer. Researchers asked the athletes to run on treadmills, at a moderate intensity for 30 minutes with high-intensity 30 second intervals and then until they couldn't run any longer, after eating a meal either 6 hours or 3 hours beforehand. The athletes ran significantly longer if they had eaten the meal 3 hours before training compared with 6 hours.

If you leave too long an interval between eating and training, you will be at risk of hypoglycaemia – low blood glucose – and this will certainly compromise your performance. You will fatigue earlier and, if you feel light-

Does exercise first thing in the morning burn more body fat?

If fat loss is your main goal, exercising on an empty stomach – such as first thing in the morning – may encourage your body to burn slightly more fat for fuel. According to University of Connecticut researchers, insulin levels are at their lowest and glucagen levels are at their highest after an overnight fast. This increases the amount of fat that leaves your fat cells and travels to your muscles, where the fat is burned. On the downside, you may fatigue sooner or drop your exercise intensity and therefore end up burning fewer calories – and less body fat! On the other hand, if performance is your main goal, exercising in a fasted state will almost certainly reduce your endurance. And if strength and muscle mass are important goals, you will be better off exercising after a light meal. After an overnight fast, when muscle glycogen and blood glucose levels are low, your muscles will burn more protein for fuel. So you could end up losing hard-earned muscle!

headed, risk injury too. On the other hand, training with steady blood glucose levels will allow you to train longer and harder.

How much carbohydrate?

Most studies suggest 2.5 g carbohydrate/kg of body weight about 3 hours before exercise. Researchers at Loughborough University found that this pre-exercise meal improved endurance running capacity by 9% compared with a no-meal trial (Chryssanthopoulos et al, 2002). So, for example, if you weigh 70 kg that translates to 175 g carbohydrate. You may need to experiment to find the exact quantity of food or drink and the timing that works best for you.

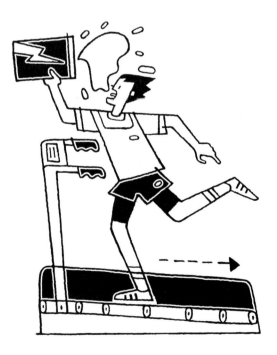

What are the best foods to eat before exercise?

Whether to eat high GI or low GI foods pre-exercise has long been a controversial area. Many experts recommend a low GI meal based on the idea that such a meal would supply sustained energy during exercise. Indeed, a number of good studies carried out at the University of Sydney have supported this recommendation. For example, the researchers found that when a group of cyclists ate a low GI pre-exercise meal of lentils (GI = 29) 1 hour before exercise, they managed to keep going considerably longer than when they consumed high GI foods (glucose drink, GI = 100; or baked potatoes, GI = 85) (Thomas et al., 1991). Remember that you can make a low glycaemic meal either by eating carbohydrate foods with a low glycaemic index – apples, oranges, milk or yoghurt – or by eating carbohydrate with protein and/or healthy fat – cereal with milk, chicken sandwich, baked potato with cheese. The boxes below give you some suggestions for pre-exercise snacks and meals.

In more recent studies (Thomas et al., 1994; DeMarco et al., 1999), the researchers have taken blood samples at regular intervals from the cyclists and found that low GI meals produce higher blood sugar and fatty acid levels during the latter stages of exercise, which is clearly advantageous for endurance sports. In other words, the low GI meals produce a sustained source of carbohydrate throughout exercise and recovery.

This isn't necessarily rule of thumb as other studies have found that the GI of the pre-exercise meal has little effect on performance, with cyclists managing to keep going for the same duration whether they ate lentils (low GI) or potatoes (high GI) (Febbraio & Stewart, 1996).

It's certainly not a clear-cut case but what you have to consider is the timing of your pre-exercise meal. High GI foods are more 'risky' to your performance, particularly if you are sensitive to blood sugar fluctuations (Burke et al., 1998). Get the timing wrong and you may be starting exercise with mild hypoglycaemia – remember they produce a rapid rise in blood sugar and, in some people, a short-lived dip

Pre-workout meals

2–4 hours before exercise:
- Sandwich/roll/bagel/wrap filled with chicken, fish, cheese, egg or peanut butter and salad
- Jacket potato with beans, cheese, tuna, coleslaw or chicken
- Pasta with tomato-based pasta sauce and cheese and vegetables
- Chicken with rice and salad
- Vegetable and prawn or tofu stir fry with noodles or rice
- Pilaff or rice salad
- Mixed bean hot pot with potatoes
- Chicken and vegetable casserole with potatoes
- Porridge made with milk
- Wholegrain cereal (e.g. bran or wheat flakes, muesli or Weetabix) with milk or yoghurt
- Fish and potato pie

Pre-workout snacks

1–2 hours before exercise:
- Fresh fruit
- Dried apricots, dates or raisins
- Smoothie (home made or ready-bought)
- Yoghurt
- Shake (homemade or a meal replacement shake)
- Energy or nutrition bar
- Cereal bar or breakfast bar
- Fruit loaf or raisin bread
- Diluted fruit juice

afterwards. The safest strategy may be to stick with low GI pre-exercise and then top up with high GI carbohydrate during exercise if you are training for more than 60 minutes.

DURING EXERCISE

For activities lasting less than an hour, drinking anything other than water is unnecessary. However, if you are exercising for more than 60 minutes at a moderate–high intensity (equivalent to more than 70% VO_2max), consuming carbohydrate during your workout can help delay fatigue and enable you to perform at a higher intensity. It may also help you to continue exercising when your muscle glycogen stores are depleted.

During that first hour of exercise, most of your carbohydrate energy comes from muscle glycogen. After that, muscle glycogen stores dwindle quite significantly, so the exercising muscles must use carbohydrate from some other source. That's where blood sugar (glucose) comes into its own. As you continue exercising hard, the muscles take up more and more glucose from the bloodstream. Eventually, after 2–3 hours, your muscles will be fuelled entirely by blood glucose and fat.

Sounds handy, but, alas, you cannot keep going indefinitely because blood glucose supplies eventually dwindle. Some of this blood glucose is derived from certain amino acids and some comes from liver glycogen. So when liver glycogen stores run low, your blood glucose levels will fall, and you will be unable to carry on exercising at the same intensity. That's why temporary hypoglycaemia is common after 2–3 hours of exercise without consuming carbohydrate. In this state, you would feel very fatigued and light-headed, your muscles would feel very heavy and the exercise would feel very hard indeed. In other words, the depletion of muscle and liver glycogen together with low blood sugar levels would cause you to reduce exercise intensity or stop completely. This is sometimes called 'hitting the wall' in marathon running

Clearly, then, consuming additional carbohydrate would maintain your blood sugar levels and allow you to exercise longer.

How much carbohydrate?

An intake of between 30–60 g carbohydrate/hour is recommended by leading researchers, Andrew Coggan and Edward Coyle at the University of Texas in Austin (1991). This matches the maximum amount of carbohydrate that can be taken up by the muscles from your bloodstream during aerobic exercise. Consuming more carbohydrate will not improve your energy output nor reduce fatigue.

It is important to begin consuming carbohydrate *before* fatigue sets in. Coggan and Coyle stress that it takes at least 30 minutes for the carbohydrate to be absorbed into the bloodstream. The best strategy is to begin

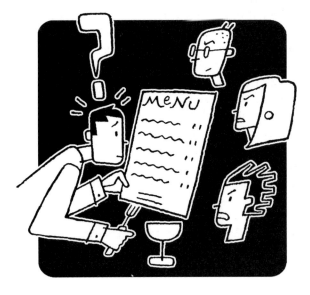

consuming carbohydrate soon after the start of your workout, certainly within the first 30 minutes.

While consuming carbohydrate during exercise can delay fatigue, perhaps by up to 45 minutes, it will not allow you to keep exercising hard indefinitely. Eventually, factors other than carbohydrate supply will cause fatigue.

Which foods or drinks are best?

It makes sense that the carbohydrate you consume during exercise should be easily digested and absorbed. You need it to raise your blood sugar level and reach your exercising muscles rapidly. Thus, high or moderate GI carbohydrates are generally the best choices (*see* Table 2.4). Whether you choose solid or liquid carbohydrate makes little difference to your performance, provided you drink water with solid carbohydrate (Mason et al., 1993). Most athletes find liquid forms of carbohydrate (i.e. sports drinks) more convenient. Carbohydrate-containing drinks have a dual benefit because they provide fluid as well as fuel, which reduces dehydration and fatigue. Obviously, you do not have to consume a commercial drink; you can make your own from fruit juice, or sugar, or squash, and water (*see* Chapter 6).

If you prefer to consume food as well as drinks during exercise, energy or 'sports nutrition' bars, sports gels, ripe bananas, raisins or fruit bars are all suitable. Have a drink of water at the same time. Whether you choose liquid or solid carbohydrate, aim to consume at least 1 litre fluid per hour.

Recent studies have suggested that consuming a drink containing protein as well as carbohydrate during exercise may minimise protein breakdown following exercise, and improve recovery. Researchers at the University of Connecticut found that skimmed milk produces a more favourable hormonal environment immediately following exercise compared with a carbohydrate sports drink (Miller *et al*, 2002). This, they suggest, may spare body protein and encourage protein anabolism during recovery.

Table 2.4	Suitable foods and drinks to consume during exercise	
Food or drink	Portion size providing 30 g carbohydrate	Portion size providing 60 g carbohydrate
Isotonic sports drink (6 g/100 ml)	500 ml	1000 ml
Glucose polymer drink (12 g/100 ml)	250 ml	500 ml
Energy bar	½–1 bar	1–2 bars
Diluted fruit juice (1:1)	500 ml	1000 ml
Raisins or sultanas	1 handful (40 g)	2 handfuls (80 g)
Cereal or breakfast bar	1 bar	2 bars
Energy gel	1 sachet	2 sachets
Bananas	1–2 bananas	2–3 bananas

AFTER EXERCISE

The length of time that it takes to refuel depends on four main factors:
- how depleted your glycogen stores are after exercise
- the extent of muscle damage
- the amount and the timing of carbohydrate you eat
- your training experience and fitness level.

Depletion

The more depleted your glycogen stores, the longer it will take you to refuel, just as it takes longer to refill an empty fuel tank than one that is half-full. This, in turn, depends on the intensity and duration of your workout.

The higher the *intensity*, the more glycogen you use. For example, if you concentrate on fast, explosive activities (e.g. sprints, jumps or lifts) or high-intensity aerobic activities (e.g. running), you will deplete your glycogen stores far more than for low-intensity activities (e.g. walking or slow swimming) of equal duration. The minimum time it would take to refill muscle glycogen stores is 20 hours (Coyle, 1991). In practice, it may take up to 7 days.

The *duration* of your workout also has a bearing on the amount of glycogen you use. For example, if you run for one hour, you will use up more glycogen than if you run at the same speed for half an hour. If you complete 10 sets of shoulder presses in the gym, you will use more glycogen from your shoulder muscles than if you had completed only 5 sets at the same weight. Therefore, you need to allow more time to refuel after high-intensity or long workouts.

Muscle damage

Certain activities which involve eccentric exercise (e.g. heavy weight training, plyometric training or hard running) can cause muscle fibre

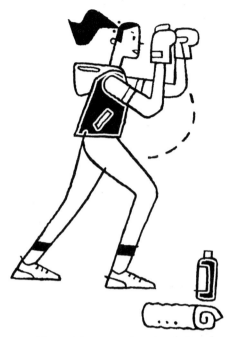

damage. Eccentric exercise is defined as the forced lengthening of active muscle. Muscle damage, in turn, delays glycogen storage and complete glycogen replenishment could take as long as 7–10 days.

Carbohydrate intake

The higher your carbohydrate intake, the faster you can refuel your glycogen stores. Figure 2.3(a) shows how glycogen storage increases with carbohydrate intake.

This is particularly important if you train on a daily basis. For example, cyclists who consumed a low-carbohydrate diet (250–350 g/day) failed to replenish fully their muscle glycogen stores (Costill et al., 1971). Over successive days of training, their glycogen stores became progressively lower. However, in a further study, cyclists who consumed a high-carbohydrate diet (550–600 g/day) fully replaced their glycogen stores in the 22 hours between training sessions (Costill, 1985) (*see* Fig. 2.3(b)).

Figure 2.3(a) Glycogen depends on carbohydrate intake

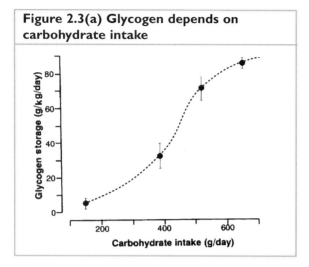

Figure 2.3(b) A low carbohydrate intake results in poor refuelling

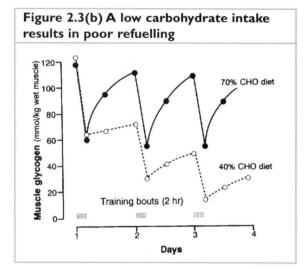

Therefore, if you wish to train daily or every other day, make sure that you consume enough carbohydrate. If not, you will be unable to train as hard or as long, you will suffer fatigue sooner and achieve smaller training gains.

Training experience

Efficiency in refuelling improves automatically with training experience and raised fitness levels. Thus, it takes a beginner longer to replace his glycogen stores than an experienced athlete eating the same amount of carbohydrate. That's why élite sportspeople are able to train almost every day while beginners cannot and should not!

Another adaptation to training is an increase in your glycogen storing capacity, perhaps by as much as 20%. This is an obvious advantage for training and competition. It is like upgrading from a 1-litre saloon car to a 3-litre sports car.

How soon should I eat carbohydrate after exercise?

The best time to start refuelling is as soon as possible after exercise, as glycogen storage is faster during this post-exercise 'window' than at any other time. Research has shown that glycogen storage following exercise takes place in three distinct stages. During the first 2 hours, replenishment is most rapid – at approximately 150% (or one-and-a-half times) the normal rate (Ivy et al., 1988). During the subsequent 4 hours the rate slows but remains higher than normal; after this period glycogen manufacture returns to the normal rate. Therefore, eating carbohydrate during this time speeds glycogen recovery. This is most important for those athletes who train twice a day.

There are two reasons why glycogen replenishment is faster during the post-exercise period. Firstly, eating carbohydrate stimulates insulin release, which, in turn, increases the amount of glucose taken up by your muscle cells from the bloodstream, and stimulates the action of the glycogen-manufacturing enzymes. Secondly, post-exercise, the muscle cell membranes are more permeable to glucose so they can take up more glucose than normal.

How much carbohydrate?

Most researchers recommend consuming 1 g/kg body weight during the 2-hour post-exercise period (Ivy et al., 1988). So, for example, if you weigh 75 kg you need to consume 75 g carbohydrate within 2 hours of exercise (*see* Table 2.5). Even if you finish training late in the evening, you still need to start the refuelling process, so do not go to bed on an empty stomach! For efficient glycogen refuelling, you should continue to eat at least 50 g carbohydrate every 2 hours until your next main meal. Therefore, plan your meals and snacks at regular intervals. If you leave long gaps without eating, glycogen storage and recovery will be slower.

Which foods are best for recovery?

Since you want to get glucose into your bloodstream and muscle cells fast, choose carbohydrates with a moderate or high GI. Indeed, a number of studies have shown that you get faster glycogen replenishment during the first 6 hours after exercise (and, in particular, the first 2 hours) with moderate and high GI carbohydrates compared with low GI (Burke et al., 1993).

However, the difference between high GI and low GI is probably less important for you if you do not train every day. Danish researchers

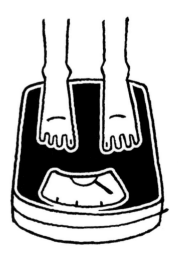

discovered that, after 24 hours, muscle glycogen storage is about the same on a high GI as on a low GI diet (Kiens et al., 1990). In other words, high GI foods post-exercise get your glycogen recovery off to a quick start but low GI foods will result in the same level of recovery 24 hours after exercise.

The bottom line is that *if you are training intensely every day or twice a day, make sure you consume high GI foods during the first 2 hours after exercise.*

It makes no difference to the glycogen storage rate whether you consume liquid or solid forms of carbohydrate (Keizer et al., 1986). Combining carbohydrate with protein has been shown to be more effective in promoting glycogen recovery than carbohydrate alone. A study at the University of Texas at Austin found that a carbohydrate-protein drink (112 g carbohydrate, 40 g protein) increased glycogen storage by 38% compared with a carbohydrate-only drink (Zawadski et al., 1992). Other studies subsequently have noted similar results (Ready et al., 1999; Tarnopolsky et al., 1997).

More recently, researchers at the University of Texas at Austin measured significantly greater muscle glycogen levels 4 hours after 2.5 hours intense cycling when cyclists consumed a protein-carbohydrate drink (80 g carbohydrate, 28 g protein, 6 g fat) compared with a carbohydrate-only drink (80 g carbohydrate, 6 g fat).

Consuming a protein-carbohydrate drink also appears to enhance recovery following resistance exercise. According to researchers at Ithaca College, New York, consuming a protein-carbohydrate drink immediately after resistance exercise promotes more efficient muscle tissue growth as well as faster glycogen refuelling, compared with a carbohydrate-only drink or a placebo (Bloomer et al., 2000). In this study, the researchers measured higher levels of anabolic hormones such as testosterone and lower levels of catabolic hormones such as cortisol for 24 hours after a weights workout when the volunteers consumed a protein-carbohydrate drink. Canadian researchers measured an increased protein uptake in the muscles after volunteers drank a protein-carbohydrate drink following resistance exercise (Gibala, 2000).

The combination of protein and carbohydrate promotes the release of insulin, which stimulates muscle glycogen replenishment as well as the transport of amino acids into muscle cells – thereby promoting protein synthesis – and blunts the rise in cortisol that would otherwise follow exercise. Cortisol suppresses the rate of protein synthesis and stimulates protein catabolism.

Post-exercise snacks

To be eaten within 2 hours after exercise:

- A meal replacement shake (a balanced mixture of maltodextrin, sugar and whey protein together with vitamins and minerals)
- 1–2 portions of fresh fruit with a drink of milk
- 1 or 2 cartons of yoghurt
- A smoothie (crushed fresh fruit whizzed in a blender)
- A homemade milkshake (milk with fresh fruit or yoghurt)
- A yoghurt drink
- A sports bar (containing carbohydrate and protein)
- A sandwich/bagel/roll/wrap filled with lean protein – tuna, chicken, cottage cheese, peanut butter or egg
- A handful of dried fruit and nuts
- A few rice cakes with jam or peanut butter and cottage cheese
- A bowl of wholegrain cereal with milk
- A bowl of porridge made with milk
- Jacket potato with tuna, baked beans or cottage cheese

The optimal post-workout meal or drink, it seems, should include 20–40 g protein and 60–120 g carbohydrate, whether from solid food or commercial sports drinks or bars. Carboydrate should be the foundation of your post-workout meal, with protein and some healthy fat supporting your recovery. This will lead to optimal glycogen recovery and muscle rebuilding or growth – depending on your training mode – between training sessions.

Which foods are best between workouts?

After you have taken advantage of the 6-hour post-exercise window, when and what carbohydrates you eat for the rest of the day are still important for glycogen recovery. To optimise glycogen replenishment, you should ensure a relatively steady supply of carbohydrates into the bloodstream. In practice, this means eating carbohydrates in small meals throughout the day. Researchers at the Human Performance Laboratory of Ball State University have shown that slowly digested carbohydrate – that is, meals with a low GI – cause much smaller rises and falls in blood sugar and insulin and create the ideal environment for the replenishment of steady glycogen stores (Costill, 1988). Avoid consuming large, infrequent meals or lots of high GI meals as they will produce large fluctuations in blood sugar and insulin. This means there will be periods of time when blood sugar levels are low, so glycogen storage will be minimal. Surges of blood sugar and insulin are more likely to result in fat gain.

Are there any other benefits of a low GI daily diet?

A low GI daily diet has been shown to increase satiety (feelings of satisfaction after eating), improve appetite and make it easier to control

Training and immunity

During periods of intense training or competition, many athletes find that they become more susceptible to colds and infections. While moderate training boosts your immune system, intense training appears to depress immune cell production. It is thought that the increased levels of stress hormones, such as adrenaline and cortisol, associated with intense exercise, inhibit the immune system. Here are some practical ways of combating exercise-related suppression of immunity.

- Match your calorie intake and expenditure – under eating will increase cortisol levels.
- Ensure you're consuming plenty of foods rich in immunity-boosting nutrients – vitamins A, C, and E, vitamin B_6, zinc, iron and magnesium. Best sources are fresh fruit, vegetables, whole grains, beans, lentils, nuts and seeds.
- Avoid low carbohydrate diets. Low glycogen stores are associated with bigger increases in cortisol levels and bigger suppression of your immune cells.
- Consume a sports drink (approximately 6 g carbohydrate/100 ml, providing 30–60 g carbohydrate per hour) during intense exercise lasting longer than one hour. This can reduce stress hormone levels and the associated drop in immunity following exercise (Bishop, 2002).
- Drink plenty of fluid. This increases your saliva production, which contains anti-bacterial proteins that can fight off air-borne germs.
- A modest antioxidant supplement or a vitamin C supplement may help to reduce the risk of upper respiratory tract infection following intense training (Peters et al., 2001). In one study of ultra-marathon runners, those who took daily vitamin C supplements (1500 mg) 7 days prior to a race had lower levels of stress hormones following the race, which suggests greater protection against infection.
- Glutamine supplements may reduce the risk of infections. Glutamine levels can fall by up to 20 % following intense exercise (Antonio, 1999), putting the immune system under greater strain.
- Echinacea taken for up to 4 weeks during a period of hard training may boost immunity by stimulating the body's own production of immune cells.

food intake and body weight. Studies have shown that the lower the GI of a meal the more satisfied and less hungry you are likely to be during the following 3 hours (Holt, 1992). What's more, low GI diets are beneficial in lowering total and LDL cholesterol levels. This is due to the lower insulin levels – high insulin levels stimulate cholesterol manufacture in the liver. Total cholesterol may drop by as much as 15 % on a low GI diet (Jenkins et al., 1987).

CARBOHYDRATE LOADING

Carbohydrate loading is a technique originally devised in the 1960s to increase the muscles' glycogen stores above normal levels. With more glycogen available, you may be able to exercise longer before fatigue sets in. This is potentially advantageous in endurance events lasting longer than 90 minutes (e.g. long distance running or cycling) or for events that involve several heats or matches over a short period (e.g. tennis tournaments or swimming galas). It is unlikely to benefit you if your event lasts less than 90 minutes as muscle glycogen depletion would not be a limiting factor to your performance. The classical 6-day regimen involved 2 bouts of glycogen-depleting exercise separated by 3 days of low-carbohydrate intake and followed by 3 days of high carbohydrate intake and minimal exercise (Ahlborg et al., 1967; Karlsson & Saltin,

1971) (Table 2.5). The theory behind this 2-phase regimen is that glycogen depletion stimulates the activity of glycogen synthetase, the key enzyme involved in glycogen storage, resulting in above-normal levels of muscle glycogen.

But this regimen had a number of drawbacks. Not only did it interfere with exercise tapering, but the low-carbohydrate diet left athletes weak, irritable and tired. Worse, many failed to achieve high glycogen levels even after 3 days of high carbohydrate intake.

Researchers at Ohio State University, Ohio, US developed a 6-day carbohydrate loading regimen that resulted in similar increases in glycogen levels but without the disadvantages described above (Sherman et al., 1981). This required tapering training on 6 consecutive days while following a normal diet during the first 3 days followed by a carbohydrate-rich diet during the next 3 days (Table 2.6).

More recently, researchers at the University of Western Australia, the have found that equally high levels of glycogen can be achieved by taking in 10 g of carbohydrate per kilogram of bodyweight over the course of a single day following a 3 minute bout of high-intensity exercise (Fairchild et al., 2002; Bussau, et al., 2002)). It appears that the rate of glycogen storage is greatly increased following such a workout. The advantage of this new regimen is that only one instead of 6 days is needed to achieve high glycogen levels, and very little change to your usual training programme needs to be made.

The original method involved 3 days of glycogen depletion (through exhaustive exercise on day 1 and a low-carbohydrate diet) followed by 3 days of glycogen loading (through reduced training and a high-carbohydrate diet) (Karlsson & Saltin, 1971). The theory behind this two-phase programme is that muscle glycogen depletion stimulates the activity of glycogen synthetase, the key enzyme in glycogen manufacture, causing an 'over-compensation' of muscle glycogen storage (*see* Table 2.5).

While this original method improved the performance of endurance athletes, it also proved to have a number of drawbacks. The depletion phase can leave you feeling excessively weak and drained, hypoglycaemic, irritable, and unable to train. Many athletes fail to load sufficient carbohydrate over the next 3 days.

Table 2.5 — Carbohydrate loading (classical regimen)

Normal training	Exhaustive prolonged exercise	Taper training	Taper training	Taper training	Taper training	Taper training	
Day 1	Day 2	Day 3	Day 4	Day 5	Day 6	Day 7	Competition
Normal diet	Low-carbohydrate diet	Low-carbohydrate diet	Low-carbohydrate diet	High-carbohydrate diet	High-carbohydrate diet	High-carbohydrate diet	

Table 2.6 — Carbohydrate loading (modified regimen)

Endurance training	Taper training	Taper training	Taper training	Taper training	Taper training	Taper training	
Day 1	Day 2	Day 3	Day 4	Day 5	Day 6	Day 7	Competition
Normal diet	Moderate-carbohydrate diet	Moderate-carbohydrate diet	Moderate-carbohydrate diet	High-carbohydrate diet	High-carbohydrate diet	High-carbohydrate diet	

Table 2.7	Carbohydrate loading (1 day regimen)						
Taper training	Taper training	Taper training	Taper training	Taper training	Taper training	Warm-up & 3 min high intensity exercise (sustained sprint)	
Day 1	Day 2	Day 3	Day 4	Day 5	Day 6	Day 7	Competition
Normal diet	Low-carbohydrate diet	Low-carbohydrate diet	Low-carbohydrate diet	High-carbohydrate diet	High-carbohydrate diet	High-carbohydrate diet 10 g carbohydrate/kg bodyweight	

More recent research has found that you can achieve equally good results by omitting the depletion phase and eating a high-carbohydrate diet for the 3 days prior to competition (Sherman et al., 1981). It appears that neither the 3-day depletion phase nor the low-carbohydrate diet is necessary to achieve maximum glycogen storage.

Table 2.7 shows a recommended programme for carbohydrate loading. On day 1, carry out endurance training for about 1 hour to reduce the amount of glycogen in your liver and muscles. For the following 3 days, taper your training and eat a moderate-carbohydrate diet (5–7 g carbohydrate/kg body weight). For the final 3 days, continue your exercise taper, or rest,

Table 2.8	Summary – what, when, and how much carbohydrate?			
	Before exercise	During exercise lasting > 60 min	After exercise	Between workouts
How much	2.5 g/kg of body weight	30–60 g/hour	1 g/kg body weight	5–10 g/kg body weight, or 60% of energy
Time period	2–4 hours before exercise	Begin after 30 min; regular intervals	Up to 2 hours; then every 2 hours	4–6 meals/snacks
GI	Low	High	High or low	Low
Examples	• Jacket potato with beans, chicken or cheese • Pasta with tomato based sauce and salad • Porridge • Rice with chicken and vegetables	• 500–1000 ml isotonic drink or diluted fruit juice (6 g/100 ml) • Energy bar with water • 1–2 handfuls of raisins (40–80 g) • 1–2 bananas	• Meal replacement shake • Fresh fruit with milk or yoghurt • Sports bar • Tuna or cottage cheese sandwich	• Pasta or rice with beans/chicken/fish • Noodles with tofu/poultry/seafood • Beans on toast • Jacket potato with cottage cheese/tuna

and increase your carbohydrate intake to 8–10 g/kg body weight.

Since glycogen storage is associated with approximately 3 g water for each 1 g of glycogen, carbohydrate loading can produce a weight increase of 1–2 kg. This may or may not affect your performance.

If you decide to try carbohydrate loading, rehearse it during training to find out what works best for you. Never try anything new before an important competition. You may need to try the technique more than once, adjusting the types and amounts of foods you eat.

PUTTING IT TOGETHER: WHAT, WHEN AND HOW MUCH

Table 2.8 summarises the recommendations on carbohydrate intake covered in this chapter. The simplest way to plan your daily food intake is to divide the day into four 'windows': before, during, and after exercise, and between training sessions. You can then work out how much and what type of carbohydrate to consume during each 'window' to optimise your performance and recovery.

SUMMARY OF KEY POINTS

- The amount, type and timing of carbohydrate intake in relation to training are important considerations for maximising glycogen storage and improving performance.
- The glycaemic index (GI) is a more useful way of categorising carbohydrates for athletes than the traditional 'complex' versus 'simple' classification.
- Carbohydrates with a high GI produce a rapid rise in blood sugar; those with a low GI produce a slow rise in blood sugar.

- Low GI foods consumed 2–4 hours before exercise may help improve endurance and delay fatigue. High GI foods consumed pre-exercise benefit some athletes but may produce temporary hypoglycaemia at the start of exercise in those athletes sensitive to blood sugar fluctuations
- The pre-exercise meal should contain approx. 2.5 g carbohydrate/kg body weight.
- For moderate–high intensity exercise lasting more than 60 minutes, consuming 30–60 g moderate or high GI carbohydrate (in solid or liquid form) during exercise can help maintain exercise intensity for longer and delay fatigue.
- Glycogen recovery takes, on average, 20 hours but depends on the severity of glycogen depletion, extent of muscle damage and the amount, type and timing of carbohydrate intake.
- Glycogen replenishment is faster than normal during the 2-hour post-exercise period. To kick-start recovery, it is recommended to consume 1 g moderate–high GI carbohydrate/kg body weight during this period.
- High or moderate GI carbohydrates produce faster glycogen replenishment for the first 6 hours post-exercise and is most important for athletes who train twice a day.
- Combining carbohydrate with protein has been shown to be more effective in promoting muscle glycogen recovery and muscle tissue growth compared with carbohydrate alone.
- A low GI daily diet comprising 4–6 small meals and supplying 5–10 g/kg body weight (depending on training hours and intensity) will optimise muscle glycogen stores.
- A modified form of carbohydrate loading – omitting the depletion phase and increasing carbohydrate during the 7 days prior to competition – will help improve endurance.

PROTEIN - THE POWERHOUSE

The importance of protein – and the question of whether extra protein is necessary – for sports performance is one of the most hotly debated topics among sports scientists, coaches and athletes and has been contended ever since the time of the Ancient Greeks. Protein has long been associated with power and strength, and as the major constituent of muscle, it would seem logical that an increased protein intake would increase muscle size and strength.

Traditionally, scientists have held the view that athletes do not need to consume more than the RDA for protein and that consuming anything greater than this amount would produce no further benefit. However, research since the 1980s has cast doubt on this view. There is considerable evidence that the protein needs of active individuals are consistently higher than those of the general population.

This chapter will help to give you a fuller understanding of the role of protein during exercise, and enable you to work out how much you need. It will show how individual requirements depend on the sport concerned and the training programme, and also how they are related to carbohydrate intake. An example of a daily menu is given to show how to meet your own protein requirements, and to provide a basis for developing your own menu. As more athletes are giving up meat and choosing a vegetarian diet, this chapter explains how you can obtain sufficient protein and other nutrients for peak performance on a meat-free diet.

Protein supplementation is discussed in detail in Chapter 5 (*see* pp. 63–65).

WHY DO I NEED PROTEIN?

Protein makes up part of the structure of every cell and tissue in your body, including your muscle tissue, internal organs, tendons, skin, hair and nails. On average, it comprises about 20 % of your total body weight. Protein is needed for the growth and formation of new tissue, for tissue repair and for regulating many metabolic pathways, and can also be used as a fuel for energy production. It is also needed to make almost all of the body enzymes as well as various hormones (such as adrenaline and insulin) and neurotransmitters. Protein has a role in maintaining optimal fluid balance in tissues, transporting nutrients in and out of cells, carrying oxygen and regulating blood clotting.

What are amino acids?

The 20 amino acids are the building blocks of proteins. They can be combined in various ways to form hundreds of different proteins in the body. When you eat protein, it is broken down in your digestive tract into smaller molecular units – single amino acids and dipeptides (two amino acids linked together).

Twelve of the amino acids can be made in the body from other amino acids, carbohydrate and nitrogen. These are called dispensable, or non-essential, amino acids (DAAs). The other eight are termed indispensable, or essential, amino acids (IAAs) meaning they must be supplied in the diet. All 20 amino acids are listed in Table 3.1. Branched-chain amino acids (BCAAs) include the three IAAs with a branched molecular configuration: valine, leucine and

Table 3.1	Indispensable and dispensable amino acids	
Indispensable (essential) amino acids (IAAs)	**Dispensable (non-essential) amino acids (DAAs)**	
Isoleucine	Alanine	
Leucine	Arginine	
Lysine	Asparagine	
Methionine	Aspartic acid	
Phenylalanine	Cysteine	
Threonine	Glutamic acid	
Tryptophan	Glutamine	
Valine	Glycine	
	Histidine*	
	Proline	
	Serine	
	Tyrosine	

*Histidine is essential for babies (not for adults)

isoleucine. They make up one-third of muscle protein and are a vital substrate for two other amino acids, glutamine and alanine, which are released in large quantities during intense aerobic exercise. Also they can be used directly as fuel by the muscles, particularly when muscle glycogen is depleted. Strictly speaking, the body's requirement is for amino acids rather than protein.

These are then re-assembled into new proteins containing hundreds or even thousands of amino acids linked together.

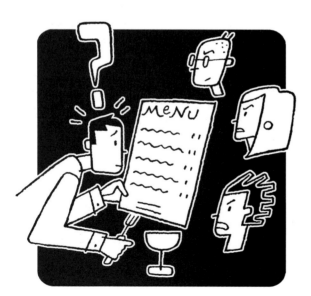

What types of protein are there?

There are four types of protein commonly used as food supplements. The advantages of each type are detailed in chapter 5, pp. 64–65.

1 whey protein
2 casein
3 soy protein
4 egg protein.

Whey protein is one of the two major types of protein found in milk (the other is casein). It is formed when milk is curdled (as in cheese manufacture), separating the curd (which

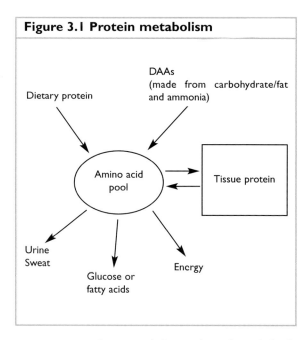

Figure 3.1 Protein metabolism

Dietary protein

DAAs
(made from carbohydrate/fat and ammonia)

Amino acid pool

Tissue protein

Urine
Sweat

Glucose or
fatty acids

Energy

Protein metabolism

Tissue proteins are continually broken down (catabolised), releasing their constituent amino acids into the 'free pool', which is located in body tissues and the blood. For example, half of your total body protein is broken down and replaced every 150 days. Amino acids absorbed from food (IAAs) and dispensable amino acids (DAAs) made in the body from nitrogen and carbohydrate can also enter the free pool. Once in the pool, amino acids have four fates. They can be used to build new proteins, they can be oxidised to produce energy and they can be converted in glucose via gluconeogenesis or they can be converted into fatty acids. During energy production, the nitrogen part of the protein molecule is excreted in urine, or possibly in sweat.

contains mainly casein) from the whey (which contains lactalbumin protein, lactose and fat).

Casein is the other major milk protein. It is basically the curd, formed when milk is separated into curds and whey. Low-fat cottage cheese is mostly casein protein together with a little lactose and calcium.

Soy protein is extracted from soybeans.

Egg protein refers to the proteins found in whole egg.

PROTEIN AND EXERCISE

How does exercise affect my protein requirement?

Numerous studies involving both endurance and strength exercise have shown that the current recommended protein intake of 0.75 g/kg body weight/day is inadequate for people who participate in regular exercise or sport. Additional protein is needed to compensate for the increased breakdown of protein during and immediately after exercise, and to facilitate repair and growth. Exercise triggers the activation of an enzyme that oxidises key amino acids in the muscle, which are then used as a fuel source. The greater the exercise intensity and the longer the duration of exercise, the more protein is broken down for fuel.

Your exact protein needs depend on the type, intensity and duration of your training. How these needs differ for endurance athletes and strength and power athletes are discussed in detail below.

Endurance training

Prolonged and intense endurance training increases your protein requirements for two reasons. Firstly, you will need more protein to compensate for the increased breakdown of protein during training. When your muscle glycogen stores are low – which typically occurs after 60–90 minutes of endurance exercise – certain amino acids, namely, the BCAAs (see p. 33) can be used for energy. One of the BCAAs, leucine, is converted into another amino acid, alanine, which is converted in the liver into glucose. This glucose is released back into the bloodstream and transported to the exercising muscles where it is used for energy. In fact, protein may contribute up to 15% of your energy production when glycogen stores are low. This is quite a substantial increase, as protein contributes less than 5% of energy needs when muscle glycogen stores are high. Secondly, additional protein is needed for the repair and recovery of muscle tissue after intense endurance training.

Strength and power training

Strength and power athletes have additional needs as protein provides an enhanced stimulus for muscle growth. To build muscle, you must be in 'positive nitrogen balance'. This means the body is retaining more dietary protein than is

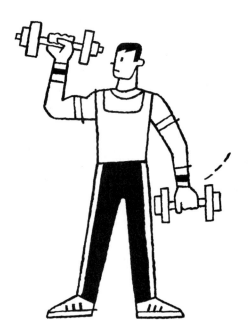

excreted or used as fuel. A sub-optimal intake of protein will result in slower gains in strength, size and mass, or even muscle loss, despite hard training. In practice the body is capable of adapting to slight variations in protein intake. It becomes more efficient in recycling amino acids during protein metabolism if your intake falls over a period of time. The body can also adapt to a consistently high protein intake by oxidising surplus amino acids for energy.

It is important to understand that a high-protein diet alone will not result in increased strength or muscle size. These goals can only be achieved when an optimal protein intake is combined with heavy resistance (strength) training.

Do beginners need more or less protein than experienced athletes?

Contrary to popular belief, studies have shown that beginners have slightly higher requirements for protein per kg body weight. When you begin a training programme your protein needs rise due to increases in protein turnover (Gontzea et al., 1975). After about 3 weeks of training, the body adapts to the exercise and becomes more efficient at recycling protein. Broken down protein can be built up again from amino acids released into the amino acid pool. The body also becomes more efficient in conserving protein. One study has shown that the requirements per kg body weight of novice bodybuilders can be up to 40% higher than those of experienced bodybuilders (Tarnopolsky, 1988).

Can I minimise protein breakdown during exercise?

Protein is broken down in increased quantities when muscle glycogen stores are low. Thus, during high-intensity exercise lasting longer than 1 hour, protein can make a substantial contribution to your energy needs (up to 15%). Clearly, it is advantageous to start your training session with high muscle-glycogen stores. This will reduce the contribution protein makes to your energy needs at any given point during training.

If you are on a weight/fat loss programme, make sure you do not reduce your carbohydrate too drastically otherwise protein will be used as an energy source making it unavailable for tissue growth. Aim to maintain 60% of your calorie intake from carbohydrate by reducing your calorie intake from carbohydrate in proportion to your calorie reduction (see Chapter 8 on weight/fat loss).

How much protein do I need for maximum performance?

Table 3.2 summarises the daily protein requirements for different types of athletes.

At low–moderate exercise intensities (<50% VO_2max), it appears there is no significant increase in protein requirements (Hergreaves & Snow, 2001).

For an endurance athlete, the recommended range is 1.2–1.4 g/kg body weight/day (Lemon, 1998; Williams & Devlin, 1992; Williams, 1998; ACSM, 2000).

Many recent studies show that strength and power athletes have a greater daily requirement for protein than most endurance athletes. The current consensus recommendation is an intake between 1.4 and 1.8 g/kg body weight/day (Williams, 1998; Tarnopolsky et al., 1992; Lemon et al., 1992). The American Dietetic Association and ACSM recommend 1.6–1.7 g/kg body weight per day. So, for example, a distance runner weighing 70 kg would need 84–98 g/day. A sprinter or bodybuilder with the same body weight would need 98–126 g/day.

In practice, protein intakes generally reflect total calorie intake, which is why the International Consensus Conference on Foods, Nutrition and Performance in Lausanne (1991) stated that protein should comprise 12–15% of total energy intake. This assumes that your calorie intake matches your calorie requirements.

HOW CAN I MEET MY PROTEIN NEEDS?

Protein intake is usually proportional to total calorie intake so the more food you eat, the greater the chances of meeting your protein needs. If you reduce your calories, you may find it more difficult to meet your protein needs so a few dietary adjustments may be needed. Additionally, if you eat a vegan diet or eat very few animal sources of protein, it may be more

Table 3.2	Protein requirements of athletes
Type of athlete	Daily protein requirements per kg body weight (g)
Endurance athlete – moderate or heavy training	1.2–1.4
Strength and power athlete	1.4–1.8
Athlete on fat-loss programme	1.6–2.0
Athlete on weight-gain programme	1.8–2.0

Source: William & Devlin, 1992; Williams, 1998; Tarnopolsky et al., 1992; Lemon et al., 1992

Table 3.3	Good sources of protein		
Food	Portion size	Protein (g)	Kcal
Meat and Fish			
Beef, fillet steak, grilled, lean	2 slices 105 g	31	197
Chicken breast, grilled meat only	1 breast 130 g	39	191
Turkey, light meat, roasted	2 slices 140 g	47	214
Cod, poached	1 fillet 120 g	25	113
Mackerel, grilled	1 fillet 150 g	31	359
Tuna, canned in brine	1 small tin (100 g)	24	99
Dairy products and eggs			
Cheese, cheddar	1 thick slice (40 g)	10	165
Cottage cheese	1 small carton (112 g)	15	110
Skimmed milk	1 glass (200 ml)	7	66
Low-fat yoghurt, plain	1 carton (150 g)	8	84
Low-fat yoghurt, fruit	1 carton (150 g)	6	135
Fromage frais, fruit	1 small carton (100 g)	7	131
Eggs	1, size 2	8	90
Nuts and seeds			
Peanuts, roasted and salted	1 handful (50 g)	12	301
Peanut butter	on 1 slice bread (20 g)	5	125
Cashew nuts, roasted and salted	1 handful (50 g)	10	306
Walnuts	1 handful (50 g)	7	344
Sunflower seeds	2 tbsp (32 g)	6	186
Sesame seeds	2 tbsp (24 g)	4	144
Pulses			
Baked beans	1 small tin (205 g)	10	166
Red lentils, boiled	3 tbsp (120 g)	9	120
Red kidney beans, boiled	3 tbsp (120 g)	10	124
Chick peas, boiled	3 tbsp (140 g)	12	169
Soya products			
Soya milk, plain	1 glass (200 ml)	6	64
Soya mince	2 tbsp dry weight (30 g)	13	79
Tofu	Half a pack (100 g)	8	73
Tofu burger	1 burger 60 g	5	71

	Food	Portion size	Protein (g)	Kcal
Table 3.3	**continued**			

Food	Portion size	Protein (g)	Kcal
Quorn products			
Quorn mince	4 tbsp (100 g)	12	86
Quorn chilli	1 bowl (200 g)	9	163
Quorn korma	1 bowl (200 g)	8	280
Grains and cereals			
Wholemeal bread	2 slices (76 g)	6	164
White bread	2 slices (72 g)	6	156
Pasta, boiled	1 bowl (230 g)	7	198
Brown rice, boiled	1 bowl (180 g)	5	254
White rice, boiled	1 bowl (180 g)	5	248

difficult to meet your needs. Table 3.3 lists a wide range of foods containing protein. Animal sources generally provide a better amino acid profile but some foods (such as meat and cheese) are high in saturated fat. Keep these to a minimum and choose lean and low-fat versions. Use the table to estimate your current intake of protein and use the eating plans detailed in Chapter 12 as a basis for developing your personal nutrition programme.

To ensure your protein requirements are adequate you can estimate how much protein you should eat per day in one of two ways:

1 From your energy intake

Calculate your energy intake (your maintenance calorie intake) either from your actual food intake over 3–7 consecutive days using food tables, or using the formulae based on your resting metabolic rate (RMR) (*see* Chapter 8, steps 1–4, p. 118). Multiply your energy intake by 12% and 15%, then divide by 4 to give you your recommended protein intake in grams.

Example:

Energy intake = 3000 kcal
Calories from protein
$\quad$ = (a) $3000 \times 12\% = 360$
$\quad$ = (b) $3000 \times 15\% = 450$
Protein intake
$\quad$ = (a) $360 \div 4 = 90$ g
$\quad$ = (b) $450 \div 4 = 112.5$ g
$\quad$ i.e. between 90–112.5 g/day

2 From your body weight

Calculate your daily protein requirement from your body weight by using the guidelines in Table 3.2.

Examples:

(a) For an endurance athlete weighing 70 kg
$\quad$ $70 \times 1.2 = 84$ g
$\quad$ $70 \times 1.4 = 98$ g
$\quad$ i.e. between 84–98 g/day

(b) For a strength or power athlete weighing 70 kg
$\quad$ $70 \times 1.4 = 98$ g
$\quad$ $70 \times 1.8 = 126$ g
$\quad$ i.e. between 98–126 g/day

Is more better?

A protein intake above your optimal requirement will not result in further muscle mass and strength gains. In a study carried out at McMaster University, Ontario, strength athletes were given either a low-protein diet (0.86 g/kg body weight/day – similar to the RDA), a medium-protein diet (1.4 g/kg body weight/day) or a high-protein diet (2.3 g/kg body weight/day) for 13 days (Tarnopolsky et al., 1992). The low-protein diet, which was close to the RDA for sedentary people, caused the athletes to lose muscle mass. Both the medium- and high-protein diets resulted in an increased muscle mass, but the amount of the increase was the same for the two groups. In other words, no further benefits were gained by increasing the protein intake from 1.4 g to 2.4 g/kg body weight/day.

Similar findings were reported at Kent State University, Ohio. Researchers gave 12 young volunteers either a protein supplement (total daily protein was 2.62 g/kg body weight) or a carbohydrate supplement (total daily protein was 1.35 g/kg body weight) for 1 month during which time they performed intense weight training 6 days a week (Lemon et al., 1992). Nitrogen balance measurements were carried out after each diet and the researchers found that an intake of 1.4–1.5 g/kg body weight/day was needed to maintain nitrogen balance, although strength, muscle mass and size were the same with either level of protein intake. The researchers concluded two main points. First, strength training approximately doubles your

What is bioavailability?

Bioavailability refers to the 'usefulness' of the protein food or supplement. Foods that contain all eight IAAs are traditionally called 'complete' proteins. These include dairy products, eggs, meat, fish, poultry and soya. Various plant foods, such as cereals and pulses, contain high amounts of several IAAs, but only very small amounts (or none) of the others. The IAA that is missing or in short supply is called the *limiting* amino acid.

The ratio of IAAs to DAAs and the amounts of specific amino acids is what determines the bioavailability of the protein food or supplement. For example, the content of glutamine and the BCAAs (leucine, isoleucine and valine) determine the extent the protein is absorbed and utilised for tissue growth.

The bioavailability of a particular protein is often measured by its *biological value* (BV), which indicates how closely matched the proportion of amino acids are in relation to the body's requirements. It is a measure of the percentage of protein that is retained by the body for use in growth and tissue maintenance. In other words, how much of what is consumed is actually used for its intended purpose.

An egg has a BV of 100, which means, out of all foods, it contains the most closely matched ratio of IAAs and DAAs to the body's needs. Therefore a high percentage of the egg protein can be used for making new body proteins. Dairy products, meat, fish, poultry, quorn and soya have a relatively high BV (70–100); nuts, seeds, pulses and grains have a relatively low BV (less than 70).

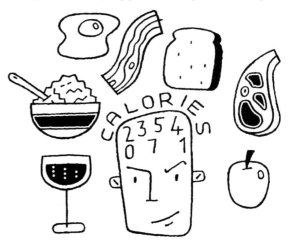

protein needs (compared with sedentary people). Secondly, increasing your protein intake does not enhance your strength, mass or size in a linear fashion. Once your optimal intake has been reached, additional protein is not converted into muscle.

Is too much protein harmful?

Consuming more protein than you need certainly offers no advantage in terms of health or physical performance. Once your requirements have been met, additional protein will not be converted into muscle, nor will it further increase muscle size, strength or stamina.

The nitrogen-containing amino group of the protein is converted into a substance called urea in the liver. This is then passed to the kidneys and excreted in the urine. The remainder of the protein is converted into glucose and used as an energy substrate. It may either be used as fuel immediately or stored, usually as glycogen. If you are already eating enough carbohydrate to refill your glycogen stores, excess glucose may be converted into fat. However, in practice this does not occur to a great extent. Fat gain is usually the result of excessive calorie consumption, in particular of fats. Recent studies have shown that eating protein increases the metabolic rate, so a significant proportion of the protein calories are oxidised and given off as heat (*see* Chapter 8). Thus, a slight excess of protein is unlikely to be converted into fat.

It was once thought that excess protein may cause liver or kidney damage as it places an undue stress on these organs. This has never been demonstrated in healthy people, though so it remains only a theoretical possibility. Those with liver or kidney problems, however, are advised to consume a low-protein diet.

It has also been claimed that eating too much protein leads to dehydration because extra water is drawn from the body's fluids to dilute and excrete the increased quantities of urea. Indeed, a study reported at the 2002 Experimental Biology meeting in New Orleans found that a high protein diet (246 g daily) consumed for 4 weeks caused dehydration in trained athletes. Their blood urea nitrogen – a clinical test for proper kidney function – reached abnormal levels and they produced more concentrated urine. According to the researchers at the University of Connecticut, this could have been avoided by increasing their fluid intake. This is unlikely to be a problem if you drink enough fluids.

Finally, there is some evidence dating from studies conducted in the early 1980s that high-protein diets cause an excessive excretion of calcium, increasing the risk of osteoporosis. However, a more recent study at the University of Maastrict, Belgium, found that a 21% protein diet produced no negative effect on calcium status compared with a 12% protein diet (Pannemans et al., 1997).

In conclusion, eating too much protein is unlikely to be harmful but it certainly offers no advantages.

Should I consume more protein if I am on a fat-loss programme?

When cutting calories to lose body fat you risk losing muscle mass as well. A higher protein intake can offset some of the muscle-wasting effects associated with any weight-reducing programme. Most researchers recommend increasing your protein intake a further 0.2 g/kg body weight. Thus, an endurance athlete would need as much as 1.6 g/kg body weight/day; and a strength athlete would need up to 2.0 g/kg body weight/day. For example, a 70 kg endurance athlete would need to consume $70 \times 1.6 = 112$ g protein/day. If you are consuming 2000 kcal a day, that would be equivalent to 22% of your total calories (i.e. 112×4 divided by 2000).

VEGETARIAN ATHLETES

Can vegetarian athletes meet their protein requirements?

Contrary to popular belief, a well-planned vegetarian diet that excludes meat, poultry and fish can provide sufficient protein for athletes and fitness participants. You do not have to eat meat to gain strength or lean body mass. It may be more difficult to obtain the 1.4–1.8 g/kg body weight daily to support muscle growth and strength, however, you can achieve this by including sufficient low-fat dairy products and protein-rich plant sources in your diet. While plant sources are generally lower in protein and contain smaller amounts of IAAs, this need not be a problem. The key is to eat the right *combination* of plant-based protein foods each day.

So how should vegetarians combine protein foods?

To get enough amino acids from a vegetarian diet, choose foods that complement each other. In other words, eat a mixture of protein foods so that the shortfall of amino acids in one is complemented by higher amounts in the other. For example, lysine is the limiting amino acid in cereals and methionine is the limiting amino acid in beans. By combining the two foods, as in baked beans on toast, you end up with a well-balanced mixture of amino acids.

In essence, you can achieve protein complementation by combining plant foods from two or more of the following categories:

1 pulses: beans, lentils, peas
2 grains: bread, pasta, rice, oats, breakfast cereals, corn, rye
3 nuts and seeds: peanuts, cashews, almonds, sunflower seeds, sesame seeds, pumpkin seeds

4 quorn and soya products: soya milk, tofu, tempeh (fermented soya curd similar to tofu but with a stronger flavour), soya mince, soya burgers, quorn mince, quorn fillets, quorn sausages.

Examples of other suitable combinations include:
• tortillas filled with re-fried beans
• pasta with chick peas
• bean and vegetable hot pot with rice
• quorn chilli with rice
• peanut butter sandwich
• lentil soup with a roll
• quorn korma with naan bread
• stir-fried tofu and vegetables with rice
• tofu burger in a roll.

If you eat dairy products and eggs, it's not essential to combine these with other protein foods to achieve a complete protein. The protein in dairy products and eggs contains all the IAAs in proportions closely matched to the body's needs. However, some of these foods are high in fat so eat these in small quantities or choose low-fat versions.

Are there any special dietary guidelines for vegetarian athletes?

As with any dietary change, it is important to plan your diet well and gain as much knowledge about vegetarian diets as possible. Some athletes adopt a vegetarian or vegan diet in order to lose body fat in the belief that such diets are automatically lower in calories. Many do not substitute suitable foods in place of meat and fail to consume enough protein and other nutrients to support their training. Athletes with disordered eating often omit meat from their diet but this is certainly not a consequence of vegetarianism!

Table 3.4	How to meet your nutritional requiremets on a vegetarian diet	
Nutrient	**Sources**	**Advice**
Protein	Milk, cheese, yoghurt, eggs, beans, lentils, peas, nuts, seeds, soya products (e.g. soya 'milk', soya mince, tofu, tempeh), quorn.	Eating a mixture of plant-protein foods over the day will ensure an adequate intake of all IAAs (protein complementation). Choose low-fat versions of dairy products to reduce fat intake.
Iron	Wholemeal bread, wholegrains, nuts, pulses, green vegetables (e.g. broccoli, watercress), fortified soya products, fortified breakfast cereals, seeds, dried fruit.	Eating vitamin C-rich foods (e.g. fruit, vegetables, fruit juice) at the same time as iron-rich foods greatly improves iron absorption.
Vitamin B$_{12}$	Dairy products, eggs, fortified foods (e.g. soya products, breakfast cereals, yeast extract).	As vitamin B$_{12}$ is found naturally only in animal products, vegans should include B$_{12}$-fortified products in their diet or take a supplement.
Calcium	Dairy products, sunflower and sesame seeds, spinach, broccoli, almonds, brazils, fortified soya products (e.g. tofu), figs.	Vegan diets are often low in calcium so more careful planning is required.
Zinc	Wholegrains, wholemeal bread, pulses, nuts, seeds, eggs.	Avoid bran and bran-enriched foods as fibre can bind zinc and reduce its absorption.

A very bulky vegetarian diet that includes lots of high-fibre foods (e.g. beans, wholegrains) may be too filling if you have high energy needs. To ensure you eat enough calories, you may need to include more compact sources of carbohydrate (e.g. dried fruit, fruit juice) or include a mixture of both wholegrain and refined grain products (e.g. wholemeal and white bread) in your diet.

See Table 3.4 for nutritional guidelines for vegetarian diets.

SUMMARY OF KEY POINTS

- Protein is needed for the maintenance, replacement and growth of body tissue. The body also uses protein to make the many enzymes and hormones that regulate the metabolism, maintain fluid balance, and transport nutrients in and out of cells.
- Athletes require more than the current RDA for protein of 0.75 g/kg body weight/day for the general population.
- Additional protein is needed to compensate for the increased breakdown of protein during intense training and for the repair and recovery of muscle tissue after training.
- Strength and power athletes have additional needs to facilitate muscle growth.
- For endurance athletes, the recommended intake is 1.2–1.4 g/kg body weight/day. For strength and power athletes, the recommended intake is 1.4–1.8 g/kg body weight/day.
- Protein breakdown is increased when muscle glycogen stores are low, e.g. during intense exercise lasting more than 1 hour, or during a calorie/carbohydrate-restricted programme.
- Protein intake above your optimal requirement will not result in further muscle mass or strength gains.
- Athletes should be able to meet their protein needs from a well-planned diet that matches their calorie needs. Low-fat protein sources are advised.
- Vegetarian athletes can meet their protein needs from low-fat dairy products and protein-rich plant sources eaten in the right combinations so that protein complementation is achieved.

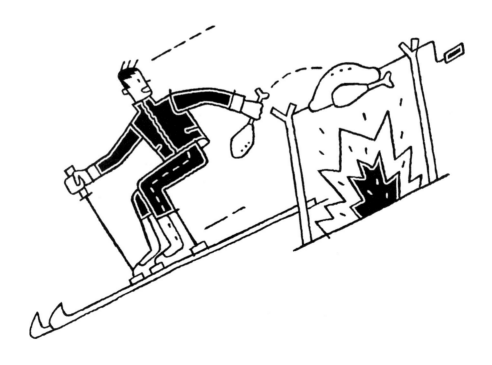

VITAMINS, MINERALS AND ANTIOXIDANTS

Vitamins and minerals are often equated with vitality, energy and strength. Many people think of them as health enhancers, a plentiful supply being the secret to a long and healthy life.

In fact, vitamins and minerals do not in themselves provide energy. Nor does an abundant supply automatically guarantee bounce and vigour or optimal health.

The truth is that vitamins and minerals are needed in certain quantities for good health, as well as for peak physical performance. However, it is the *balance* of vitamins and minerals in the diet that is most important.

For sportspeople, it is tempting to think that extra vitamins lead to better performance. Because a small amount is 'good for us', more would surely be better. Or would it?

This chapter explains what vitamins and minerals do, where they come from, and how exercise affects requirements. Do athletes need extra amounts; and should they take supplements?

The functions, sources, requirements and upper safety levels of vitamins and minerals are given in the Glossary of Vitamins and Minerals (Appendix 2). The table also examines the claims made for supplementation of vitamins and minerals and whether they could benefit athletic performance.

What are vitamins?

Vitamins are required in tiny amounts for growth, health and physical well-being. Many form the essential parts of enzyme systems that are involved in energy production and exercise performance. Others are involved in the functioning of the immune system, the hormonal system and the nervous system.

Our bodies are unable to make vitamins, so they must be supplied in our diet.

What are minerals?

Minerals are inorganic elements that have many regulatory and structural roles in the body. Some (such as calcium and phosphorus) form part of the structure of bones and teeth. Others are involved in controlling the fluid balance in tissues, muscle contraction, nerve function, enzyme secretion and the formation of red blood cells. Like vitamins, they cannot be made in the body and must be obtained in the diet.

How much do I need?

Everyone has different nutritional requirements. These vary according to age, size, level of physical activity and individual body chemistry. It is, therefore, impossible to state an intake that would be right for everyone. To find out your exact requirements you would have to undergo a series of biochemical and physiological tests.

However, scientists have studied groups of people with similar characteristics, such as age and physical activity, and have come up with some estimates of requirements. The Reference Nutrient Intake (RNI) is the measure used in the UK but the RNI value for a nutrient can vary from country to country. European Union (EU) regulations require Recommended Daily Amounts (RDAs) to be shown on food and supplement labels. RDAs are said to apply to 'average adults' and are only very rough guides.

RNI values are derived from studies of the physiological requirements of healthy people. For example, the RNI for a vitamin may be the amount needed to maintain a certain blood concentration of that vitamin. The RNI is not the amount of a nutrient recommended for optimum nutrition nor for athletic performance. Some guidelines for optimal intakes have been produced by reputable scientists but none have yet been adopted by the government.

WHAT ARE DIETARY REFERENCE VALUES (DRVs)?

In 1991 the Department of Health published *Dietary Reference Values for Food Energy and Nutrients for the United Kingdom*. A Dietary Reference Value (DRV) is a generic term for various daily dietary recommendations and covers three values that have been set for each nutrient:

1 the **Estimated Average Requirement** (**EAR**) is the amount of a nutrient needed by an average person, so many people will need more or less.

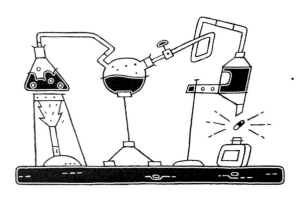

2 the **Reference Nutrient Intake** (**RNI**) is the amount of a nutrient that should cover the needs of 97% of the population. It is more than most people require, and only a very few people (3%) will exceed it.
3 the **Lower Reference Nutrient Intake** (**LRNI**) is for a small number of people who have low needs (about 3% of the population). Most people will need more than this amount.

In practice, the majority of the general population are somewhere in the middle. Athletes and sportspeople may exceed the upper limits as they have the highest requirements.

How are DRVs set?

It is not easy to set a DRV. First of all, scientists have to work out what is the minimum amount of a particular nutrient that a person needs to be healthy. Once this has been established, scientists usually add on a safety margin, to take account of individual variations. No two people will have exactly the same requirement. Next, a storage requirement is assessed. This allows for a small reserve of the nutrient to be kept in the body.

Unfortunately, scientific evidence of human vitamin and mineral requirements is fairly scanty and contradictory. A lot of scientific guesswork is inevitably involved, and results are often extrapolated from animal studies.

In practice, DRVs are arrived at through a compromise between selected scientific data and good judgement. They vary from country to country and are always open to debate.

Should I plan my diet around RNI?

The RNI is not a target intake to aim for – it is only a guideline. It should cover the needs of most people but, of course, it is possible that some athletes may need more than the RNI, due to their higher energy expenditure.

In practice, if you are eating consistently less than the RNI, you may be lacking in that nutrient.

Can a balanced diet provide all the vitamins and minerals I need?

Most athletes eat more food than the average sedentary person. With the right food choices, this means you should automatically achieve a higher vitamin and mineral intake. However, in practice many athletes do not plan their diets well enough, or they restrict their calorie intake so it can be difficult to obtain sufficient amounts of vitamins and minerals from food. Vitamin losses also occur during food processing, preparation and cooking, thus further reducing your actual intake. Intensive farming practices have resulted in crops with a lower nutrient content. For example, the use of agro-chemicals has depleted the mineral content of the soil so plants have a smaller mineral content. EU pricing policy, which keeps prices artificially high, has resulted in mountains of cauliflowers, cabbages and many other produce, which remain in storage for up to a year before being sold in supermarkets. Obviously, considerable vitamin losses may have occurred during that time. See 'How does exercise increase my requirements for vitamins and minerals?' (p. 50) for more details.

The best sort of diet is one that provides enough vitamins and minerals to meet your needs. They should come from a wide variety of foods. In the UK, the Department of Health has produced a guide describing a balanced diet centred around the five main food groups (*see* Table 4.1).

When may vitamin and mineral supplements be useful?

Eating a balanced diet may not always be easy in practice, particularly if you travel a lot, work shifts or long hours, train at irregular times, eat on the run or are unable to purchase and prepare your own meals. Planning and eating a well-balanced diet requires considerably more effort under these circumstances, so you may not be getting all the vitamins and minerals you need. A deficient intake is also likely if you are on a restricted diet (e.g. eating less than 1500 calories a day for a period of time or excluding a food group from your regular diet).

A number of surveys have shown that many sportspeople do not achieve an adequate intake of vitamins and minerals from their diet (Short & Short, 1983; Steen & McKinney, 1986; Bazzare et al., 1986). Low intakes of certain minerals and vitamins are more common

Table 4.1	Achieving a balanced diet
Foods	Portions/day
Cereals and starchy vegetables	5–11
Fruit and vegetables	> 5
Milk and dairy products	2–3
Meat, fish and vegetarian alternatives	2–3
Oils and fats	0–3

Source: Department of Health, 1994.

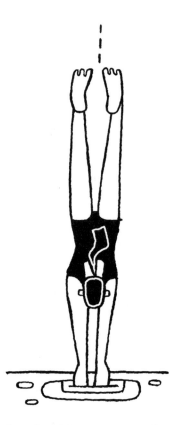

among female athletes compared with males. A study of 60 female athletes found that calcium, iron and zinc intakes were less than 100% of the RDA (Cupista et al., 2002). US researchers also measured low intakes of vitamin E, calcium, iron, magnesium, zinc and phosphorus in US national figure skaters (Ziegler, 1999). This was correlated with lower than recommended intakes of fruit, vegetables, dairy and high-protein foods. Study of US elite female hept-athletes by researchers at the University of Arizona found that while average nutrient intakes were greater than 67% of the RDA, vitamin E intakes fell below this minimum level (Mullins, 2001). However, more than half of the athletes were taking vitamin and mineral supplements, which would boost their overall intake.

Who may benefit from taking supplements?

Research shows that one in three people take some form of vitamin supplement – the most popular being multivitamins (Gallup, 2000). A study of 411 university athletes found that over half routinely took supplements (Krumbach, 1999). The most common reasons were to "improve performance" and "build muscle". Obviously, supplements are not a substitute for poor, or lazy, eating habits. If you think you may be lacking in vitamins and minerals, try to adjust your diet to include more vitamin- and mineral-rich foods.

As a temporary measure, you may benefit from taking supplements if:
• you have erratic eating habits
• you eat less than 1500 kcal a day
• you are pregnant (folic acid)
• you eat out a lot/rely on fast foods
• you are a vegan (vitamin B12 and possibly other nutrients)
• you are anaemic (iron)
• you have a major food allergy or intolerance (e.g. milk)
• you are a heavy smoker or drinker
• you are ill or convalescing.

How does exercise increase my requirements of vitamins and minerals?

Regular, intense exercise increases your requirements for a number of vitamins and minerals, particularly those involved in energy metabolism, tissue growth and repair, red blood cell manufacture and free radical defence.

Vitamin E is a powerful antioxidant (*see* p. 51), which prevents the oxidation of fatty acids in cell membranes and protects the cell from damage. Indeed, a study with élite cyclists showed that vitamin E supplementation reduced the amount of free radical (*see* p. 54) damage following prolonged intense cycling to exhaustion, compared with a placebo (Rokitzki et al., 1994).

Vitamin C has several exercise-related functions. It is required for the formation of connective tissue and certain hormones (e.g. adrenaline), which are produced during exercise; it is involved in the formation of red blood cells, which enhances iron absorption; it is a powerful antioxidant, which, like vitamin E, can also protect against exercise-related cell damage.

A vitamin C supplement may be useful if you are involved in prolonged high-intensity training because it may stabilise cell membranes and protect against viral attack. One study (Peters et al., 1993) found a reduced incidence in upper respiratory tract infections in ultra-marathon runners after taking 600 mg vitamin C for 21 days prior to the race. Another study at the University of Cape Town found that vitamin C supplements and combined vitamin C/vitamin E/beta-carotene supplements halved the incidence of post-race infections.

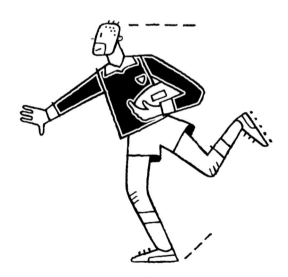

The B vitamins thiamin (B_1), riboflavin (B_2) and niacin (B_3), are involved in releasing energy from food. Since requirements for these are based on the amount of carbohydrate and calories consumed, athletes do need more than sedentary people. In general, it is easy to obtain these vitamins from wholegrain carbohydrate-rich foods such as bread, breakfast cereals, oatmeal and brown rice. However, if you use carbohydrate supplements, such as glucose polymer drinks and bars, you may need to take supplements. If you are restricting your calorie intake (e.g. on a fat-loss programme) or you eat lots of refined carbohydrates you may also be missing out on B vitamins. To compensate for any shortfall, you should take a multivitamin supplement that contains at least 100% of the RDA of the B vitamins.

Vitamin B_6 is involved in protein and amino acid metabolism. It is needed for making red blood cells and new proteins so the right amount of vitamin B_6 is very important to athletes.

Pantothenic acid (vitamin B_5) is necessary for making glucose and fatty acids from other metabolites in the body. It is also used in the manufacture of steroid hormones and brain chemicals. Obviously, a deficiency would be detrimental to health and athletic performance.

Folic acid and vitamin B_{12} are both involved with red blood cell production in the bone marrow. They are also needed for cell division, and protein and DNA manufacture. Clearly, exercise increases all of these processes and therefore your requirements for folic acid and vitamin B_{12}. Vegans, who eat no animal products, must obtain vitamin B_{12} from fortified foods such as Marmite and breakfast cereals or fermented foods such as tempeh and miso. Taking a multivitamin supplement is a good insurance.

Beta-carotene is one of 600 carotenoid pigments which give fruit and vegetables their yellow, orange and red colours. They are not vitamins but act as antioxidants by protecting cells from free radical damage. Beta-carotene enhances the antioxidant function of vitamin E, helping to regenerate it after it has disarmed free radicals. However, carotenoids function most effectively together so it is best to take these nutrients packaged together, in a supplement or in food.

Calcium is an important mineral in bone formation, but it also plays an important role in muscle growth, muscle contraction and nerve transmission. While the body is able to increase or decrease the absorption of this mineral according to its needs, extra calcium is recommended for female athletes with low oestrogen levels (*see* Chapter 10, pp. 148–9). Weight-bearing exercise, such as running and weight training, increases bone mass and calcium absorption so it is important to get enough calcium in your diet.

Iron is important for athletes. Its major function is in the formation of haemoglobin (which transports oxygen in the blood) and myoglobin (which transports oxygen in the muscle cells). Many muscle enzymes involved in energy metabolism require iron. Clearly, athletes have higher requirements for iron compared with sedentary people. Furthermore, iron losses may occur during exercise that involves pounding of the feet, such as running, aerobics and step aerobics. Also at risk of iron-deficiency are women who have been pregnant in the last year (lower iron stores) and athletes who eat less than about 2000 kcal a day. Athletes who tend to avoid red meat, a rich source of iron, need to ensure they get iron from other sources or supplements. Iron deficiency and sports anaemia are discussed in detail in Chapter 10 (*see* pp. 149–51).

Can vitamin and mineral supplements improve your performance?

Many studies have been carried out over the years using varying doses of supplements. In the vast majority of cases, scientists have been unable to measure significant improvements in the performance of healthy athletes. Where a beneficial effect has been observed, for example increased endurance, this has tended to be in athletes who started with a sub-optimal vitamin or mineral status. Taking supplements simply restored the athletes' nutrient stores to 'normal' levels.

In other words, low body stores or deficient intakes can adversely affect your performance, but vitamin and mineral supplements taken in excess of your requirements will not necessarily produce a further improvement in performance. More does not mean better!

To find out if your diet is deficient in any nutrient, you should consult a qualified nutritionist (look for the initials BSc or SRD) for a dietary analysis. He or she will then be able to advise you about your diet and supplementation.

Can supplements be harmful?

Some vitamins and minerals taken in high doses can be harmful. The fat-soluble vitamins A and D, as well as several minerals, can be stored in organs and fatty tissues (e.g. the liver, adipose tissue) and, therefore, accumulate over time.

Excess vitamin A can cause nausea, skin changes such as flakiness, liver damage and birth defects in unborn babies. Pregnant women are advised to avoid vitamin A supplements, fish liver oils and concentrated food sources of vitamin A such as liver and liver paté. Too much vitamin D from supplements can cause high blood pressure and kidney stones. Excessive doses of vitamin B_6 may lead to numbness, persistent pins and needles and unsteadiness (a type of neuropathy). High doses of iron can cause constipation and discomfort through an upset or bloated stomach.

Vitamin C and the B vitamins are water soluble and are therefore not stored in the body. Excessive intakes are excreted in the urine, although extremely high intakes from supplements may have minor adverse effects.

Vitamin E, unlike the other fat-soluble vitamins, appears to be safe even at doses 10–100 times the recommended intake. There is evidence that supplements of up to 80 mg/day (i.e. the EU RDA) may be beneficial in preventing heart disease.

Except perhaps in the case of doses of vitamin A from liver (owing to modern animal feeding practices), it is almost impossible to overdose on vitamins and minerals from food. Problems are more likely to arise from the indiscriminate use of supplements, so always follow the guidelines on the label or the advice of a nutritionist. As a rule of thumb, never take more than 10 times the RDA of the fat-soluble vitamins A and D, and no more than the RDA for any mineral.

Can supplements cause imbalances?

Taking single vitamins or minerals can easily lead to imbalances and deficiencies. Many interact with each other, competing for absorption, or enhancing or impairing each other's functions. For example, iron, zinc and calcium share the same absorption and transport system, so taking large doses of iron can reduce the uptake of zinc and calcium. For healthy bones, a finely tuned balance of vitamin D, calcium, phosphorus, magnesium, zinc, manganese, fluoride, chloride, copper and boron is required. Vitamin C enhances the absorption of iron, converting it from its inactive ferric form to the active ferrous form. Most of the B vitamins are involved in energy metabolism, so a short-term shortage of one may be compensated for by a larger than normal use of another.

If in doubt about supplements, it is safest to choose a multivitamin and mineral formulation rather than individual supplements. Single supplements should only be taken upon the advice of your doctor or nutritionist.

Are 'natural' vitamin supplements better than synthetic?

There is no proof that so-called 'natural' or 'food state' vitamin supplements are better absorbed than synthetic vitamins. The majority have an identical chemical structure. In other words, they are the same thing and such terms on supplement labels are meaningless. Tests have shown that a relatively new type of supplement called 'food form' vitamins and minerals are more readily absorbed than synthetic vitamins. 'Food form' vitamins and minerals are micronutrients that are grown from food-based (yeast) cultures in the lab and are therefore intricately bound to protein, in a similar way as naturally occurring vitamins in food. That means you need to take lower doses for maximum effect.

Are time-release supplements better than normal synthetic supplements?

Time-release vitamins are coated with protein and embedded in micropellets within the supplement. In theory, the supplement should take longer to dissolve, with the protein coating slowing down vitamin absorption. However, there is little evidence that this is the case or that they are better for you. Some may not even dissolve fully and end up passing straight through the digestive tract. If you take any supplement with a meal, the absorption of the vitamins and minerals is retarded anyway by the carbohydrate/fat/ protein in the food. So, it is not worth paying extra money for time-release supplements.

How should I choose a multi-vitamin/mineral supplement?

Here are some basic guidelines.

- Choose a multivitamin/mineral supplement which highlights its antioxidant content.
- Check it contains at least 23 vitamins and minerals.
- The amounts of each vitamin should be between 100 and 1000% of the RDA stated on the label, but below the safe upper limit (*see* Appendix 2).
- Avoid supplements containing more than the RDA of any mineral as these nutrients compete for absorption and can be harmful in doses that are higher than the RDA.
- Choose beta-carotene rather than vitamin A – it is a more powerful antioxidant and has no harmful side effects in high doses.
- Avoid supplements with unnecessary ingredients such as sweetners, colours, artificial flavours and talc (a bulking agent).
- Choose 'food form' if possible – the supplement is better absorbed.
- Choose low-dose supplements, designed to be taken in 2 or more doses daily, rather than mega-doses.
- Take with food and water.

ANTIOXIDANTS

What are antioxidants?

Antioxidants are enzymes and nutrients in the blood that 'disarm' free radicals (*see* below) and render them harmless. They work as free radical scavengers by donating one of their own electrons to 'neutralise' the free radicals. Fortunately, your body has a number of natural defences against free radicals. They include various enzymes (e.g. superoxide dismutase, glutathione, peroxidase) which have minerals such as manganese, selenium and zinc incorporated in their structure; vitamins C and E, as well as hundreds of other natural substances in plants, called phytochemicals. These include carotenoids (such as beta-carotene), plant pigments, bioflavanoids and tannins.

What are free radicals?

Free radicals are atoms or molecules with an unpaired electron and are produced all the time in our bodies as a result of normal metabolism and energy production. They can easily generate other free radicals by snatching an electron from any nearby molecule, and exposure to cigarette smoke, pollution, exhaust fumes, UV light and stress can increase their formation.

In large numbers, free radicals have the potential to wreak havoc in the body. Free radical damage is thought to be responsible for heart disease, many cancers, ageing and post-exercise muscle soreness, as unchecked, free radicals can damage cell membranes and genetic material (DNA), destroy enzymes, disrupt red blood cell membranes, and oxidise LDL cholesterol in the bloodstream, thus also increasing the risk of atherosclerosis or the furring of arteries – the first stage of heart

The good side of free radicals

Not all free radicals are damaging. Some help to kill germs, fight bacteria and heal cuts. The problem arises when too many are formed and cannot be controlled by the body's defence system.

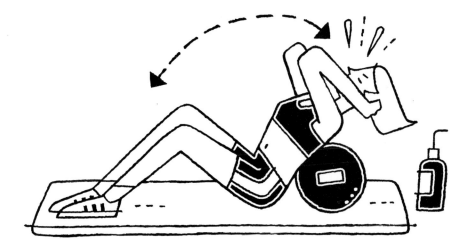

disease. Recent studies have demonstrated increased levels of free radicals following exercise and these have been held responsible for muscle soreness, pain, discomfort, oedema (fluid retention) and tenderness post-exercise.

How does exercise affect free radical levels?

Because exercise increases oxygen consumption, there is an increased generation of free radicals. No one knows exactly how or why exercise does this but it is thought to be connected to energy metabolism. During the final steps of ATP production (from carbohydrates or fats) electrons (the negative particles of atoms) sometimes get off course and collide with other molecules, creating free radicals. Exercise increases ATP production and so creates more free radicals.

Another source is the damage done to muscle cell membranes during high-intensity eccentric exercise, such as heavy weight training or plyometrics exercise causes minor tears and injury to the muscles that result in the production of free radicals.

Other factors such as increased lactic acid production, increased haemoglobin breakdown, and heat generation may be involved too. In essence, the more you exercise the more free radicals you generate (Halliwell & Gutteridge, 1985).

What are the best sources of antioxidants?

The best source of antioxidants is the natural one: food! There are hundreds of natural substances in food called phytochemicals. These substances, which are found in plant foods, have antioxidant properties which are not present in supplements. Each appears to have a slightly different effect and to protect against different types of cancer and other degenerative diseases. For example, the phytochemicals in soya beans may prevent the development of hormone dependent cancers, such as breast, ovarian and prostate cancer, while those in garlic can slow down tumour development. It is therefore wise to obtain as wide a range of phytochemicals from food as possible.

Table 4.2 lists the food sources for the various types of antioxidants.

How much do you need?

There are few official guidelines for daily intakes of antioxidants, and debate between scientists about optimal intakes for athletes. See Chapter 5, pp. 60–2 for further details.

Antioxidant tips

- Eat at least 5 portions of fresh fruit and vegetables a day.
- Include nuts and seeds regularly in your diet.
- Eat more fresh fruit for snacks.
- A daily tipple of red wine (1–2 glasses) may be beneficial.
- Add a side salad to your meals.
- Store vegetable oils in a cool dark place and do not re-use heated oil.

Table 4.2	Good sources of antioxidants
Antioxidant	Source
Vitamins	
Vitamin C	Most fruit and vegetables, especially blackcurrants, strawberries, oranges, tomatoes, broccoli, green peppers, baked potatoes
Vitamin E	Sunflower/safflower/corn oil, sunflower seeds, sesame seeds, almonds, peanuts, peanut butter, avocado, oily fish, egg yolk
Minerals	
Selenium	Wholegrains, vegetables, meat
Copper	Wholegrains, nuts, liver
Manganese	Wheatgerm, bread, cereals, nuts
Zinc	Bread, wholegrain pasta, grains, nuts, seeds, eggs
Carotenoids	
Beta-carotene	Carrots, red peppers, spinach, spring greens, sweet potatoes, mango, cantaloupe melon, dried apricots
Alpha- and gamma-carotene	Red coloured fruit, red and green coloured vegetables
Canthaxanthin and lycopene	Tomatoes, watermelon
Flavanoids	
Flavanols and polyphenols	Fruit, vegetables, tea, coffee, red wine, garlic, onions

SUMMARY OF KEY POINTS

- Vitamin and mineral requirements depend on age, body size, activity level and individual metabolism.
- DVRs should be used as a guide for the general population; they are not targets and do not take account of the needs of athletes.
- Regular and intense exercise increases the requirements for a number of vitamins and minerals. However, there are no official recommendations for athletes.
- Low intakes can adversely affect health and performance. However, high intakes exceeding requirements will not necessarily improve performance.
- Vitamins A, D and B_6 and a number of minerals may be toxic in high doses (more than $10 \times$ RNI). Indiscriminate supplementation may lead to nutritional imbalances and deficiencies.
- Due to an erratic lifestyle or restricted food intake, many athletes consume sub-optimal amounts of vitamins and minerals. Therefore a supplement containing a broad spectrum of vitamins and minerals would benefit their long-term health and performance.
- A well-formulated supplement should contain between 100–1000% of the RDA for vitamins (but below the safe upper limit); and no more than 100% of the RDA for minerals.
- Optimal doses of certain antioxidants have been suggested by scientists but have not yet been adopted by the UK government.

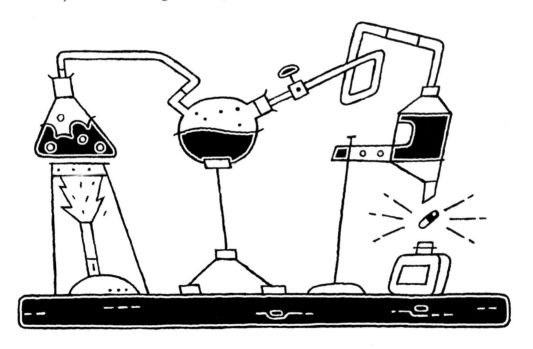

SPORTS SUPPLEMENTS

5

Athletes are always searching for that magic ingredient that will give them the competitive edge and help them achieve their best. The most effective way to develop your natural sports ability and achieve your fitness goals is through efficient training combined with optimal nutrition. However, to get the very best out of your training programme it may be worth considering certain nutritional supplements. There is a huge variety of products on the market, including pills, powders, drinks and bars. Such supplements are sometimes classed as ergogenic aids, meaning substances which 'increase work'.

The purpose of sports supplements is to enhance performance. Many claim to increase muscle tissue, increase endurance, promote fat burning or improve strength.

Most athletes believe supplements are an essential component for sports success and it has been estimated that the majority of Olympic athletes are using some form of performance-enhancing agent. Certainly the use of supplements has increased dramatically since the 1980s. An increasing variety of products are readily available through the internet as well as from mail order companies, health food stores and sports shops.

Sifting through the multitude of products on offer can be an overwhelming task for athletes. It can be hard to pinpoint which ones work, especially when advertising claims sound so persuasive. Scientific research may be exaggerated or used selectively by manufacturers trying to sell a product. Testimonials from well-known athletes are also a common ploy that is used to hype products. Figure 5.1 gives you guidelines for evaluating the claims of supplements.

This chapter examines some of the most popular supplements and focuses on those which have been the subject of scientific studies. These include:

- antioxidant supplements
- protein supplements
- branched-chain amino acid (BCAA) supplements
- meal replacement products
- creatine
- glutamine
- HMB
- DHEA
- pro-hormones
- ephedrine
- caffeine.

It explains what they are, how they work, their possible benefits to athletes, suggested doses, possible side effects and whether they are allowed by the IOC. Banned supplements have only been included where their popularity merits special mention. The chapter also provides a 'Fact file' for each supplement, which gives you the essential facts at a glance.

Vitamin and mineral supplementation is examined in Chapter 4. The background to the use of some of the supplements covered in this chapter has already been dealt with in earlier chapters: for antioxidants and BCAA supplements, *see* Chapter 4; for protein supplements, *see* Chapter 3; for creatine, *see* Chapter 1.

Figure 5.1 Protein metabolism

Guidelines for evaluating the claims of sports supplements*

1 How valid is the claim?
- Does the claim made by the manufacturer of the product match the science of nutrition and exercise, as you know it? If it sounds too good to be true, then it probably isn't valid.
- Does the amount and form of the active ingredient claimed to be present in the supplement match that used in the scientific studies on this ergogenic aid?
- Does the claim make sense for the sport for which the claim is made?

2 How good is the supportive evidence?
- Is the evidence presented based on testimonials or scientific studies?
- What is the quality of the science? Check the credentials of the researchers (look for University-based or independent) and the journal in which the research was published (look for a peer-reviewed journal reference). Did the manufacturer sponsor the research?
- Read the study to find out whether it was properly designed and carried out. Check that it contains phrases such as 'double-blind placebo controlled', i.e. that a 'control group' was included in the study and that a realistic amount of the ergogenic substance/placebo was used.
- The results should be clearly presented in an unbiased manner with appropriate statistical procedures. Check that the results seem feasible and the conclusions follow from the data.

3 Is the supplement safe and legal?
- Are there any adverse effects?
- Does the supplement contain toxic or unknown substances?
- Is the substance contraindicated in people with a particular health problem?
- Is the product illegal or banned by any athletic organizations?

*Adapted from ACSM/ADA/DC (2000), Butterfield (1996), Clark (1995).

What is the evidence for antioxidants?

Exercise causes an increased generation of free radicals (*see* p. 55) although there is unequivocal evidence whether this causes increased damage (peroxidation) to cell membranes. Researchers have found that regular exercise enhances athletes' natural antioxidant defences; in other words, the body produces more antioxidant enzymes as free radical levels rise (Robertson et al., 2001). A study of elite Alpine ski racers found no direct evidence of free radical damage, but measured a drop in the skiers' antioxidant status over a period of intense training (Subudhi et al.,

2001). It is possible, then, that antioxidant supplements will bolster the body's defences against increased free radical attack and prevent subsequent tissue damage. Certainly there is plenty of evidence that antioxidant supplements protect against age-related diseases such as heart disease, certain forms of cancer and cataracts.

Studies using antioxidants supplements with athletes have produced mixed results (Goldfarb, 1999). Researchers at Loughborough University found that daily vitamin C supplementation (200 mg) for 2 weeks reduced muscle soreness and improved recovery following intense exercise (Thompson et al., 2001).

In summary, it seems as if antioxidant mixtures rather than single nutrients (e.g. vitamin E) work best and that greater benefits are to be had during high intensity training (Kanter M. M. & Eddy D. M. (1992); Kanter M. M. et al. (1993). While recommendations specifying types and doses of antioxidants are difficult to make, it seems likely that regular exercisers and athletes would benefit from antioxidant supplementation (Sen, 2001).

Although antioxidants won't give you dramatic gains in strength, speed or mass, the evidence suggests that it's worth taking them for their long-term effect against free radicals (Sen, 2001, Faff, 2001). (*See also* box 'Antioxidant supplements and exercise', p. 62.)

How much should you take?

Fruit and vegetables supply a vast array of antioxidants, particularly beta-carotene, vitamin C and folic acid, as well as other protective substances called phytochemicals. Scientists at the American Institute for Cancer Research say that eating at least 5 portions of fruit and vegetables each day can prevent 20% of all cancers. The best advice is to get as many antioxidants as possible from food. The Department of Health and the World Health Organisation advises a minimum of 400 g or 5 portions of fruit and vegetables a day. The average UK intake is just 2.8 portions a day (Food Standards Agency, 2002). Tables 5.1 and 5.2 list the food sources of antioxidants that assist in protecting against cancer and heart disease.

Recommended daily amounts have only been set by the EU for vitamin C (60 mg) and vitamin E (10 mg). These are levels judged sufficient to support health; they are not optimal amounts for athletic performance or heart disease prevention. A number of scientists believe the UK and US recommended intakes are too low. Professor Anthony Diplock, from the University

Antioxidants

Antioxidant fact file

What are they?
Substances that quench free radicals; they include enzymes, vitamins, minerals and phytochemicals.

What are the benefits?
Help reduce the symptoms and risks associated with high levels of free radicals generated during exercise, protect against age-related diseases, slow down the effects of ageing.

Who could they benefit?
Anyone involved in regular exercise or sport.

How much?
Not certain, but levels around 15–25 mg beta-carotene, up to 1000 mg vitamin C, 250–500 mg vitamin E and 50–100 mg selenium advised by leading scientists.

Any side effects?
No toxic effects from large doses of antioxidant vitamins but doses of selenium over 900 mg can be toxic (cause nausea, vomiting).

Are they legal?
Yes.

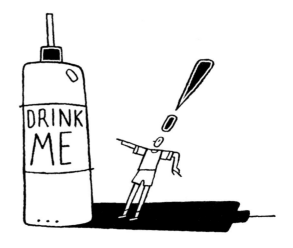

Table 5.1	Anti-cancer phytochemicals
Antioxidant	**Food source**
Beta-carotene	Carrots, red peppers, spinach, spring greens mangoes, apricots
Alpha- and gamma-carotene	Red coloured fruit, red and green coloured vegetables
Canthaxanthin	Tomatoes, watermelon
Coumaric acid	Green peppers, tomatoes, carrots
Allicin saponins	Onions, garlic, leeks
Glucosinolates	Broccoli, cabbage, cauliflower, brussel sprouts
Sulphoramine	Broccoli
Lycopene	Tomatoes
Lutein	Green vegetables
D-limonene	Pith of citrus fruits
Ellagic acid	Grapes, strawberries, cherries

Table 5.2	Heart disease protection
Antioxidant	**Food source**
Folate	Spinach, broccoli, curly kale, green cabbage and other green leafy vegetables
Quercetin	Onions, garlic, apples, grapes
Phenols	Grapes
Resveratrol	Grape skins, red wine

of London at Guy's Hospital, for example, has proposed optimal intakes which would give greater protection from disease. For beta-carotene, the optimal level would be 15–25 mg, for vitamin E 50–80 mg and for vitamin C 100–150 mg, all of which are considerably greater than current daily RNIs intake. On the other hand, Professor Mel Williams, of the Dept of Exercise Science, Physical Education and Recreation at Old Dominion University, Virginia, advises 500–1000 mg vitamin C, 250–500 mg vitamin E and 50–100 mg selenium.

However, it is doubtful whether athletes can get the intakes of antioxidant vitamins and minerals recommended by Diplock and Williams from food alone. For example, to get 80 mg vitamin E, you would need to consume 162 g (about 15 tbsp) of sunflower oil (one of the richest sources of vitamin E) daily. To obtain 25 mg beta-carotene, you would need to eat 333 g carrots (that's 6 carrots) daily. Therefore, it makes sense to take a daily antioxidant supplement.

Antioxidant supplements and exercise

A study by German researchers (Rokitzki et al., 1994) looked at the effects of vitamin E on the performance of 30 top racing cyclists. The volunteers were divided into two groups. Half were given 330 mg vitamin E (approx. 60 times the average dietary intake) and half were given a placebo for five months. At the end of this period, the supplemented cyclists had considerably greater blood levels of vitamin E. All cyclists were then instructed to cycle until exhaustion on a stationery bike. The resistance was increased every five minutes.

Those who had taken supplements had fewer signs of free radical damage, e.g. less leakage of muscle cell enzymes into the blood. The researchers concluded that vitamin E helped to protect the cells from free radical damage although it had no immediate effect on their performance.

Another study by researchers at the University of Goteborg, Sweden, and the Polish Academy of Sciences tested the effect of a general antioxidant supplement (a pollen extract) on post-exercise soreness (Krotkiewski et al., 1994). Fifty sedentary volunteers were given either the antioxidant supplement or a placebo for four weeks. They then performed an exercise test, which included a combination of stepping and cycling at 60–70% of VO_2max. Those who took the antioxidant supplement had less free radical damage and reported less pain, oedema, discomfort and tension in their muscles after exercise.

Researchers concluded that the antioxidant supplement had a beneficial effect as it reduced post-exercise soreness.

Are there any side effects?

No toxic effects have been found for the antioxident vitamins. Large doses of carotenoids consumed in the form of food or supplements can turn your skin orange, but this effect is harmless and will gradually go away. Large doses of vitamin C (over 2000 mg) can cause diarrhoea and flatulence but can obviously be corrected by reducing your supplement dose. Vitamin E, despite being a fat-soluble vitamin and capable of being stored, appears safe even at levels 50 times higher than the RDA.

However, you should be careful with selenium supplements because the margin of safety between a healthy dose of selenium (up to 200 µg a day) and a toxic dose (as little as 900 µg) is very small. Toxic symptoms include nausea, vomiting, hair loss and loss of fingernails.

The other antioxidant minerals – zinc, magnesium and copper – may produce toxic symptoms in high doses so stick to the upper safe limits given in Appendix 2.

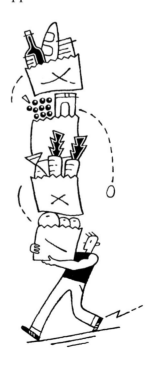

Protein-based supplements

Protein supplements fact file

What are they?
Shakes and bars containing whey casein or soy protein.

What are the benefits?
Help meet daily protein needs; well-absorbed; may have immune-enhancing and muscle sparing properties.

Who could they benefit?
Strength and power athletes with high protein and calorie needs; athletes on below-maintenance calorie intakes, vegan and vegetarian athletes.

How much?
Enough to make up any shortfall in your diet.

Any side effects?
Unlikely.

Are they legal?
Yes.

What is the evidence for protein supplements?

Many studies show that strength and power athletes have a greater daily requirement for protein than most endurance athletes. For example, Tarnopolsky et al. (1992) and Lemon et al. (1992) recommend that strength trainers need between 1.3–2.0 g/kg body weight/day. In essence, the harder and more intensively you train, the more important dietary protein is for maximising your results. Protein supplements are not a substitute for a poorly planned diet but may offer you a convenient and easy way to make up the shortfall in your diet. They are more likely to benefit you if you have particularly high protein requirements, you are on a calorie-restricted diet or you cannot consume enough protein from food alone (e.g. a vegetarian or vegan diet). Supplements are most appropriate, therefore, for strength and power athletes; athletes on a fat-loss programme; athletes undergoing very heavy training; and possibly vegans and vegetarians. Estimate your daily protein intake from food and compare that with your protein *requirement*. If there is a consistent shortfall, consider adding a supplement. For example, a strength athlete weighing 80 kg may need as much as 144 g protein a day. This may be difficult to get from food alone.

Do protein supplements have additional benefits?

Yes, because as well as meeting your protein requirement there may be other benefits, such as the immune-enhancing or muscle-sparing properties from whey protein isolates (see below). In addition, many protein supplements contain other nutrients (e.g. vitamins, minerals, amino acids, carbohydrates, essential fatty acids). In other words, you get protein along with a package of other nutrients.

When is the best time to take protein supplements?

Including protein in your post-workout meal, together with carbohydarate can enhance recovery (*see* pp. 29–30, Chapter 2). Researchers at the University of Texas, Austin, have found that a ratio of about 1 part protein to 3 parts carbohydrate promotes faster glycogen refuelling, muscle repair and growth compared with carbohydrate alone. For example, consume a protein shake with a couple of bananas or a bowl of cereal.

Are there any side effects?

No side effects of protein supplementation have been reported although, clearly, excess protein offers no further benefits. Fears about high protein intakes causing liver and kidney damage, dehydration or calcium loss have not been proven (*see* Chapter 3, p. 43 'Is too much protein harmful?').

What type of protein is best?

Protein-based supplements may contain one or more of the four types of protein:

• whey
• casein
• soy
• egg.

Each type of protein has its particular merits, which are discussed in detail below.

What are the advantages of whey protein?

Whey proteins are extracted from curdled milk using either a process called micro-filtration (the whey proteins are physically extracted by a microscopic filter) or by ion-exchange (the whey proteins are extracted by taking advantage of their electrical charges).

Isolated whey protein has a *higher* BV than any wholefood source; manufacturers claim BVs up to 159, which is considerably higher than egg (100) – the 'gold standard' protein. That means it has an amino acid profile that is better matched to muscle proteins than any other food. It is also extremely easy to digest. It produces a relatively rapid increase in blood levels of amino acids, so may be the best type of protein to have immediately after training.

Another advantage is that it has an especially high concentration of IAAs (around 50%), about half of which are BCAAs (23–25%), compared with other protein sources. This empowers a 'muscle-sparing effect' on whey, which means it minimises muscle protein breakdown during high-intensity exercise. BCAAs make up a high proportion of muscle tissue and are the first to be broken down for energy during high-intensity, prolonged exercise, so the more BCAAs you have around, the less likely it is that you will break down existing muscle tissue.

Another key feature of whey is its *immune-enhancing* capability. Research at McGill University in Canada shows that the unique amino acid make-up of whey protein can stimulate glutathione production in the body (Bounous and Gold, 1991). Glutathione is a powerful antioxidant and also helps support the immune system. This is particularly useful during periods of intense training when the immune system is suppressed.

Whey protein may also help to stimulate muscle growth, by increasing *insulin-like growth factor-1* (IGF-1) production – a powerful ana-bolic hormone made in the liver that enhances protein manufacture in muscles.

What are the advantages of casein?

Casein has a high BV (77) relative to food sources of proteins, which means a relatively high percentage of the amino acids are utilised for tissue growth.

Casein has a particularly high content of the amino acid glutamine (around 20%) compared to other protein sources. A high glutamine intake can help spare muscle mass during intense exercise and prevent exercise-induced suppress-ion of the immune system (see section on glutamine supplements later in this chapter).

Casein also travels through the gut more slowly than whey protein. This slow transit means that the amino acids and peptides could be absorbed more thoroughly, in other words, a greater percentage of the protein ends up being absorbed.

Whether a single meal of slowly digested casein would result in greater lean body mass gains than frequent small meals of whey protein is a hotly debated issue. French scientists examined the protein balance – a measure of whole body anabolism – after consuming various combinations of casein and whey protein and found that frequent whey meals were better than a single larger meal of casein (Dangin, 2000). In reality, the choice of casein or whey depends on the flexibility of your daily schedule. Whey protein based meals may be better immediately after a workout to get a faster uptake of protein into your system. Casein may be better before bedtime or anytime you know you won't be able to eat a meal for several hours.

What are the advantages of soy protein?

The soy protein powder used in soy supplements has a higher protein content and nutritional quality than the soy protein found in soymilk, tofu and meat analogues. It undergoes a more detailed extraction process that eliminates more of the fat and carbohydrate and improves the protein fractions. It appears on the ingredients panel either as soy protein isolates or under the trademark name, 'Supro'.

Soy protein isolate has the highest concentration of the key amino acids that are important for muscle growth: BCAAs (leucine, valine and isoleucine), glutamine and arginine. These amino acids make up 36% of the soy protein. The glutamine content (19%) is similar to that of casein, so it's a good protein for sparing muscle tissue during intense exercise.

Some studies have shown that soy protein isolate may enhance the production of thyroid hormones (Forsythe, 1995). These are important for regulating the metabolic rate.

What are the advantages of egg protein?

Egg protein has a BV of 100, higher than any wholefood source, and has long been considered the highest quality protein available out of all wholefood proteins. It is still used as the gold standard protein against which the BV of all other proteins is compared. However, technology has brought us 'new' proteins (the whey isolates) that have even higher BVs.

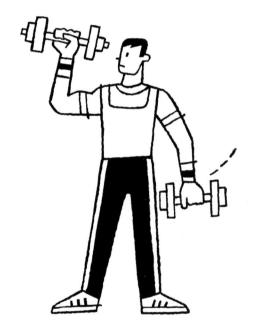

Branched-chain amino acid (BCAA) supplements

BCAA fact file

What are they?
Three IAAs that have a branched molecular configuration: valine, leucine and isoleucine.

What are the benefits?
May decrease protein breakdown during intense exercise but may not offer any advantage over carbohydrate supplementation.

Who could they benefit?
Athletes on a fat-loss programme who are consuming inadequate carbohydrate.

How much?
4 g taken during and after exercise.

Any side effects?
BCAAs are relatively safe as they are normally found in protein in the diet. Excessive intakes may reduce the absorption of other amino acids into the body.

Are they legal?
Yes.

What are they?

The BCAAs include the three IAAs with a branched molecular configuration: valine, leucine and isoleucine. They make up one-third of muscle protein.

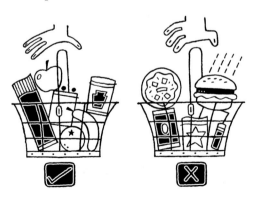

What do they do?

The theory behind BCAA supplements is that they can help prevent the break down of muscle tissue during intense exercise. They are converted into two other amino acids – glutamine and alanine – which are released in large quantities during intense aerobic exercise. Also they can be used directly as fuel by the muscles, particularly when muscle glycogen is depleted.

What is the evidence for BCAAs?

Studies at the University of Guelph, Ontario, suggest that taking 4 g BCAA supplements during and after exercise can reduce muscle breakdown (MacLean et al., 1994). They appear to be effective in preserving muscle in athletes on a low-carbohydrate diet (Williams, 1998). However, it is not clear whether chronic BCAA supplementation benefits performance. Studies with long distance cyclists at the University of Virginia found that supplements taken before and during a 100 km bike performance test did not improve performance compared with a carbohydrate drink (Madsen et al., 1996). In other words, BCAAs may not offer any advantage over carbohydrate drinks taken during exercise.

Who could benefit from BCAAs?

BCAAs are found in good amounts in most protein supplements (especially whey protein supplements) and meal replacement products so it probably is not worth taking them if you already use one of these products.

Meal replacement products (MRPs)

MRP fact file

What are they?
Shakes and bars containing protein, carbohydrate, vitamins, minerals, and small amounts of other nutrients.

What are the benefits?
Provide a balanced and convenient alternative to real food.

Who could they benefit?
Regular exercisers.

How much?
Just enough to top up your regular food aintake and make up any shortfall in your diet.

Any side effects?
High intakes are unlikely to be harmful, although they provide no further benefit either.

Are they legal?
Yes. Check the ingredients for banned substances such as caffeine or ephedrine.

What are MRPs?

MRPs include multinutrient powders – which mix with water or milk to produce a 'shake' – and bars. They are designed to provide a good balance of protein (usually whey and/or casein and/or other milk proteins), carbohydrate (usually maltodextrin and/or various sugars), vitamins and minerals.

Some MRPs contain other ergogenic nutrients such as creatine (*see* pp. 68–72) and glutamine (see pp. 72–4).

Why take MRPs instead of food?

MRPs should be regarded as *supplement* meals, rather than *substitute* meals. The two biggest advantages of MRPs over food are 'completeness' and convenience. They generally have a good nutritional profile and are relatively low in calories and fats. They are quick and easy to prepare, portable and convenient for consuming on the go. They will not have any amazing effect on your strength, stamina or performance. Instead they may help meet your nutritional needs and save valuable time when you cannot prepare meals and snacks from scratch.

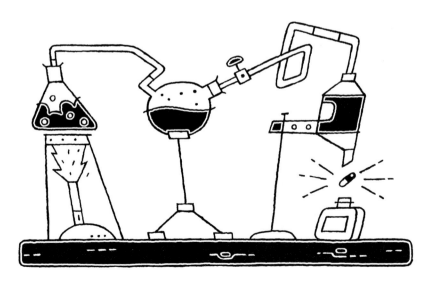

Creatine

Creatine fact file

What is it?
A protein made from 3 amino acids (arginine, glycine and methionine) in the body, but can also be found in meat and fish,m or taken as a supplement. Stored mostly as phosphocreatine (PC) in muscles. PC generates rapid energy during high-intensity activity.

What are the benefits?
Prolongs maximal power output, speeds recovery between high-intensity sets, increases lean and total body mass, buffers build-up of lactic acid in muscles.

Who could it benefit?
Athletes involved in high-intensity and anaerobic-based sports may benefit. But creatine doesn't work for everyone.

How much?
Either a loading dose of 20 g (4 × 5 g) per day for 5 days followed by 2 g a day maintenance; or a daily 3–6 g divided dose for 30 days.

Any side effects?
Weight gain (as water and/or lean mass). Long-term effect not proven.

Is it legal?
Yes.

What does creatine supplementation do?

Increasing the muscle stores of PC through creatine supplementation would theoretically increase the ability to maintain power output during brief periods of intense exercise and promote recovery between short bursts of exercise. This would result in more efficient training gains and give athletes the competitive edge.

Creatine supplementation raises PC stores by 10–40% (typically around 20%) (Hultman et al., 1996). Theoretically, elevated creatine stores would allow athletes to maintain greater training volumes, particularly if involved in repeated short bursts of activity (e.g. weight training, sprinting, football, rugby). Creatine supplementation may help athletes by one or more of the following mechanisms:

- boosts the short-term energy store of PC so the duration of maximal exercise can be increased, e.g. perform more reps or sets
- speeds recovery between 'sets' (i.e. regeneration) so it is beneficial for repeated high-intensity bursts
- promotes protein manufacture and muscle hypertrophy (by drawing water into the cells), increasing lean body mass
- reduces muscle acidity (it buffers excess hydrogen ions), thus allowing more lactic acid to be produced before fatigue sets in
- reduces muscle protein breakdown following intense exercise.

What's the evidence for creatine?

Anaerobic performance

Hundreds of studies have measured the effects of creatine supplements on anaerobic performance. Just over half of these report a positive effect on performance; the remainder show no real effect (Volek and Kraemer, 1996; Volek et al., 1997).

Studies reviewed in the Journal of Strength and Conditioning Research (Volek and Kraemer, 1996) found the best results were with:

- 1 rep-max bench press
- number of repetitions (70% of 1 rep-max.) performed to fatigue
- jump-squat peak power
- cycle power of ten 6-second bouts (better maintained)
- isokinetic knee extensions (produce less fatigue).

Aerobic performance

There is less evidence for the use of creatine with aerobic-based sports, only a few laboratory studies have shown an improvement in performance. This is probably due to the fact that the PC energy system is less important during endurance activities. However, one study at Louisiana State University suggests creatine supplements may be able to boost athletes' lactate threshold and therefore prove beneficial for certain aerobic-based sports (Nelson et al., 1997).

Body mass and composition

The vast majority of studies show that short-term creatine supplementation increases body mass. This effect occurs in males, females, trained and sedentary people, élite and non-élite athletes. Longer term studies lasting up to 12 weeks on well-trained athletes also demonstrate considerable increases in lean body mass.

Professor Kreider of the University of Memphis estimates athletes can gain up to 1.5 kg during the first week of a loading dose and up to 4.5 kg after 6 weeks. Dozens of studies show significant increases in lean mass and total mass, typically between 1–3% lean body weight (approx. 0.8–3 kg) after a 5-day loading dose, compared with controls.

The observed gains in weight are due partly to an increase in cell volume and partly to muscle synthesis.

1 Creatine is an osmotically active substance, which means it can cause water to move across cell membranes. When muscle cell creatine concentration goes up, water is drawn into the cell, an effect that boosts the thickness of muscle fibres by around 15%. The water content of muscle fibres stretches the cells' outer sheaths – a mechanical force that can trigger anabolic reactions. This may

Creatine supplementation

According to a Canadian study, relatively low doses of creatine supplementation can significantly improve weight-training performance to the same extent as higher doses (Burke et al., 2000). Volunteers who took 7.7 g creatine daily for 21 days were able to perform more repetitions on the bench press and maintain maximum power longer than those who took a placebo. They also gained significantly more muscle mass (2.3% versus a 1.4% increase with placebo).

Creatine appears to enhance performance in both men and women. Researchers at McMaster University, Ontario gave 12 male and 12 female volunteers either creatine supplements or a placebo before a high intensity sprint cycling test (Tarnopolsky & McLennan, 2000). Creatine improved the performance equally in both sexes.

stimulate protein synthesis and result in increased lean tissue (Haussinger et al., 1996).

2 Creatine may have a direct effect on protein synthesis. In studies at the University of Memphis, athletes taking creatine gained more body mass than those taking the placebo yet both groups ended up with the same body water content (Kreider et al., 1996; Clark, 1997.)

3 If creatine improves the quality of resistance training over time, this would lead to faster gains in mass, strength and power.

Who could benefit from creatine?

Creatine supplements are more likely to benefit the performance of those involved in sports or activities involving repeated high-intensity bursts, such as weight training, sprinting, football and rugby. Bodybuilders and those wishing to gain muscle mass and strength may benefit from creatine. Researchers at the Australian Institute of Sport found that creatine improved sprint times and agility run times in football players (Cox et al., 2002). Another study found that creatine supplements improved performance in events lasting 90–300 seconds in elite kayakers (McNaughton et al., 1998). However, not all studies have demonstrated positive results with creatine. Creatine supplements failed to improve sprint swim performance in a group of 20 competitive swimmers (Mujika et al., 1996).

Does creatine work for everyone?

For some reason, not everyone responds well to creatine. In some people (approx. two out of every 10), creatine concentrations increase only very slightly. It may be partly due to differences in muscle fibre types. Fast-twitch (FT) fibres tend to build up higher concentrations of creatine than slow-twitch (ST) fibres. This means that athletes with a naturally low FT fibre composition may experience smaller gains from creatine supplements. Taking creatine with carbohydrate may help solve the problem as carbohydrate raises insulin, which, in turn, helps creatine uptake by muscle cells.

What is the best form of creatine?

Creatine monohydrate is the most widely available form of creatine. It is a white powder that dissolves readily in water and is virtually tasteless. It is the most concentrated form available commercially and the least expensive. Creatine monohydrate comprises a molecule of creatine with a molecule of water attached to it so it is more stable.

Although other forms of creatine such as creatine serum, creatine citrate and creatine phosphate are available there is no evidence that they are better absorbed, produce higher levels of phosphocreatine in the muscle cells or result in greater increases in performance or muscle mass.

Can muscle creatine levels be enhanced further?

Studies have shown that insulin helps shunt creatine faster in to the muscle cells (Green et al., 1996; Steenge et al., 1998). Taking creatine along with carbohydrate – which stimulates insulin release – will increase the uptake of creatine by the muscle cells and raise levels of PC. The exact amount of carbohydrate needed to produce an insulin spike is debatable but estimates range from 35 g to around 100 g.

Some scientists recommend taking creatine with or shortly after eating a meal. The idea is to take advantage of the post-meal rise in insulin to get more creatine into the muscle cells. Taking plain creatine monohydrate is the least expensive way to achieve this. Creatine drinks and supplements containing carbohydrate are expensive and may add a lot of unwanted calories to your diet.

Creatine uptake is also greater immediately after exercise so adding creatine to the post-exercise meal will help to boost muscle creatine levels.

Canadian researchers have suggested that muscle creatine levels may be enhanced when alpha-lipoic acid (an antioxidant) is given at the same time (Burke et al., 2001a). And researchers at St Francis Xavier University, Nova Scotia found that those who supplemented with whey protein and creatine achieved greater increases in strength (bench press) and muscle mass compared with those who took only whey protein or placebo (Burke et al., 2001b).

How much should you take?

The most common creatine-loading protocol used in the creatine studies of the 1990s was to take 4×5–7 g doses per day over a period of 5 days, i.e. 20–25 g daily. That's the strategy many manufacturers still recommend for fastest results. It works but that doesn't mean it's the best way to load up. In fact, it's a pretty inefficient and costly way of getting creatine into your muscles.

The truth is that around two-thirds of this creatine ends up in your urine and only one-third ends up in your cells. The key to efficient creatine supplementation is to take small quantities at a time – and to slow down the speed of absorption from the gut. That gives the maximum chance of all the creatine consumed ending up in your muscle cells and not your urine

Roger Harris (1998) recommends taking only 0.5–1 g at a time with a total daily dose of 6 g (i.e. 6×1 g doses) and sprinkling it on your food so it reduces the absorption rate. Over a 5 or 6 day period that will produce results that are equivalent to taking 20 g a day. After that, a maintenance dose of 2 g a day will keep muscle creatine levels high enough. The loading strategy can be repeated in 8–12 weeks. Alternatively, you can load up with 3 g a day over 30 days. This technique also results in saturation of your muscles with creatine, and should produce the least water retention (Hultman et al., 1996).

Muscle has a maximal creatine storage capacity of 150–160 mmol/kg (normal is 125 mmol/kg), which makes supplementation over the quantities recommended above a waste of time and money (Harris et al., 1992).

Are there any side effects?

The main side effect of creatine supplementation appears to be weight gain due mostly to water retention. There have been anecdotal reports

Long-term safety of creatine

To date, short-term studies lasting up to 63 days (Robinson et al., 2000; Mihic et al., 2000) as well as studies lasting up to a year (Kreider, 2000) have failed to show any adverse effects of creatine supplements.

A longer-term study at Truman State University, Kirksville, US involved 23 American football players who had been using creatine supplements for up to 5 years (Mayhew et al., 2002). The researchers found no correlation between blood levels of various metabolites relating to liver and kidney function (such as albumin, bilirubin and creatinine) and the dose or duration of supplementation. They concluded that there appears to be no adverse effects of long-term supplementation on liver or kidney functions.

about muscle cramping, gastrointestinal discomfort, dehydration, muscle injury and kidney and muscle damage. However, there is no clinical data to support these statements (Williams et al., 1999).

There is concern that the water retention resulting from creatine supplementation can cause dehydration via fluid shifts into the muscle cells. While this has not been proven, most manufacturers recommend taking extra fluids while taking creatine.

Richard Kreider, from the University of Memphis and one of the world's leading creatine researchers, found that reports of gastrointestinal distress were actually less among creatine users compared to athletes taking a placebo. Provided you do not exceed the recommended dose, creatine should not produce any gastrointestinal symptoms.

Several studies have evaluated the effects of creatine supplementation on biochemical markers of kidney and muscle stress. They measured levels of creatinine, the normal breakdown product of creatine, in the urine and blood. High levels would indicate muscle or kidney damage. However, neither short- or long-term studies have found any abnormality in creatinine levels. In summary, there is no evidence for kidney or muscle damage (Poortmans & Francaux, 1999).

In conclusion, all the studies since the early 1990s indicate that there are no health risks associated with creatine supplements.

When would creatine be a disadvantage?

Body weight gain attributable to creatine could be considered a disadvantage in certain sports where the body has to be moved efficiently from A to B. For example, in distance running creatine supplementation could impair performance because more energy is required to move a heavier body weight. In swimmers, a heavier body weight may cause more drag and reduce swim efficiency. It's a matter of weighing up the potential advantage of increased maximal power and/or lean mass against the possible dis-

advantage of increased weight.

Water retention appears to be far less of a problem with the new, more moderate loading strategy.

What happens when I stop taking creatine supplements?

When you stop taking supplements, elevated muscle creatine stores will drop very slowly to normal levels over a period of four weeks (Greenhaff, 1997). During supplementation your body's own synthesis of creatine is depressed but this is reversible. In other words, you automatically step up creatine manufacture once you stop supplementation. Certainly, fears that your body permanently shuts down normal creatine manufacture are unfounded. You may experience weight loss and there are anecdotal reports about athletes experiencing small reductions in strength and power, although not back to pre-supplementation levels.

It has been proposed that creatine is best taken in cycles, such as 3–5 months followed by a one-month break.

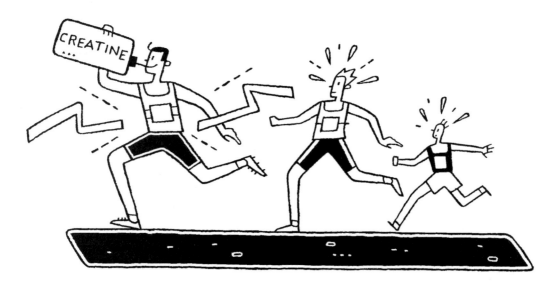

Glutamine

Glutamine fact file

What is it?
Dispensable amino acid (DAA) found in muscle cells; the major fuel of the immune system.

What are the benefits?
May help prevent muscle breakdown and suppress exercise-induced immune depression, but the evidence is not conclusive.

Who could it benefit?
Although studies are conflicting it may benefit athletes during periods of intense training or immediately after prolonged intense exercise (e.g. major competition).

How much?
100 mg/kg body weight (i.e. 7 g for 70 kg athlete) during 2-hour post-exercise period.

Any side effects?
None proven to date.

Are it legal?
Yes.

What is it?

Glutamine is a DAA. It can be made in the muscle cells from other amino acids (glutamic acid, valine and isoleucine) and is the most abundant free amino acid in muscle cells. It is essential for cell growth and is a critical source of energy for immune system cells called lymphocytes.

How could glutamine supplements benefit athletes?

The interest in glutamine stems from the observation that after intense prolonged exercise or during periods of heavy training, blood and muscle glutamine levels tend to fall quite dramatically. There is also a drop in the activity of immune cells, making athletes more susceptible to infection during this time. In other words, without adequate fuel (glutamine), immune cell activity is impaired.

The idea behind glutamine supplementation is to prevent the post-exercise drop in glutamine levels and maintain the immune system. Theoretically, glutamine may also prevent the muscle breakdown normally associated with hard training. That's because it helps draw water into the muscle cells, increasing the cell volume. This inhibits enzymes from breaking down muscle proteins.

What is the evidence?

Studies at Oxford University with marathon runners and ultra-marathon runners have shown that glutamine supplements taken immediately after running and again two hours later appeared to lower the risk of infection and boost immune cell activity (Castell & Newsholme, 1997). Only 19% of those taking glutamine became ill during the week following the run while 51% of those taking a placebo became ill. However, not all studies have managed to replicate these findings.

While some studies have suggested that supplements may reduce the risk of infection and promote muscle growth (Parry-Bollings et al., 1992; Rowbottom et al., 1996), others have failed to show any effect on performance, body composition or muscle breakdown (Haub, 1998). According to a Canadian study, glutamine produces no increase in strength or muscle mass compared with a placebo (Candow et al., 2001). After 6 weeks weight training, those taking glutamine achieved the same gains in strength and muscle mass as those taking a placebo.

How much should you take?

The case for glutamine is not clear. Studies have used doses of around 100 mg glutamine per kg body weight during the 2 hours following a strenuous workout or competition (Bledsoe, 1999). That's equivalent to a 7 g dose in a 70 kg athlete. But that doesn't mean you will get any benefit.

Many protein and meal replacement supplements contain glutamine.

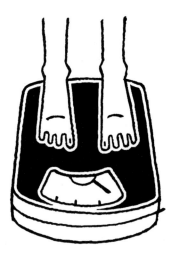

HMB

HMB fact file

What is it?
A metabolite of the amino acid, leucine.

What are the benefits?
May reduce muscle damage, repair and build muscle after exercise, increase muscle strength and reduce body fat.

Who could benefit?
Many novices – strength and power athletes, athletes wishing to gain lean mass, possibly serious endurance athletes.

How much?
38.1 mg/kg body weight/day – approximately 3 g (men) or 2 g (women) daily.

Any side effects?
In animal tests no adverse effects have been found even at very high doses. As it is water soluble, excess HMB ends up being excreted in urine.

Is it legal?
Yes.

What is HMB?

HMB (beta-hydroxy beta-methylbutyrate) is made in the body from the BCAA, leucine. You can also obtain it from a few foods such as grapefruit, alfalfa and catfish. The supplement has been on the market since 1995.

What does it do?

HMB assists with the immune system and has also been shown to build muscle size and strength, decrease body fat and lower blood cholesterol. No one knows exactly how HMB works but it is thought to be involved in cellular repair. HMB is a precursor to an important component of cell membranes, that helps with growth and repair of muscle tissue. There is data to show that HMB protects muscle protein from excessive breakdown and accelerates repair. Thus, HMB helps build muscle and repair tissue more rapidly after exercise.

What is the evidence?

Several studies suggest that HMB may increase strength and muscle mass and reduce muscle damage after resistance exercise. Studies at Iowa State University have shown muscle mass gains of 1.2 kg and strength gains of 18% after three weeks, compared with a 0.45 kg muscle gain and 8% strength gain from a placebo (Nissen et al., 1996; Nissen et al., 1997). However, this degree of improvement hasn't been found in all HMB studies.

It appears to have little effect in experienced athletes (Kreider et al., 2000). One study at the Australian Institute of Sport failed to find strength or mass improvements in 22 athletes taking 3 g per day for 6 weeks (Slater et al., 2001). Researchers at the University of Queensland in Australia found no beneficial effect on reducing muscle damage or muscle soreness following resistance exercise (Paddon-Jones et al., 2001).

HMB may boost muscle mass more effectively when taken together with creatine (Jowko et al., 2001).

Who could benefit from HMB?

HMB may benefit strength and power athletes looking to gain muscle mass and strength but probably only for the first two months of training. No long-term studies have been carried out to date – it is unlikely to benefit more experienced athletes. It has also been suggested that HMB may speed recovery in endurance athletes during intense training periods.

How much should you take?

If you decide to try HMB, try the doses used in the studies: 3 g daily for men usually divided into two or three equal doses. For women, researchers recommend around 2 g daily. This equates to 38.1 mg per kg of body weight per day. Higher doses do not offer any further benefits.

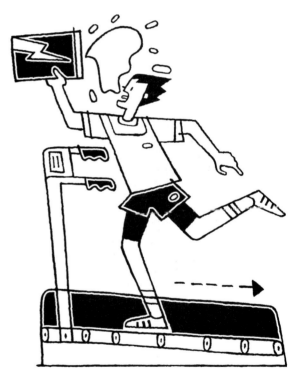

ZMA
(Zinc monomethionine aspartate and magnesium aspartate)

ZMA fact file

What is it?
Zinc monomethionine aspartate and magnesium aspartate (ZMA) is a supplement that combines zinc and magnesium.

What are the benefits?
May boost anabolic hormone levels (testosterone and IGF-I) by correcting a zinc and magnesium deficiency (Brilla & Conte, 2000).

Who could it benefit?
Strength and power athletes during periods of intense training – but only if dietary levels of zinc and magnesium are low.

How much?
No recommended dose.

Any side effects?
High levels of zinc – more than 50 mg – can interfere with the absorption of iron and other minerals, leading to iron-deficiency. Check the zinc content of any other supplement you may be taking.

Is it legal?
Yes.

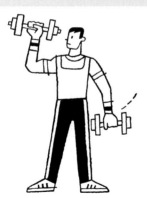

Pro-hormones

Pro-hormone fact file

What are they?
Inactive substances which are converted into testosterone – including androstenedione – in the body.

What are the benefits?
Supplement advertisements claim they increase testosterone production, strength and muscle mass. In practice, there is no scientific proof for their purported effects.

Who could they benefit?
Despite aggressive marketing to strength and power athletes, there is a lack of evidence on which to recommend them.

How much?
Manufacturers recommend daily doses between 50 and 100 mg amounts that have no proven effect.

Any side effects?
Raise oestrogen levels and decrease HDL. May contain illegal steriods.

Are they legal?
Legal to buy, but may result in a positive doping test. Banned by the I.O.C.

What are pro-hormones?

Pro-hormones – including androstenedione (or andro for short) and dehydroepiandrosterone (DHEA) – are weak androgenic steroid compounds capable of being converted to testosterone. They are produced naturally in the body. The theory behind pro-hormone supplements is that because they are precursors to the production of testosterone, supplemental doses should increase levels of testosterone, muscle mass and strength.

What is the evidence?

Current research does not support supplement manufacturers' claims. Studies show that andro supplements and DHEA have no significant testosterone-raising effects, and no effect on muscle mass or strength (King et al., 1999; Broeder et al., 2000; Powers, 2002). A study at Iowa State University found that 8 weeks of supplementation with andro, DHEA, saw palmetto, Tribulus terrestris and chrysin combined with a weight training programme failed to raise testosterone levels or increase muscle strength or mass – in spite of increased levels of androstenedione – compared with a placebo (Brown et al., 2000).

Are there side effects?

There are a number of serious risks associated with pro-hormone use. Andro supplements can increase oestrogen and decrease HDL (good cholesterol) levels (King et al., 1999). Clearly, this is undesirable as raised oestrogen can lead to gynecomastia (breast development), enlarged prostate and lowered libido in men. Reduced HDL carries a greater heart disease risk.

Supplement manufacturers claim that dihydroxyflavone (chrysin) can block the effects of oestrogen but this has been disproved by researchers at Iowa State University (Brown et al., 2000).

Are pro-hormones legal?

Most athletic associations, including the International Olympic Committee, ban pro-hormones. There is a risk of achieving an inadvertent positive doping test. A number of reports have found that some pro-hormone supplements are incorrectly labelled and contain illegal steroids without any indication on the label.

In an analysis of 634 supplements carried out by the International Olympic Committee, 15% contained substances – including nandrolone – that would lead to a failed drugs test. Nineteen per cent of UK samples were contaminated. In another study, researchers from Olympic Analytical Laboratory at the University of California found the some brands of androstenedione are grossly mislabelled and contained the illegal anabolic steroid, testosterone (Catlin et al., 2000). Men who took either 100 mg or 30 mg of androstenedione for one week tested positive for 10-norandrostenrone, a metabolic by-product of nandrolone. In another report, Swiss researchers found different substances than those declared on the labels, including testosterone, in seven out of 17 pro-hormone supplements, i.e. 41% of the supplements (Kamber, 2001)! European Sports Ministers have called for a stricter labelling of supplements in light of these findings.

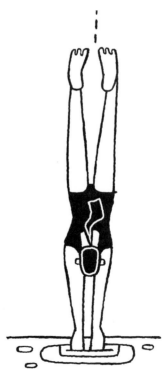

Ephedrine

Ephedrine fact file

What is it?
A stimulant substance derived from the ephedra or mahuang plant.

What are the benefits?
Increases alertness, arousal and motivation to train; increases thermogenesis (heat production) and helps fat loss.

Who could it benefit?
Not recommended to anyone in drug-tested sports; but it is commonly taken by endurance and strength athletes to increase workout intensity and duration and to aid weight loss.

How much?
Up to 25 mg in one dose is considered safe in cold remedies; higher doses (around 150 mg) would be needed to produce a stimulant effect.

Any side effects?
Anxiety, heart palpitations, insomnia, hypertension, when taken in high doses; can be fatal.

Is it legal?
Legal to buy but banned by the IOC.

What is ephedrine?

Ephedrine, also known as mahuang, is, strictly, a drug rather than a nutritional supplement. It is a common ingredient in 'energy boosters', 'fat burners' and weight loss supplements. It is also used at low concentrations in cold and flu remedies (pseudoephedrhe). It comes from the dried young branches of the Ephedra sinica plant, an Asian shrub commonly called ephedra or mahuang.

What does ephedrine do?

Ephedrine is chemically similar to amphetamines which act on the brain and the central nervous system. Athletes use it because it increases arousal, physical activity and the potential for neuromuscular performance. It is often combined with caffeine, which enhances the effects of ephedrine.

What is the evidence for ephedrine?

Ephedrine is a proven stimulant. However, research studies generally show it has little effect on strength and endurance. This is probably because relatively low doses were used. What is more likely is that these products have a 'speed-like' effect; they make you feel more awake and alert, more motivated to train hard and more confident.

There is some evidence that ephedrine helps fat loss: partly due to an increase in thermogenesis (heat production), partly because it suppresses your appetite and partly because it makes you more active.

When taken as a 'caffeine–ephedrine stack', or a 'caffeine–ephedrine–aspirin stack', it is thought that ephedrine has a greater effect in terms of thermogenesis and weight loss. In one study, volunteers who took a combination of caffeine and ephedrine before a cycle sprint (anaerobic exercise) achieved a better performance than those who took caffeine only, ephedrine only or a placebo (Bell, 2001).

Are there any side effects?

Ephedrine is judged to be safe in doses containing around 18–25 mg, that's the amount used in decongestants and cold remedies. Taking too much can have serious side effects. These include increased heart rate, increased blood pressure, palpitations, anxiety, nervousness, insomnia, nausea, vomiting and dizziness. Very high doses (around 3000 mg) cause heart attacks and can even be fatal. Caffeine–ephedrine stacks produce adverse effects at even lower doses. A case of a sportsman who suffered an extensive stroke after taking high doses of 'energy pills' (caffeine–ephedrine) has been reported in the Journal of Neurology, Neurosurgery and Psychiatry (Vahedi, 2000).

In 2002, the American Medical Association called for a ban on ephedrine due to concerns over its side effects.

Is it legal?

Ephedrine is classed as a banned substance by the IOC. Despite being an ingredient in over-the-counter remedies it is not permitted even at low levels.

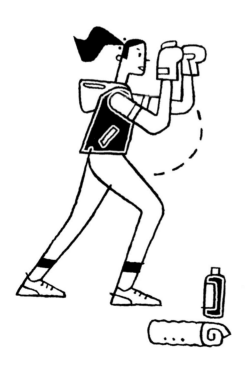

Caffeine

Caffeine fact file

What is it?
A stimulant.

What are the benefits?
Increases alertness, concentration and endurance.

Who could it benefit?
Athletes involved in both high-intensity short-term activities and endurance activities may benefit. Not recommended in pharmacological doses to athletes in drug-tested sports.

How much?
Doses between 210–1050 mg will have an ergogenic effect – varies between individuals.

Any side effects?
Varies but may induce or exacerbate anxiety and sleeplessness. Diuretic action may cause dehydration without extra fluids consumed.

Is it legal?
Legal to buy but banned by IOC at levels above 12 μg/ml in the urine.

What is caffeine?

Caffeine has a pharmacological action on the body so is classed as a drug rather than a nutrient. It is found in certain drinks such as coffee (50–100 mg per cup), tea (30–60 mg per cup), cola (50 mg per 330 ml can), herbs such as guarana (54 g) and chocolate (40 mg per 54 g bar). It is also added to a number of energy drinks and sports drinks (around 100 mg per 250 ml can).

The amounts used in research range from 3–15 mg/kg body weight, which is equivalent to 210–1050 mg for a 70 kg athlete. Studies normally used caffeine pills rather than drinks.

What does caffeine do?

Caffeine acts on the central nervous system, increasing alertness and concentration, which could be considered advantageous in many sports. It also stimulates adrenaline release and – in doses above 5 mg/kg body weight – mobilises fatty acid release. This means more fatty acids are used for energy and less glycogen. This could be advantageous for many sports as it would spare glycogen and increase endurance. Caffeine can also affect muscle contraction positively by releasing calcium from its storage sites in muscle cells. This could be advantageous for both anaerobic and aerobic activities.

What is the evidence for caffeine?

There is a huge amount of research evidence that caffeine improves performance (Dodd, 1993; Graham & Spriet, 1991). It has proved beneficial in both short-term high-intensity activities, such as 100 m sprint runs or swims, as well as aerobic activities, such as long distance swimming and running (Spriet, 1995). Positive effects have even been shown for doses within the legal limit.

In runners, caffeine can improve performance by as much as 40% (Graham & Spriet, 1991). One study with swimmers showed a 23 second improvement in a 21-minute swim (MacIntosh, 1995). Researchers at RMIT University, Victoria, Australia found that caffeine improved performance by 4–6 seconds in competitive rowers during a 2000 m row (Anderson et al., 2000). However, not all studies have shown positive results. Researchers at the University of Stirling, UK, and the University of Cape Town, South Africa found that caffeine had no effect on performance during a 100 km cycling time trial (Hunter et al., 2002).

Are there any side effects?

Caffeine's side effects include anxiety, trembling and sleeplessness. Some people are more susceptible to these than others.

Although caffeine is a diuretic, a daily intake of less than 300 mg caffeine results in no larger urine output than water. At this level, caffeine is considered safe and unlikely to have any detrimental effect on performance or health (Armstrong, 2002). Taking caffeine regularly (e.g. drinking coffee) builds up your caffeine tolerance so you experience smaller diuretic effects.

According to a study from Ohio State University, caffeine taken immediately before exercise does not promote dehydration (Wemple, 1997). Six cyclists consumed a sports drink with or without caffeine over a 3 hour cycle ride. Researchers found that there was no difference in performance or urine volume during exercise. Only at rest was there an increase in urine output.

In another study, when 18 healthy men consumed 1.75 litres of three different fluids at rest, the caffeine-containing drink did not change their hydration status (Grandjean, 2000).

Researchers at the University of Maastrict found that cyclists were able to rehydrate after a long cycle equally well with water or a caffeine-containing cola drink (Brouns, 1998). Urine output was the same after both drinks. However, large doses of caffeine – over 600 mg, enough to cause a marked ergogenic effect – may result in a larger fluid loss.

If you do decide to use caffeine, make sure that you are well hydrated before training or competition. Cutting down on caffeine for several days prior to competition may result in a more marked ergogenic effect. Then, immediately before exercise, take approximately 150–200 mg of caffeine from drinks, such as coffee (1–2 strong cups) or an energy/sports drink (1–2 cans). This may help you to keep exercising longer and harder.

Is caffeine legal?

The IOC classes caffeine as a stimulant, but as it is a constituent of drinks it is permitted in doses that produce a level less than 12 mg/ml in the urine. The amount needed to reach this legal limit varies from one person to the next, but on average, it's equivalent to 8 cups of coffee or 16 cans of cola.

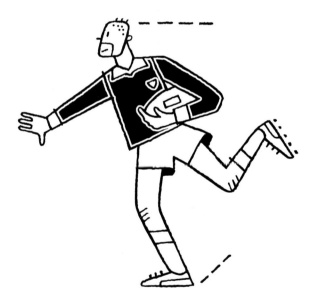

Fat burners
(ephedrine-free)

Fat burners fact file

What is it?
The most popular fat-burner supplements include citrus aurantium (synephrine or bitter orange extract), green tea extract (which contains among other antioxidants, epigallocatechin gallate) and forskolin extract (a herb). They claim to produce similar effects to ephedrine.

What are the benefits?
All claim to boost the metabolism and enhance fat loss. Green tea extract may boost levels of the hormone, norepinephrine, which curbs appetite and stimulates metabolism. But the overall calorie-burning effect is small compared with total energy expenditure; in studies, volunteers burned only an extra 64 calories a day, equivalent to a small plain biscuit! (Dulloo et al., 1999). The doses used in some brands may be too small to provide a measurable effect.

Who could it benefit?
Those wishing to lose body fat – although the overall benefit may only be small. Careful eating and exercise are likely to produce better results in the long term.

How much?
A daily dose that provides 100–300 mg of EGCG – equivalent to a minimum of six cups of green tea – may have an effect.

Any side effects?
Generally safer than ephedrine but high doses may cause side effects. Citrus aurantium can increase blood pressure. High doses of forskolin may cause heart disturbances.

Is it legal?
Yes.

SUMMARY OF KEY POINTS

- Antioxidant supplementation provides many health benefits, and helps reduce the risks and symptoms associated with the high levels of free radicals that are generated during exercise. Short-term benefits to performance are not clear but, in the long term, it could promote faster recovery in athletes during periods of hard training.
- Protein supplements based on whey protein have a superior amino acid profile compared with food sources, have additional functional properties, and would be most beneficial to strength and power athletes.
- Meal replacement or multinutrient supplements are formulated to provide balanced amounts of protein, carbohydrate, vitamins and minerals. They are convenient 'snacks' and may benefit those with high nutritional needs.
- Creatine may benefit athletes involved in high-intensity activities, especially those involving sprinting, multiple high-effort events and weight training. Dietary supplementation can improve the capacity to sustain maximum power output, speed recovery between sets and increases lean and total body mass. However, it does not work for everyone.
- Glutamine may be useful for athletes during periods of intense training, or immediately after prolonged intense exercise but the studies are not conclusive. Theoretically, it may help prevent muscle breakdown and suppress exercise-induced immune depression.
- HMB may promote muscle growth and accelerating muscle repair after intense exercise in novices, but again, the evidence is inconclusive.
- Pro-hormones, including 'andro' and DHEA **do not** increase testosterone production, strength or muscle mass contrary to manufacturers claims. They should be avoided in drug-tested sports due to the risk of an inadvertent positive drugs test.
- Ephedrine-containing supplements are popular fat-loss aids and performance-enhancers, but they are associated with a number of side effects and many athletic bodies prohibit their use.
- Caffeine increases alertness, concentration, and endurance and, taken in pharmacological doses, could benefit performance in both high-intensity and endurance activities.

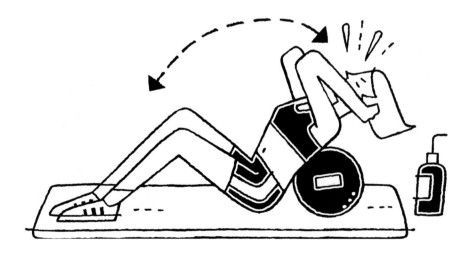

DRINK AND BE MERRY!

6

Exercise is thirsty work.

Whenever you exercise you lose fluid, not only through sweating but also as water vapour in the air that you breathe out. Your body's fluid losses can be very high and, if the fluid is not replaced quickly, dehydration will follow. This will have an adverse effect on your physical performance and health. Exercise will be much harder and you will suffer fatigue sooner.

This chapter explains why it is important to drink fluids to avoid dehydration, when is the best time to drink, and how much to drink. It deals with the timing of fluid intake: before, during and after exercise, and considers the science behind the formulation of sports drinks. Do they offer an advantage over plain water; and can they improve performance? Finally, this chapter looks at the effects of alcohol on performance and health, and gives a practical, sensible guide to drinking.

Why do I sweat?

First, let us consider what happens to your body when you exercise. When your muscles start exercising, they produce extra heat. In fact, about 75% of the energy you put into exercise is converted into heat, and is then lost. This is why exercise makes you feel warmer. Extra heat has to be dissipated to keep your inner body temperature within safe limits – around 37–38°C. If your temperature rises too high, normal body functions are upset and eventually heat stroke can result.

The major method of heat dispersal during exercise is sweating. Water from your body is carried to your skin via your blood capillaries

and as it evaporates you lose heat. For every litre of sweat that evaporates you will lose around 600 kcal of heat energy from your body. (You can lose some heat through convection and radiation, but it is not very much compared with sweating.)

How much fluid do I lose?

The amount of sweat that you produce and, therefore, the amount of fluid that you lose, depends on:

- how hard you are exercising
- how long you are exercising for
- the temperature and humidity of your surroundings
- individual body chemistry.

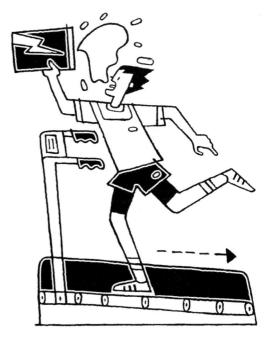

The harder and longer you exercise, and the hotter and more humid the environment, the more fluid you will lose. During 1 hour's exercise an average person could expect to lose around 1 litre of fluid – and even more in hot conditions. During more strenuous exercise in warm or humid conditions (e.g. marathon running) you could be losing as much as 2 litres an hour.

Some people sweat more profusely than others, even when they are doing the same exercise in the same surroundings. This depends partly on body weight and size (a smaller body produces less sweat), your fitness level (the fitter and better acclimatised to warm conditions you are, the more readily you sweat due to better thermoregulation), and individual factors (some people simply sweat more than others!). In general, women tend to produce less sweat than men, due to their smaller body size and their greater economy in fluid loss. The more you sweat, the more care you should take to avoid dehydration.

You can estimate your sweat loss and, therefore, how much fluid you should drink by weighing yourself before and after exercise. Every 1 kg decrease in weight represents a loss of approximately 1 litre of fluid.

What are the dangers of dehydration?

An excessive loss of fluid (dehydration) impairs performance and has an adverse effect on health (Below et al., 1995; McConnell et al., 1997). As blood volume decreases and body temperature rises, it places extra strain on the heart, lungs and circulatory system, which means the heart has to work harder to pump blood round your body. The strain on your body's systems means that exercise becomes much harder, and your performance drops.

A loss of just 2% in your weight will affect your ability to exercise, and your maximal aerobic

Figure 6.1 Fluid loss reduces exercise capacity

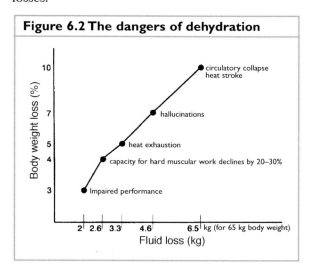

capacity will fall by 10–20% (i.e. your performance will deteriorate). If you lose 4%, you may experience nausea, vomiting and diarrhoea. At 5% your aerobic capacity will decrease by 30%, while an 8% drop will cause dizziness, laboured breathing, weakness and confusion (*see* Fig. 6.1). Greater drops have very serious consequences (Montain & Coyle, 1992; Noakes, 1993). Figure 6.2 shows the danger of dehydration with progressively greater fluid losses.

Figure 6.2 The dangers of dehydration

Ironically, the more dehydrated you become, the less able your body is to sweat. This is because dehydration results in a smaller blood volume (due to excessive loss of fluid), and so a compromise has to be made between maintaining the blood flow to muscles and maintaining the blood flow to the surface of the skin to carry away heat. Usually the blood flow to the skin is reduced, causing your body temperature to rise.

If you carry on exercising without replacing fluids you become more and more dehydrated. Your body temperature will increase more and more, and a vicious circle will be set up, resulting eventually in fatigue or heat stroke.

Can I minimise my fluid loss?

You cannot prevent your body from losing fluid. After all, this is a natural and desirable way to regulate body temperature. On the other hand, you can prevent your body from becoming dehydrated by offsetting fluid losses as far as possible. The best way to do this is to make sure you are well hydrated before you start exercising, and to drink plenty of fluids during and after exercise to replace losses (see 'When and how much should I drink?' and 'What should I drink?' overleaf).

Are you dehydrated?

Many people, both athletes and non-athletes, suffer chronic mild dehydration without realising. Dehydration is cumulative which means you can easily become dehydrated over successive days of training or competition if you fail to rehydrate fully between workouts. Symptoms of dehydration include sluggishness, a general sense of fatigue, headaches, loss of appetite, feeling excessively hot, light headedness and nausea.

From a practical point of view, you should be producing a dilute pale-coloured urine. Concent-

rated, dark-coloured urine of a small volume indicates you are dehydrated and is a signal that you should drink more before you exercise.

Indeed, many coaches and trainers advise their players or athletes to monitor their urine output and colour as this is a surprisingly accurate way of assessing hydration status. University of Connecticut researchers found that urine colour correlated very accurately with hydration status – as good as measurements of specific gravity and osmolality of the urine (Armstrong et al., 1998). Urine described as 'very pale yellow' or 'pale yellow' indicates you are within 1% of optimal hydration.

How do sweat suits affect fluid loss?

Many athletes use sweat suits, plastic, neoprene and other clothing to 'make' weight for competition. This is definitely not a good idea! By preventing sweat evaporation, the clothing prevents heat loss. This will cause body temperature to rise more and more. In an attempt to expel this excess heat your body will continue to produce more sweat, thus losing increasing amounts of fluid. You will become dehydrated, with the undesirable consequences this entails.

As mentioned above, your ability to exercise will be impaired – you will suffer fatigue much sooner and will have to slow down or stop altogether. Obviously, this is not a good state in which to train or compete.

Losing weight through exercise in sweat suits is not only potentially dangerous, but has no effect whatsoever on fat loss. Any weight loss will simply be fluid, which will immediately be regained when you next eat or drink. The exercise may seem harder because you will be sweating more, but this will not affect the body's rate of fat breakdown. If anything, you are likely to lose less fat, because you cannot exercise as hard or for as long when you wear a sweat suit.

WHEN AND HOW MUCH SHOULD I DRINK?

1 Before exercise

It is clear that if you begin a training session or competition in a dehydrated state your performance will suffer and you will be at a competitive disadvantage. For example, in one study, runners performed a 5000 m run and a 10,000 m run in either a normally hydrated or slightly dehydrated condition (Armstrong et al., 1985). When dehydrated by 2% of body weight their running speed dropped substantially (6–7%) in both events.

Obviously, prevention is better than cure. Make sure you are well hydrated before you begin exercising, especially in hot and humid weather. In a joint position statement, the American College of Sports Medicine (ACSM) and the American Dietetic Association and Dietitians of Canada recommend drinking *400–600 ml of fluid about 2 hours before exercise* to promote hydration and allow enough time for excretion of excess water (ACSM/ADA/DC, 2000).

The larger the volume of fluid in your stomach, the faster it is emptied into the intestines, and the faster it replaces fluid losses in your body. That's why it is best to drink as much as you comfortably can early on in your workout, and then continue topping up with frequent drinks. Obviously, this is easier to do during activities such as cycling, swimming or weight training, where the body is supported or impact is kept to a minimum.

Can you 'hyperhydrate' before competition?

'Loading up' with fluid before an event seems like a good strategy if you compete in ultra-endurance events, activities during which there is little opportunity to drink, or in hot humid conditions. Unfortunately, you cannot achieve hyperhydration by simply consuming large volumes of water or sports drinks prior to the event. The body simply excretes surplus fluid and you just end up paying frequent visits to the toilet or bushes. However, there is method of hyperhydration that involves the consumption of glycerol along with fluid 2 hours before exercise. Glycerol is a hyperhydrating agent, which, through its strong osmotic activity, drags water into both the extra-cellular and intra-cellular fluid. This results in an increase in total body fluid. In theory, you will be able to maintain blood volume, increase sweating and reduce the rise in core body temperature that occurs during exercise. Studies at the Australian Institute of Sport found that by doing this athletes retained an extra 600 ml of fluid and improved performance in a time trial by 2.4% (Hitchins et al., 1999). However, a few side effects have been reported, including gastro-intestinal upsets and headaches.

2 During exercise

As soon as you start exercising you will start to lose fluid, so your aim is to offset fluid losses by *drinking early and at regular intervals*. Drink as much as you comfortably can: aim for 150–350 ml every 15–20 minutes during exercise (ACSM 2000). Clearly, the more you sweat, the more you need to drink. However, do not be guided by thirst as this is not a good indicator of your hydration status. Studies have shown that you can maintain optimal performance if you replace at least 80% of your sweat loss during exercise (Montain and Coyle, 1992).

From a practical point of view, the ACSM recommend cool drinks (15–22°C). You will also be inclined to drink more if the drink is *palatable* and in a container that makes it *easy to drink*. Studies have shown that during exercise athletes voluntarily drink more of a flavoured sweetened drink than water (Wilk and Bar-Or, 1996; Minchan, 2002). Drinks bottles with sports caps are probably the most popular containers. It is also important to make drinks readily accessible; for example, for swim training have drinks bottles at the poolside, for games played on a pitch or court (soccer, hockey, rugby, netball, tennis) have the bottles available adjacent to the pitch or court.

Why do I feel nauseous when I drink during exercise?

If you feel nauseous or experience other gastro-intestinal symptoms when you drink, the chances are you are already dehydrated! Even a fairly small degree of dehydration (around 2% of body weight) slows down stomach emptying and upsets the normal rhythmical movement of your gut. This can result in feelings of bloatedness, nausea and vomiting. Avoid this by drinking as much as you comfortably can before exercise and then continue drinking early on in your workout. Do not wait until you feel thirsty or 'save' your drink until the latter stages of your workout!

3 After exercise

In order to restore normal fluid balance after exercise, researchers recommend you should consume approximately 1.5 times (i.e. 150%) the fluid lost during exercise (Shirreffs et al., 1996).

The simplest way to work out how much you need to drink is to weigh yourself before and after training. Working on the basis that 1 litre of sweat is equivalent to a 1 kg body weight loss, you need to drink 1.5 fluid/kg weight lost. The ACSM/ADA recommend at least 450–675 ml of fluid for every 0.5 kg of body weight loss.

Clearly, you should not drink all this amount straight away. Consume as much as you feel comfortable with then drink the remainer in divided doses until you are fully hydrated.

4 Between workouts

Researchers recommend drinking 1 litre of fluid for every 1000 kcal you consume. This includes fluid in foods such as milk, fruit, soup and shakes. You will need to drink more in hot humid weather as water loss increases due to sweating. Table 6.1 gives daily fluid guidelines.

WHAT SHOULD I DRINK?

1 Before exercise

Your main priority is to ensure you are well-hydrated before exercise so you should choose a drink that delivers fluid relatively fast. Water would be fine. However, you may benefit further from a sports drink because it also provides carbohydrate. As explained in Chapter 2 ('How much carbohydrate should I consume before

Table 6.1	Daily fluid guidelines	
Daily energy expenditure	**Minimum daily fluid intake***
2000 kcal	2 litres
2500 kcal	2½ litres
3000 kcal	3 litres
3500 kcal	3½ litres
4000 kcal	4 litres

*includes food and drink

exercise?, pp. 22–3), consuming approximately 1 g carbohydrate/kg body weight about 1 hour before exercise can help to improve endurance. Therefore, a sports drink would help ensure full hydration as well as providing pre-exercise carbohydrate. Alternatively, water together with solid food would do an equally good job. *See* Chapter 2 (p. 26) for suggestions.

2 During low- or moderate-intensity exercise lasting less than 1 hour

For activities such as 'easy pace' swimming, 'easy pace' cycling, or power walking carried out for less than 1 hour, fluid losses are likely to be relatively small and can be replaced fast enough with plain water. After all, water is a very good fluid replacer. Sports drinks would increase the speed of water absorption (*see* 3 below) but there is little further benefit to be gained from drinking them during these types of activities. However, flavoured drinks are usually preferred to water and studies show that people are more likely to drink larger volumes of them during exercise (Minehan, 2002). The most important message is to drink enough water.

3 During high-intensity exercise lasting less than 1 hour

A number of studies have found that drinking a sports drink rather than water may benefit your performance during high-intensity exercise or interval training lasting less than 1 hour (Wagenmakers et al., 1996; Ball et al., 1995). Examples of these activities include a 10 km run, tennis, squash, cycling, sprint training, circuit training and weight training. *See* box opposite.

If you are exercising at a high intensity for less than 1 hour, or under very warm and humid conditions, then *rapid* fluid replacement is likely to be your priority. Therefore, a drink containing

Are sports drinks more effective than water?

Many studies since the 1970s have shown that hypotonic and isotonic sports drinks can have an erogenic effect and enhance performance during intense and/or prolonged exercise.

Researchers at the Medical School at the University of Aberdeen found that sports drinks containing glucose and sodium can delay fatigue (Galloway & Maughan, 2000). Cyclists given a dilute sports drink (2% carbohydrate) were able to keep going considerably longer (118 mins) than those drinking plain water (71 mins) or even a higher strength (15% carbohydrate) sports drink (84 mins). The success of the more dilute drink may be due to the larger volume drunk

For example, in a study carried out by researchers at Loughborough University, seven endurance runners drank similar volumes of either water, a 5.5% sports drink (5.5 g carbohydrate/100 ml) or 6.9% (6.9 g carbohydrate/100 ml) sports drink before and during a 42 km treadmill run (Tsintzas et al., 1995). Those who took the 5.5% sports drink produced running times on average 3.9 minutes faster compared with water, and 2.4 minutes faster compared with the 6.9% drink.

At Texas University, eight cyclists performed a time trial lasting approximately 10 minutes after completing 50 minutes of high-intensity cycling at 85% VO$_2$max. Those who drank a sports drink (6 g carbohydrate/100 ml) during the 50 minute cycle reduced the time taken to cycle the final trial by 6% compared with those who drank water (Below et al., 1995).

In a study at the University of South Carolina, cyclists who consumed a sports drink containing 6 g carbohydrate/100 ml knocked 3 minutes off their time during a time trial, compared with those who drank plain water (Davis et al., 1988).

up to 8 g sugar/100 ml (hypotonic or isotonic sports drink) would be best. The choice of an hypotonic or isotonic drink (see p. 86) is largely down to personal preference and how hard you are exercising. Although isotonic drinks provide more fuel and would suit high-intensity exercise, some athletes find them a little too concentrated and experience greater fullness or stomach discomfort. You may wish to dilute a ready-made isotonic drink, i.e. make it hypotonic.

4 During high-intensity exercise lasting longer than 1 hour

When you are exercising at a high-intensity for longer then 1 hour (e.g. half-marathon, football match), you will benefit from (1) rapid fluid replacement, and (2) fuel replacement. In other words, you need to avoid early glycogen depletion and low blood sugar, as well as dehydration, as all three can result in fatigue.

The ACSM (2000) recommends consuming 30–60 g carbohydrate/hour to maintain blood sugar levels and delay fatigue. Most commercial isotonic sports drinks contain 40–80 g carbohydrate/L, which corresponds to the maximum rate that fluid can be emptied from the stomach. More concentrated fluids take longer (ACSM, 1996). Therefore, you can achieve optimal carbohydrate intake by drinking approximately 1 litre per hour. During hot and humid conditions you may be losing more than 1 litre of sweat per hour. Therefore, you should increase your drink volume, if possible, and use a more dilute drink (around 20–40 g/L).

Sports drinks based on glucose polymers may be a good choice if your sweat rate is low (e.g. during cold conditions) yet you are exercising hard, because they can provide more fuel than fluid replacers as well as reasonable amounts of fluid. In practice, many athletes find that glucose polymer drinks cause stomach discomfort and that sports drinks containing 4–8 g carbohydrate/100 ml do an equally good job.

The key to choosing the right drink during exercise is to experiment with different drinks in training to find one that suits you best (*see* Table 6.2).

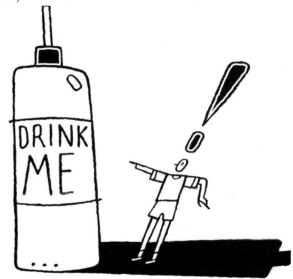

Table 6.2	Choosing the right type of drink
Exercise conditions	**Drink**
Exercise lasting <30 minutes	Nothing; water
Low–moderate intensity exercise lasting less than 1 hour	Water
High-intensity exercise lasting less than 1 hour	Hypotonic or isotonic sports drink
High-intensity exercise lasting more than 1 hour	Hypotonic or isotonic sports drink or glucose polymer drink

> ### Is it possible to drink too much water?
>
> Drinking too much water is rarely a problem as the body normally excretes any fluid not required. The only circumstance where excessive water may be a problem is during prolonged strenuous exercise (e.g. marathon running) when sweat losses are very high and only plain water is drunk. If sodium is not replaced, there will be a rapid drop in blood sodium concentration (hyponatraemia) with very 'watery' blood plasma. This can result in dizziness, mental confusion and, in severe cases, seizures, respiratory failure and even death. Hyponatraemia sometimes occurs during endurance events (e.g. ironman triathlon) in very hot conditions (Speedy et al., 1999; Barr et al., 1989). USA Track & Field advise endurance runners to drink when they are thirsty during races, rather than drinking constantly (Noaker & Martin, 2003).
>
> Therefore, if you are sweating heavily for long periods of time, drink dilute electrolyte/carbohydrate drinks rather than plain water. These will help maintain better fluid levels in the body, spare muscle glycogen and thus delay fatigue.

5 After exercise

Sports drinks may be better than water at speeding recovery after exercise, particularly when fluid losses are high or for those athletes who train or compete twice a day. The problem with drinking water is that it causes a drop in blood osmolality (i.e. it dilutes sodium in the blood), reducing your thirst and increasing urine output and so you may stop drinking before you are rehydrated (Maughan et al., 1996; Gonzalez-Alonzo et al., 1992). Sodium plays an important role in driving the thirst mechanism. A low sodium concentration in the blood signals the brain a low thirst sensation. Conversely, a high sodium concentration in the blood signals

greater thirst and thus drives you to drink. Hence, the popular strategy of putting salted peanuts and crisps at the bar to encourage customers to buy more drink to quench their thirst! Sports drinks, on the other hand, increase the urge to drink and decrease urine production.

THE SCIENCE OF SPORTS DRINKS

What are electrolytes?

Electrolytes are mineral salts dissolved in the body's fluid. They include sodium, chloride, potassium and magnesium, and help to regulate the fluid balance between different body compartments (for example, the amount of fluid inside and outside a muscle cell), and the volume of fluid in the bloodstream. The water movement is controlled by the concentration of electrolytes on either side of the cell membrane. For example, an increase in the concentration of sodium outside a cell will cause water to move to it from inside the cell. Similarly, a drop in sodium concentration will cause water to move from the outside to the inside of the cell. Potassium draws water across a membrane, so a high potassium concentration inside cells increases the cell's water content.

Why do sports drinks contain sodium?

Electrolytes in sports drinks do not have a direct effect on performance. However, sodium does have one key benefit: *it increases the urge to drink and improves palatability.* That's because an increase in sodium concentration and decrease in blood volume that accompany exercise increase your natural thirst sensation, making you want to drink. If you drink plain water it effectively dilutes the sodium, thus reducing your urge to drink before you are fully hydrated. Therefore, including a small amount of sodium (0.5–0.7 g/l) in a sports drink will encourage you to drink more fluid (ACSM, 1996; 2000).

It was originally thought that sodium also speeds water absorption in the intestines. However, research at the University of Iowa has since shown that adding sodium to a sports drink does not enhance fluid absorption (Gisolphi et al., 1995). Researchers discovered that after you have consumed any kind of drink, sodium passes from the blood plasma into the intestine where it then stimulates water absorption. In other words, the body sorts out the sodium concentration of the liquid in your intestines all by itself, so the addition of sodium to sports drinks is unnecessary.

Glucose is more important than sodium for promoting fluid absorption. That said, sodium remains an important ingredient in sports drinks. The ACSM (1996; 2000) recommends adding sodium to sports drinks, not to speed water absorption, but to enhance palatability, encourage drinking and promote fluid retention.

What does osmolality mean?

Osmolality is a measure of the number of dissolved particles in a fluid. A drink with a high osmolality means that it contains more particles per 100 ml than one with a low osmolality. These particles may include sugars, glucose polymers, sodium or other electrolytes. The osmolality of the drink determines which way the fluid will move across a membrane (e.g. the gut wall). For example, if a drink with a relatively high osmolality is consumed, then water moves from the bloodstream and gut cells into the gut. This is called *net secretion*. If a drink with a relatively low osmolality is consumed, then water is absorbed from the gut (i.e. the drink) to the gut cells and bloodstream. Thus there is *net water absorption*.

How does sugar (carbohydrate) speed up fluid replacement?

Although plain water is absorbed relatively quickly, the speed of fluid replacement can be increased by the sugar (carbohydrate) concentration of the fluid.

Relatively dilute solutions of sugar (hypotonic or isotonic) stimulate water absorption from the small intestine into the bloodstream. A sugar concentration up to approximately 8 g/100 ml accelerates water absorption, while more concentrated drinks (hypertonic) slow down the stomach emptying and therefore reduce the speed of fluid replacement.

What are glucose polymers?

Between a sugar (1–2 units) and a starch (several 100,000 units), although closer to the former, are glucose polymers (maltodextrins). These are chains of between 4 and 20 glucose molecules produced from boiling cornstarch under controlled commercial conditions.

The advantage of using glucose polymers instead of glucose or sucrose in a drink is that a higher concentration of carbohydrate can be achieved (usually between 10 and 20 g/100 ml) at a lower osmolality. That's because each molecule contains several glucose units yet still exerts the same osmotic pressure as just one molecule of glucose. So an isotonic or hypotonic drink can be produced with a carbohydrate content greater than 8 g/100 ml.

Also, glucose polymers are less sweet than simple sugars, so you can achieve a fairly concentrated drink that does not taste too sickly. In fact, most glucose polymer drinks are fairly tasteless unless they have added artificial flavours or sweeteners.

What types of sports drinks are available?

Sports drinks can be divided into two main categories: fluid replacement drinks and carbohydrate (energy) drinks.

- **Fluid replacement drinks** are dilute solutions of electrolytes and sugars (carbohydrate). The sugars most commonly added are glucose, sucrose, fructose and glucose polymers (maltodextrins). The main aim of these drinks is to replace fluid faster than plain water, although the extra sugars will also help maintain blood sugar levels and spare glycogen. These drinks may be either hypotonic or isotonic (*see* below).
- **Carbohydrate (energy) drinks** provide more carbohydrate per 100 ml than fluid replacement drinks. The carbohydrate is mainly in the form of glucose polymers (maltodextrins). The main aim is to provide larger amounts of carbohydrate but at an equal or lower osmolality than the same concentration of glucose. They will, of course, provide fluid as well. Ready-to-drink brands are generally isotonic. Powders which you make up into a drink may be made hypotonic or isotonic (*see* below).

What is the difference between hypotonic, isotonic and hypertonic drinks?

- **A hypotonic drink** has a relatively low osmolality, which means it contains fewer particles (carbohydrate and electrolytes) per 100 ml than the body's own fluids. As it is more dilute, it is absorbed faster than plain water. Typically, a hypotonic drink contains less than 4 g carbohydrate/100 ml.
- **An isotonic drink** has the same osmolality as the body's fluids, which means it contains about the same number of particles (carbohydrate and electrolytes) per 100 ml and is therefore absorbed as fast as or faster than plain water. Most commercial isotonic drinks contain between 4 and 8 g carbohydrate/100 ml. In theory, isotonic drinks provide the ideal compromise between rehydration and refuelling.
- **A hypertonic drink** has a higher osmolality than body fluids, as it contains more particles (carbohydrate and electrolytes) per 100 ml than the body's fluids, i.e. it is more concentrated. This means it is absorbed more slowly than plain water. A hypertonic drink usually contains more than 8 g carbohydrate/100 ml.

Can I make my own sports drinks?

Definitely! Commercial sports drinks work out to be very expensive if you are drinking at least 1 litre per day to replace fluid losses during exercise. (If you need to drink less than 1 litre then you probably don't need a sports drink anyway.)

Table 6.3 includes some recipes for making your own sports drink.

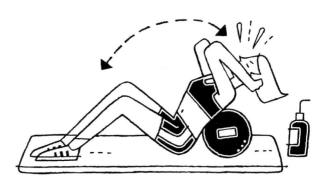

Table 6.3	DIY sports drinks
Hypotonic	**Isotonic**

• 20–40 g sucrose
  1 L warm water
  1–1.5 g (¼ tsp) salt (optional)
  Sugar-free/low-calorie squash for
  flavouring (optional)
	• 40–80 g sucrose
	  1 L warm water
	  1–1.5 g (¼ tsp) salt (optional)
	  Sugar-free/low-calorie squash for
	  flavouring (optional)

• 100 ml fruit squash
  900 ml water
  1–1.5 g (¼ tsp) salt (optional)
	• 200 ml fruit squash
	  800 ml water
	  1–1.5 g (¼ tsp) salt (optional)

• 250 ml fruit juice
  750 ml water
  1–1.5 g (¼ tsp) salt (optional)
	• 500 ml fruit juice
	  500 ml water
	  1–1.5 g (¼ tsp) salt (optional)

How does weather affect performance?

Air temperature and wind speed can both affect performance. The hotter and more humid the weather, and the less wind there is, the more fluid your body will lose and the greater the chance of dehydration occurring.

In one study, six athletes cycled on a stationary bike at a set resistance. When the surrounding temperature was 2°C they could cycle for 73 minutes before experiencing exhaustion. When the surrounding temperature increased to 33°C, they could only cycle for 35 minutes. When the athletes were given a carbohydrate drink it was found that they could keep going for longer in the cold temperature. However, the drink made no difference in the hot temperature.

In hot conditions the body's priority is to replace water rather than carbohydrate. So drink water or a dilute carbohydrate electrolyte drink rather than a more concentrated carbohydrate drink. If you exercise in cold weather and sweat only a little, you may find a more concentrated carbohydrate drink beneficial.

Should I take salt tablets in hot weather?

No, salt tablets are not a good idea, even if you are sweating heavily in hot weather. They produce a very concentrated sodium solution in your stomach (strongly hypertonic), which delays stomach emptying and rehydration as extra fluid must first be absorbed from your body into your stomach to dilute the sodium. The best way to replace fluid and electrolyte losses is by drinking a dilute sodium/carbohydrate drink (either hypotonic or isotonic) with a sodium concentration of 40–110 mg/100 ml.

OTHER NON-ALCOHOLIC DRINKS

What about ordinary soft drinks and fruit juice?

Ordinary soft drinks (typically between 9 and 20 g carbohydrate/100 ml) and fruit juices (typically between 11 and 13 g carbohydrate/100 ml) are too concentrated to be used as fluid replacers during exercise. They empty more slowly from the stomach than plain water because they must first be diluted with water from the body, thus causing a net reduction in body fluid. In fact, they can exacerbate dehydration!

If you dilute one part fruit juice with one part water, you will get an isotonic drink, ideal for rehydrating and refuelling during or after exercise (*see* Table 6.2).

What about 'diet' drinks?

'Diet' or low-calorie drinks contain artificial sweeteners in place of sugars and have a very low sodium concentration. They are, therefore, useless as fuel replacers during exercise, although they will help replace fluid at approximately the same speed as plain water. Artificial sweeteners have no known advantage or disadvantage on performance. Choose these types of drink only if you dislike the taste of water, and under the same circumstances that you would normally choose water, i.e. for low- to moderate-intensity exercise lasting less than 1 hour.

Should I choose still or carbonated drinks?

Experiments at East Carolina University and Ball State University found that carbonated and still sports drinks produced equal hydration in the body (Hickey et al., 1994). However, the carbonated drinks tended to produce a higher incidence of mild heartburn and stomach discomfort. In practice, many athletes find that carbonated drinks make them feel full and 'gassy', which may well limit the amount they drink. Others actually prefer lightly carbonated to still drinks, so it is really down to individual preference.

Are caffeinated drinks a good idea?

Coffee, tea, cola and a number of 'sports' drinks contain caffeine (or guarana), a stimulant that has been shown to improve performance in both endurance- and sprint-based activities (*see* Table 6.4). It can also improve alertness and lift your mood. The exact mechanism is not clear, but it is thought that caffeine enhances fatty acid oxidation and spares glycogen utilisation during exercise – effects desired by most athletes.

A moderate and regular intake does not dehydrate the body but in larger doses (equivalent to 300 mg) or when taken by those who are not regular caffeine-takers, it can have a marked diuretic effect. You will have to offset this effect by drinking more fluid before and during exercise. In some people caffeine produces adverse effects: shaking, anxiety and rapid heart beat. The IOC has banned caffeine at levels over 12 µg/L in the urine (equivalent to drinking 8 cups of coffee or 16 cans of cola). The safest advice is to keep off caffeinated drinks before, during and after exercise if you are sensitive to its side effects or are competing in a drug-tested competition (*see* also Chapter 5, 'Caffeine', pp. 79–81).

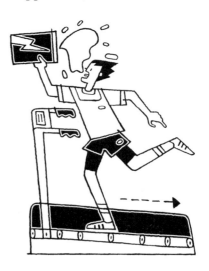

Table 6.4	Caffeine content of various drinks and foods
Drink	mg caffeine/cup
Ground coffee	80–90
Instant coffee	60
Decaffeinated coffee	3
Tea	40
Energy/sports drinks	Up to 100 (per can)
Can of cola	40
Energy gel (1 sachet)	40
Chocolate (54 g bar)	40

ALCOHOL

How does alcohol affect performance?

Drinking alcohol before exercise may appear to make you more alert and confident but, even in small amounts, it will certainly have the following negative effects:

- reduce coordination, reaction time, balance and judgement
- reduce strength, power, speed and endurance
- reduce your ability to regulate body temperature
- reduce blood sugar levels and increase the risk of hypoglycaemia
- increase water excretion (urination) and the risk of dehydration
- increase the risk of accident or injury.

Can I drink alcohol on non-training days?

There is no reason why you cannot enjoy alcohol in moderation on non-training days. The Department of Health recommends up to 4 units a day for men and 3 units a day for women as a safe upper limit (*see* Table 6.5 for 1 unit equivalent measures). The daily limits are intended to discourage binge-drinking which is dangerous to health.

In fact, research has shown that alcohol drunk in moderation reduces the risk of heart disease.

Table 6.5	Alcoholic and calorie contents of drinks	
Drink equivalent to 1 unit	% alcohol by volume	Calories
½ pint ordinary beer/lager	3.0–3.5	90
1 measure spirits	38	50
1 measure vermouth/aperitif	18	60–80
125 ml glass of wine	11	75–100
1 measure sherry	16	55–70
1 measure liqueur	40	75–100

Moderate drinkers have a lower risk of death from heart disease than teetotallers or heavy drinkers. The exact mechanism is not certain, but it may work by increasing HDL cholesterol levels, the protective type of cholesterol in the blood. HDL transports cholesterol *back* to the liver for excretion, thereby reducing the chance of it sticking to artery walls. It may also reduce the stickiness of blood platelets, thus reducing the risk of blood clots (thrombosis).

Red wine, in particular, may be especially good for the heart. Studies have shown that drinking up to two glasses a day can lower heart disease risk by 30–70%. It contains flavanoids from the grape skin, which have an antioxidant effect and thus protect the LDL cholesterol from free radical damage.

Is alcohol fattening?

Any food or drink can be 'fattening' if you consume more calories than you need. Alcohol itself provides 7 kcal/g, and many alcoholic drinks also have quite a high sugar/carbohydrate content, boosting the total calorie content further (*see* Table 6.5). Excess calories from alcoholic drinks can, therefore, lead to fat gain.

What exactly happens to alcohol in the body?

When you drink alcohol, about 20% is absorbed into the bloodstream through the stomach and the remainder through the small intestine. Most of this alcohol is then broken down in the liver (it cannot be stored as it is toxic) into a substance called acetyl CoA and then, ultimately, into ATP (energy). Obviously, whilst this is occurring, less glycogen and fat are used to produce ATP in other parts of the body.

However, the liver can only carry out this job at a fixed rate of approximately 1 unit alcohol/ hour. If you drink more alcohol than this, it is

Sensible drinking guidelines

- Intersperse alcoholic drinks with water, diluted juice or other non-alcoholic drinks.
- Extend your alcoholic drink (e.g. wine, spirits) with water, low-calorie mixers or soda water.
- Keep a tally on your alcohol intake when you go out; set yourself a safe limit.
- If you think you have drunk too much, drink plenty of water/sports drink before retiring to bed – at least 500 ml/2–3 units.
- Do not feel obliged to drink excessively, even if your friends press you: tell them you are training the next day or that you are driving.
- Do not drink on an empty stomach as this speeds alcohol absorption. Try to eat something first or reserve drinking for mealtimes. Food slows down the absorption of alcohol.

dealt with by a different enzyme system in the liver (the microsomal ethanol oxidising system, MEO) to make it less toxic to the body. The more alcohol you drink on a regular basis, the more MEO enzymes are produced, which is why you can develop an increased tolerance to alcohol – you need to drink more to experience the same physiological effects.

Initially, alcohol reduces inhibitions, increases self-confidence and makes you feel more at ease. However, it is actually a depressant rather than a stimulant, reducing your psychomotor (coordination) skills. It is potentially toxic to all of the cells and organs in your body and, if it builds up to high concentrations, it can cause damage to the liver, stomach and brain.

Too much alcohol causes hangovers – headache, thirst, nausea, vomiting and heartburn. These symptoms are due partly to dehydration and a swelling of the blood vessels in the head. Congeners, substances found mainly in darker alcoholic drinks such as rum and red wine, are also responsible for many of the hangover symptoms. Prevention is better than cure, so make sure you follow the guidelines on p. 96. The best way to deal with a hangover is to drink plenty of water or, better still, a sports drink. Avoid coffee or tea as these will make dehydration worse. Do not attempt to train or compete with a hangover!

SUMMARY OF KEY POINTS

- Dehydration causes cardiovascular stress, increases core body temperature and impairs performance.
- Fluid losses during exercise depend on exercise duration and intensity; temperature and humidity; body size; fitness level and the individual. They can be as high as 1–2 l/hour.
- Always start exercise well hydrated. Drink 500 ml fluid 2 hours before exercise.
- During exercise, start drinking early and at regular intervals; aim for 125–250 ml every 10–20 minutes.
- Aim to replace at least 80% of sweat loss during exercise.
- After exercise, replace by 150% any body weight deficit.
- Water is a suitable fluid replacement drink for low- or moderate intensity exercise lasting less than 1 hour.

- For intense exercise, lasting up to 1 hour, a sports drink containing up to 8% carbohydrate (8 g carbohydrate/100 ml) can speed up water absorption, provide additional fuel, delay fatigue and improve performance.
- Consuming 30–60 g carbohydrate/hour can maintain blood sugar levels, and improve performance in intense exercise lasting more than 1 hour.
- Hypotonic (<4%) and isotonic (4–8%) sports drinks are most suitable when rapid fluid replacement is the main priority.
- Carbohydrate drinks based on glucose polymers also replace fluids, but provide greater amounts of carbohydrate (10–20%) at a lower osmolality. They are most suitable for prolonged intense exercise (>90 minutes), when fuel replacement is a major priority or fluid losses are small.
- The main purpose of sodium in a sports drink is to increase the urge to drink and increase palatability.
- Alcohol before exercise has a negative effect on strength, endurance, co-ordination, power and speed, and increases injury risk.
- Moderate amounts of alcohol (<4 units/day for men; <3 units/day for women) in the overall diet – particularly red wine, which is rich in antioxidants – may protect against heart disease.

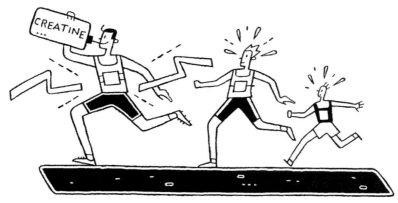

FAT MATTERS

7

As athletes in almost every sport strive to get leaner and competitive standards get higher, the relationship between body fat, health and performance becomes increasingly important. However, the optimal body composition for fitness or sports performance is not necessarily a desirable one from a health point of view. This chapter deals with different methods for measuring body fat percentage and body fat distribution, and considers their relevance to performance. It highlights the dangers of attaining very low body fat levels, as well as the risks associated with a very low-fat diet. It gives realistic guidance on recommended body fat ranges and fat intakes, and explains the difference between the various types of fats found in the diet.

Does body fat affect performance?

Carrying around excess body weight in the form of fat is a distinct disadvantage in almost every sport. It can adversely affect strength, speed and endurance. Surplus fat is basically surplus baggage. Carrying around this extra weight is not only unnecessary, but also costly in terms of energy expenditure.

For example, in endurance sports (e.g. long distance running) surplus fat can reduce speed and increase fatigue. It is like carrying a couple of shopping bags with you as you run; they make it harder for you to get up speed, slow you down and cause you to tire quickly. It is best to leave your shopping bags at home, or at least to lighten the load.

In explosive sports (e.g. sprinting/jumping), where you must transfer or lift the weight of your whole body very quickly, extra fat again is non-functional weight, slowing you down, reducing your power and decreasing your mechanical efficiency. Muscle is useful weight, whereas excess fat is not.

In weight-matched sports (e.g. boxing, karate, judo, lightweight rowing), greater emphasis is put on body weight, particularly during the competitive season. The person with the greatest percentage of muscle and the smallest percentage of fat has the advantage.

In virtually every sport, it is the leanest body that wins. Reducing your body fat while maintaining lean mass and health will result in improved performance.

Is body fat an advantage in certain sports?

Until recently it was believed that extra weight – even in the form of fat – was an advantage for certain sports in which momentum is important (e.g. discus, hammer throwing, judo, wrestling).

A heavy body can generate more momentum to throw an object or knock over an opponent, but there is no reason why this weight should be fat. It would be better if it were in the form of muscle. Muscle is stronger and more powerful than fat – although, admittedly, it is harder to acquire! If two athletes both weighed 100 kg, but one comprised 90 kg lean (10 kg fat) mass, and the other 70 kg lean (30 kg fat) mass, the leaner one would obviously have the advantage. Perhaps the only sport where fat could be considered a necessary advantage is sumo wrestling – it would be almost impossible to acquire a very large body mass without fat gain.

Table 7.1	BMI classification	
<20	Underweight	increasing health risk
20–24.9	'Normal' weight (Grade 0)	lowest health risk
25–29.9	Overweight/'plump' (Grade I)	
30–40	Moderately obese (Grade II)	increasing health risk
40+	Severely obese (Grade III)	

How can I tell if I am too fat?

Looking in the mirror is the quickest and simplest way to see if you are too fat by everyday standards, but will not give the accurate information that you need for your sport. Many women also tend to perceive themselves as fatter than they really are. It is useful, therefore, to employ some sort of measurement system so that you can work towards a definite goal.

Standing on a set of scales, reading your weight and comparing it to standard weight and height charts is easy. However, it has several drawbacks. Weights and heights given in charts are based on average weights of a sample population. They are only *average* weights for *average* people, not ideal weights, and give no indication of health risk.

To get a general picture of your health risk, you can calculate your Body Mass Index (BMI) from your weight and height measurements.

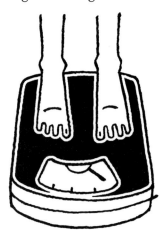

How much body fat do I really need?

A fat free body would not survive. It is important to realise that a certain amount of body fat is absolutely vital. In fact, there are two components of body fat: essential fat and storage fat. *Essential fat* includes the fat which forms part of your cell membranes, brain tissue, nerve sheaths, bone marrow and the fat surrounding your organs (e.g. heart, liver, kidneys). Here it provides insulation, protection and cushioning against physical damage. In a healthy person, this accounts for about *3% of body weight.*

Women have an additional essential fat requirement called sex-specific fat, which is stored mostly in the breasts and around the hips. This fat accounts for a further 5–9% of a woman's body weight and is involved in oestrogen production as well as the conversion of inactive oestrogen into its active form. So, this fat ensures normal hormonal balance and menstrual function. If stores fall too low, hormonal imbalance and menstrual irregularities result, although these can be reversed once body fat increases. There is some recent evidence that a certain amount of body fat in men is necessary for normal hormone production too (*see* p. 106).

The second component of body fat, *storage fat*, is an important energy reserve that takes the form of fat (adipose) cells under the skin (subcutaneous fat) and around the organs (intra-abdominal fat). Fat is used virtually all the time during any aerobic activity: while sleeping, sitting, standing and walking, as well as in most types of exercise. It is impossible to spot reduce fat selectively from adipose tissue sites by specific exercises or diets. The body generally uses fat from all sites, although the exact pattern of fat utilisation (and storage) is determined by your genetic make-up and hormonal balance. An average person has enough fat for three days and three nights of continuous running – although, in practice, you would experience fatigue long before your fat reserves ran out. So, your fat stores are certainly not a redundant depot of unwanted energy!

What is the BMI?

Doctors and researchers often use a measurement called the Body Mass Index (BMI) to classify different grades of body weight and to assess health risk. It is sometimes referred to as the Quetelet Index after the Belgian researcher who observed that for normal weight people there is more or less a constant ratio between weight and the square of height. The BMI assumes that there is no single ideal weight for a person of a certain height, and that there is a healthy weight range for any given height.

The BMI is calculated by dividing a person's weight (in kg) by the square of his or her height (in m). For example, if your weight is 60 kg and height 1.7 m, your BMI is 21.

$$\frac{60}{1.7 \times 1.7} = 21$$

How useful is the BMI?

Researchers and doctors use BMI measurements to assess a person's risk of acquiring certain health-related conditions, such as heart disease. Studies have shown that people with a BMI of between 20 and 25 have the lowest risk of developing diseases that are linked to obesity,

e.g. cardiovascular disease, gall bladder disease, hypertension (high blood pressure) and diabetes. People with a BMI of between 25 and 30 are at moderate risk, while those with a BMI above 30 are at a greater risk.

It is not true that the lower a person's BMI the better, though. A very low BMI is also not desirable; people with a BMI below 20 have a higher risk of other health problems, such as respiratory disease, certain cancers and metabolic complications.

Both those with a BMI below 20 and those above 30 have an increased risk of premature death (*see* Fig. 7.1).

The BMI has a number of limitations. It does not give information about body composition, i.e. how much weight is fat and how much lean tissue. It simply gives the desirable weight of *average* people – not *sportspeople*!

When you stand on the scales you weigh everything – bone, muscle and water, as well as fat. Therefore you do not know how fat you actually are. Someone with a lot of muscle but little fat could be classed as overweight, and vice versa – someone with a relatively high proportion of fat and little muscle could be classed as of average weight.

Figure 7.1 Relative risk of death according to BMI

Is the *distribution* of body fat important?

Yes. Scientists believe that the distribution of your body fat is more important than the total amount of fat. This gives a more accurate assessment of your risk of metabolic disorders, such as heart disease, maturity onset diabetes, high blood pressure and gall bladder disease. Fat stored mostly around the abdomen (central or android obesity) gives rise to an 'apple' or 'barrel' shape, and this carries a much bigger health risk than fat stored mostly around the hips and thighs (peripheral or gynecoid obesity) in a pear shape.

The way we distribute fat on our body is determined partly by our genetic make-up and partly by our natural hormonal balance. Men, for example, have higher levels of testosterone, which favours fat deposition around the abdomen, between the shoulder blades and close to the internal organs. Women have higher levels of oestrogen, which favours fat deposition around the hips, thighs, breasts and triceps. After the menopause, however, when oestrogen levels fall, fat tends to transfer from the hips and thighs to the abdomen, giving women more of an apple shape and pushing up their chances of heart disease.

How can I measure my body fat distribution?

You can assess your body fat distribution by two methods:

1 The *waist/hip ratio*, which is your waist measurement (in inches or centimetres) divided by your hip measurement. For women (because of their proportionately larger pelvic hip bones), it should be 0.8 or less. For men, this ratio should be 0.95 or less. For example, a woman with a waist measurement of 66 cm and hips of 91.5 cm has a W/H ratio of 0.72 (66 ÷ 91.5).

2 *Waist circumference*: Scientists at the Royal Infirmary, Glasgow, have found that a simple waist circumference measurement correlates well with intra-abdominal fat. It can also be used to predict total body fat percentage (Lean et al., 1995). A waist circumference of 94 cm or more in men, or 80 cm or more in women indicates excess abdominal fat.

Excess fat in the abdomen is a health risk. For example, a man with a W/H ratio of 1.1 has double the chance of having a heart attack as if it was below 0.95. The most likely explanation is to do with the close proximity of the intra-abdominal fat to the liver. Fatty acids from the adipose tissue are delivered into the portal vein that goes directly to the liver. The liver thus receives a continuous supply of fat-rich blood and this stimulates increased cholesterol synthesis. High blood cholesterol levels are a major risk factor for heart disease.

What does *body composition* mean?

The body is composed of two elements: lean body tissue (i.e. muscles, organs, bones and blood) and body fat (or adipose tissue). The proportion of these two components in the body is called body composition. This is more important than total weight.

For example, two people may weigh the same, but have a different body composition. Athletes usually have a smaller percentage of body fat and a higher percentage of lean weight than less physically active people. Lean body tissue is functional (or useful) weight, whereas fat is non-functional in terms of sports performance.

How can I measure body composition?

Clearly, height and weight measurements are not very accurate for assessing your body composition. To give you a more accurate idea of how much fat and how much muscle you have, there are a number of techniques for measuring body composition. These will tell you how much of your weight is muscle or fat as a percentage of your total weight.

The only method that is 100% accurate is cadaver analysis. Clearly this is impractical so indirect methods must be used.

Underwater weighing

For a long time, this method was judged to be the most accurate. Its accuracy rate averages 97–98%. However, there are other methods, such as dual energy x-ray absorptiometry and magnetic resonance imaging which produce similar, if not more accurate, results.

Underwater weighing works on the Archimedes' principle which states that when an object is submerged under water it creates a buoyant counter force that is equal to the weight of water that it has displaced. Since bone and muscle are more dense than water, a person with a higher percentage of lean mass will weigh more in water, indicating a lower percentage of fat. Since fat is less dense than water, a person with a high fat percentage will weigh less in water than on land.

In this test, the person sits on a swing-seat and is then submerged into a water tank. After expelling as much air as possible from the lungs, the person's weight is recorded. This figure is then compared with the person's weight on dry land, using standard equations on a computer, and the fat percentage calculated.

The disadvantage of this method is that the specialised equipment is expensive and bulky and found only at research institutions or laboratories, i.e. it is not readily available to the public. The person also needs to be water confident.

Skinfold callipers

The skinfold measurement method is widely available and used by many sports teams and in many health clubs. The callipers measure in millimetres the layer of fat just underneath the skin at various places on the body. This is done on three to seven specific places (such as the triceps, biceps, hip bone area, lower-back, abdomen, thigh and below the shoulder blade). Using these measurements, scientists have developed mathematical equations that account for age, sex, known body densities and estimated hidden fat that the callipers cannot measure. These equations produce a body density value, which another equation then changes into a body fat percentage.

The accuracy of this method depends almost entirely on the skill of the person taking the measurements. Also, it assumes that everyone has a predictable pattern of fat distribution as they age. Therefore, it becomes less accurate

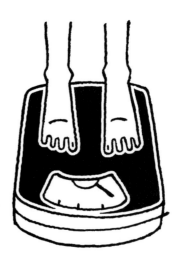

Table 7.2	Accuracy of body fat measurement methods	
Method	**Degree of inaccuracy**
DEXA	<2%
Skinfold measurement	3–4%
Underwater weighing	2–5%
Bio electrical impedence	3–4%
Near infrared interactance	5–10%

with élite athletes, as they tend to have a different pattern of fat distribution compared with sedentary people, and for very lean and obese people. There are different sets of equations which you can use to take account of these factors. For the general population (over 15% body fat) the Durnin and Womersley (1974) equations are more suitable. The Jackson–Pollock (1984) equations apply best to lean and athletic people.

Kinanthropometry is the term for the recording of skinfold thickness measurements and body girth measurements (e.g. arms, chest, legs etc.) in order to monitor changes in body composition over time. The sites of girth measurements are shown in Figure 8.2 (Chapter 8, p. 120).

An alternative is to present the body fat measurement as a 'sum of skinfolds'. This is the sum of the individual skinfold thicknesses from the seven specific sites.

Bioelectrical Impedance Analysis

In Bioelectrical Impedance Analysis (BIA) a mild electrical current is used to measure the conductivity of the body. The principle is that lean tissue is a good conductor of electricity whereas fat creates a resistance. So, by measuring the current that flows between electrodes attached to two specific points of the body (either between the hand and opposite foot, or from one foot to the other), your body fat is calculated.

The advantages are the machine is portable, simple to operate and testing takes less than one minute. The disadvantage is the poor degree of accuracy compared with other methods. For example, changes in body fluid levels and skin temperature will affect the passage of the current and therefore the body fat reading. It tends to overestimate the body fat percentage of lean muscular people by 2–5% and underestimate the body fat percentage of overweight people by the same amount. It is important that you are well-hydrated when having a BIA measurement; if you are dehydrated the current will not be conducted through your lean mass so well, giving you a higher body fat percentage reading.

Dual Energy X-ray Absorptiometry

Dual Energy X-ray Absorptiometry (DEXA) measures not only your total body fat but produces an accurate body fat map, showing exactly where your fat is distributed around the body. In this method, two types of x-rays are scanned over the whole body to measure fat, bone and muscle. The procedure takes about 5–20 minutes depending on the type of machine.

It is the most accurate method for assessing body fat. The disadvantages are the cost and size of the machine and lack of accessibility. DEXA machines are found in hospitals and research institutions. It may be possible to request a body fat analysis at your nearest site but be prepared to pay considerably more than you would for the other methods.

Table 7.2	Average body fat percentages in various sports	
Sport	Men%	Women%
Basketball	7–12	18–27
Bodybuilding (competitive)	6–7	8–10
Cycling	8–9	15–16
Football	8–18	(not available)
Gymnastics	3–6	8–18
Running	4–12	8–18
Swimming	4–10	12–23
Throwing	12–20	22–30
Tennis	12–16	22–26
Weight lifting	6–16	17–20

Near-infrared interactance

In near-infrared interactance, an infra-red beam is shone perpendicularly through the upper arm. The amount of light reflected back to the analyser from the bone depends on the amount of fat located there, which is correlated to the body fat percentage. Age, weight, height, sex and activity level are all taken into account in the calculations.

The obvious disadvantage of this method is the assumption that fat in the arm is proportional to total body fat. However, it is a very fast, easy and cheap method. The equipment is portable, and anyone can operate it.

How accurate are these methods?

DEXA and underwater weighing are regarded as the most accurate methods. Skinfold and BIA measurements – provided they are carefully carried out – can estimate body fat percentages with a 3–4% error (Houtkooper, 2000; Lohman, 1992). For example, if the actual body fat percentage is 15%, then predicted values could range from 12 to 18% (assuming a 3% error). But

if poor measurement techniques or incorrectly calibrated instruments are used, then the margin of error could be greater. Since a relatively high degree of error is associated with these indirect body fat assessment methods, it is not recommended to set a specific body fat goal for athletes (ACSM, 2000). Instead, a range of target body fat values would be more realistic.

What is a desirable body fat percentage for athletes?

Body fat percentages for athletes vary depending on the particular sport. According to scientists at the University of Arizona, the ideal body fat percentage, in terms of performance, for most male athletes lies between 6 and 15% and for female athletes, 12 and 18% (Wilmore, J. H., 1983; Table 7.2) In general, for men, middle- and long-distance runners and bodybuilders have the lowest body fat levels (less than 6%) while cyclists, gymnasts, sprinters, triathletes and basketball players average between 6 and 15% body fat (Sinning, 1998). In female athletes, the lowest body fat levels (6–15%) are observed in bodybuilders, cyclists, gymnasts, runners and triathletes (Sinning, 1998).

Physiologists recommend a minimum of 5% fat for men and 12% fat for women to cover the most basic functions associated with good health (Lohman, 1992). However, optimal body fat levels may be much higher than these minimums. The % fat associated with lowest health risk is 13–18% for men and 18–25% for women.

Clearly, there is no ideal body fat percentage for any particular sport. Each individual athlete has an optimal fat range at which their performance improves yet their health does not suffer.

HOW LOW CAN YOU GO?

Women and men who try to attain very low body fat levels, or a level that is unnatural for their genetic make-up, encounter problems. These problems can be serious, particularly for women, who may suffer long-term effects. Collectively known as the 'Female Athlete Triad' these problems are discussed in greater detail in Chapter 10.

What are the dangers for women with very low body fat levels?

One of the biggest problems for women with very low body fat levels is the resulting hormonal imbalance and amenorrhoea (absence of periods). As explained in more detail in Chapter 10, this tends to be triggered once body fat levels fall below 15–20% – the threshold level varies from one person to another. This fall in body fat, together with other factors such as low calorie intake and heavy training, is sensed by the hypothalamus of the brain, which then decreases its production of the hormone (gonadotrophin-releasing hormone) that acts on the pituitary gland. This, in turn, reduces the production of important hormones that act on

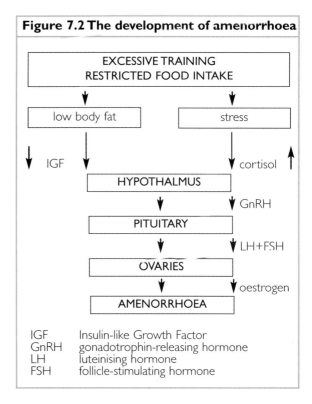

Figure 7.2 The development of amenorrhoea

EXCESSIVE TRAINING
RESTRICTED FOOD INTAKE

low body fat   stress

↓ IGF   ↓ cortisol ↑

HYPOTHALMUS

↓ GnRH

PITUITARY

↓ LH+FSH

OVARIES

↓ oestrogen

AMENORRHOEA

IGF   Insulin-like Growth Factor
GnRH   gonadotrophin-releasing hormone
LH   luteinising hormone
FSH   follicle-stimulating hormone

the ovaries (luteinising hormone and follicle-stimulating hormone), causing them to produce less oestrogen and progesterone. The end result is a deficiency of oestrogen and progesterone and a cessation of menstrual periods (see Fig. 7.2).

Low body fat levels also upset the metabolism of the sex hormones, reducing their potency and thus fertility. Therefore, a very low body fat level drastically reduces a woman's chances of getting pregnant. However, the good news is that once your body fat level increases over your threshold and your training volume is reduced, your hormonal balance, periods and fertility generally return to normal.

What are the dangers for men with very low body fat levels?

Studies on competitive male wrestlers 'making weight' for contests found that once body fat levels fell below 5%, testosterone levels decreased, causing a drastic fall in sperm count, libido and sexual activity! Studies on male runners found similar changes. Thankfully, though, testosterone levels and libido return to normal once body fat increases. Team doctors in the US recommend a minimum of 7% fat before allowing wrestlers to compete.

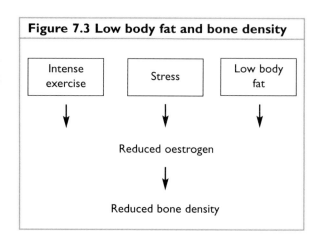

Figure 7.3 Low body fat and bone density

Can a low body fat harm your bones?

Amenorrhoea can lead to more serious problems such as bone loss. That's because low oestrogen levels result in loss of bone minerals and, therefore, bone density (*see* Fig. 7.3). In younger (premenopausal) women, this is called osteopoenia (i.e. lower bone density than normal for age), which is similar to the osteoporosis that affects post-menopausal women, where bones become thinner, lighter and more fragile. Amenorrhoeic athletes, therefore, run a greater risk of stress fractures. The British Olympic Medical Centre has reported cases of athletes in their twenties and thirties with osteoporotic-type fractures.

What are the problems with low-fat diets?

Very low fat intakes can leave you deficient in a variety of nutrients and lead to several health problems. You will certainly be missing out on the essential fatty acids (linoleic acid and linolenic acid) found in vegetable oils, seeds, nuts and oily fish (*see* pp. 108–10), and will therefore be susceptible to dull flaky skin and other dermatological problems; cold extremities;

prostaglandin (hormone) imbalance; poor control of inflammation, blood pressure, vasoconstriction and blood clotting.

Low-fat diets will be low in fat-soluble vitamins A, D and E. More importantly, fat is needed to enable your body to absorb and transport them, and to convert beta-carotene into vitamin A in the body. Although you can get vitamin D from UV light and vitamin A from beta-carotene in brightly coloured fruit and vegetables, getting enough vitamin E can be much more of a problem. It is found in significant quantities only in vegetable oils, seeds, nuts and egg yolk. Vitamin E is an important antioxidant that protects our cells from harmful free radical attack (*see* Chapter 4, pp. 54–6). It is thought to help prevent heart disease, certain cancers and even retard aging. It may also help reduce muscle soreness after hard exercise. So, cutting out oils, nuts and seeds means you are increasing your risk of free radical damage.

Chronically low-fat diets often result in a low-calorie and low-nutrient intake overall. Low-calorie diets quickly lead to depleted glycogen (carbohydrate) stores, resulting in poor energy levels, reduced capacity for exercise, fatigue, poor recovery between workouts and eventual burn-out. They can also increase protein breakdown – causing loss of muscle mass and strength or a lack of muscular development. This is just the opposite of what you should be achieving in your fitness programme.

FAT IN YOUR DIET

How much fat should I eat?

The American Dietetic Association and ACSM recommend a diet containing 20–25% energy from fat (ACSM, 2000). This range is below the current average intake of the general population (37–40% energy from fat) – higher fat intakes provide no further benefit to athletes – and above the minimum 15% recommended for optimum health (Dreon, 1999).

International Conference on Foods, Nutrition and Sports Performance (1991) recommended a fat intake of between 15 and 30% of total calorie intake for sportspeople. Both recommendations are in line with the maximum recommended by the World Health Organisation (30% of calories) and the UK government (33–35% of calories). Using the ACSM recommendations a person eating 2000 kcal would require 44–56 g fat a day. If you eat 2500 kcal, your daily fat intake should be 56–69 g; if you eat 3000 kcal, 67–83 g. Most of your fat intake should come from unsaturated fats, found in vegetable oils (e.g. olive, rapeseed, sunflower), nuts (all kinds), seeds (e. g. sunflower, sesame, pumpkin), oily fish (e.g. sardines, mackerel, salmon), peanut butter and avocado.

What are fats?

Fats and oils found in food consist mainly of *triglycerides*. These are made up of a unit of glycerol and three fatty acids. Each fatty acid is a chain of carbon and hydrogen atoms with a carboxyl group (–COOH) at one end and a

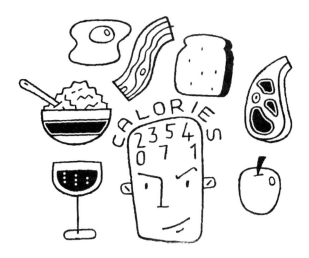

methyl group at the other end (–CH3) – chain lengths between 14 and 22 carbon atoms are most common. These fatty acids are classified in three different groups, according to their chemical structure: saturated, monounsaturated and polyunsaturated. In food, the proportions of each group determine whether the fat is hard or liquid, how it is handled by the body and how it affects your health.

What are saturated fats?

Saturated fatty acids are fully saturated with the maximum amount of hydrogen; in other words, all of their carbon atoms are linked with a single bond to hydrogen atoms. Fats containing a high proportion of saturates are hard at room temperature and mostly come from animal products such as butter, lard, cheese and meat fat. Processed foods made from these fats include biscuits, cakes and pastry. Alternatives to animal fats are palm oil and coconut oil. Also highly saturated, these are often used in margarine, as well as in biscuits and bakery products.

Saturated fatty acids are considered the culprit fat in heart disease because they can increase total cholesterol and the more harmful low-density lipoprotein (LDL) cholesterol in the blood. The Department of Health (DoH) recommend a saturated fatty acid intake of no more than 10% of total calorie intake.

To achieve peak sports performance and health, you should avoid saturated fats: they provide no positive benefit.

What are monounsaturated fats?

Monounsaturated fatty acids have *slightly less hydrogen* because their carbon chains contain one double or unsaturated bond (hence 'mono'). Oils rich in monounsaturates are usually liquid at room temperature, but may solidify at cold temperatures. The richest sources include olive, rapeseed, groundnut, hazelnut and almond oil, avocados, olives, nuts and seeds.

Monounsaturated fatty acids are thought to have the greatest health benefits. They can reduce total cholesterol, in particular LDL cholesterol, without affecting the beneficial high-density lipoprotein (HDL) cholesterol. The DoH recommend a monounsaturated fatty acid intake of up to 12% of total calorie intake.

What are polyunsaturated fats?

Polyunsaturated fatty acids have the least hydrogen – the carbon chains contain two or more double bonds (hence 'poly'). Oils rich in polyunsaturates are liquid at both room and cold temperatures. Rich sources include most vegetable oils and oily fish (and their oils).

Polyunsaturates can reduce LDL blood cholesterol levels – however they can also lower the good HDL cholesterol slightly. It is a good idea to replace some with mono-unsaturates, if you eat a lot of them. For this reason, the DoH recommend a maximum intake of 10% of total calorie intake.

What are the essential fatty acids?

A sub-category of polyunsaturated fats, called essential fatty acids, cannot be made in your body so they have to come from the food you eat. They are grouped into two series:

1 the omega-3 series, derived from alpha-linolenic acid (ALA)
2 the omega-6 series, derived from linoleic acid.

The series are called omega-3 and omega-6 because the last double bond is 3 and 6 carbon atoms from the last carbon in the chain respectively.

The omega-3 fatty acids can be further divided into two groups: long chain and short chain. The long-chain omega-3 fatty acids are eicosapentanoic acid (EPA) and docosahexanoic acid (DHA). They are found in oily fish and can also be formed in the body from ALA – the short-chain omega-3 fatty acid. EPA and DHA are then converted into hormone-like substances called prostaglandins, thromboxanes and leukotrienes. These control many key functions, such as blood clotting (making the blood less likely to form unwanted clots), inflammation (improving the ability to respond to injury or bacterial attack), the tone of blood vessel walls (widening and constriction of blood vessels) and your immune system.

Studies show that people with the highest intake of omega-3 fatty acids have a lower risk of heart attacks. This is because the prostaglandins reduce the ability of red blood cells to clot and reduce blood pressure.

The omega-6 fatty acids include linoleic acid, gamma-linolenic acid (GLA) and docosapentanoic acid (DPA) (*see* Fig. 7.4) and are important for healthy functioning of cell membranes. They are especially important for

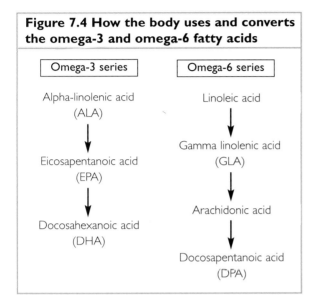

Figure 7.4 How the body uses and converts the omega-3 and omega-6 fatty acids

Omega-3 series	Omega-6 series
Alpha-linolenic acid (ALA)	Linoleic acid
↓	↓
Eicosapentanoic acid (EPA)	Gamma linolenic acid (GLA)
↓	↓
Docosahexanoic acid (DHA)	Arachidonic acid
	↓
	Docosapentanoic acid (DPA)

healthy skin. People on very low-fat diets, who are deficient in linoleic acid, often develop extremely dry, flaky skin. Omega-6 fatty acids reduce LDL cholesterol but a very high intake may also reduce HDL cholesterol. A high intake may also encourage increased free radical damage and, therefore, cancer risk. A moderate intake is recommended. Figure 7.4 shows how the body converts the two series of fatty acids.

What are the best food sources of essential fatty acids?

Oily fish such as mackerel, fresh tuna (not tinned), salmon and sardines are undoubtedly the richest sources of DHA and EPA, but don't worry if you are a vegetarian or do not eat fish, because you can also get reasonably good amounts of ALA from certain plant sources. The best are linseeds (flax seeds), linseed (flax) oil, pumpkin seeds, walnuts, rapeseed oil and soybeans. The dark green leaves of leafy vegetables (e.g. spinach, curly kale) and sweet potatoes also contain small amounts. Other good

sources include omega-3 enriched foods such as 'Columbus' eggs (achieved by feeding hens on omega-3 enriched feed) and 'Nutribread Wholemeal Loaf For the Family' bread. It is easier to meet your requirement for omega-6 fatty acids because they are found in more commonly eaten foods: vegetable oils, polyunsaturated margarine and many dishes and processed foods made from these oils and fats (e.g. fried foods, cakes, stir-fry, sandwiches spread with margarine, biscuits, crisps, cakes).

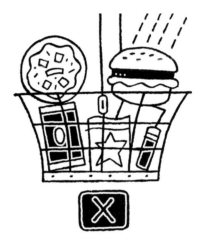

How much do I need?

We need both omega-3s and omega-6s to be healthy but our diets are more often deficient in omega-3s. Most people have a far greater intake of omega-6 compared with omega-3; we tend to get most of our unsaturated fats from margarines and oils, processed foods containing vegetable oils, and oily fish. Experts recommend shifting this balance in favour of omega-3s.

The right balance between omega-3 and omega-6 fatty acids is the most important factor if you are to get enough EPA and DHA. That's because both ALA (omega-3) and linoleic acid (omega-6) compete for the same enzymes to metabolise them. If you eat a lot of linoleic acid in relation to ALA, that puts you at risk of not getting as much EPA and DHA as you need. The best way to correct this is to eat more oily fish or take supplements.

The DoH recommends a minimum of 200–300 g oily fish each week, which is equivalent to about two servings, and a minimum of 0.2% total energy as linolenic acid. This will supply about 4–5 g omega-3 fatty acid. In 1999 at the XX1st Congress of the European Society of Cardiology in Barcelona, scientists concluded that lower intakes of fish oils – 0.9 g omega-3 fatty acids/day – do just as good a job at lowering blood fats and heart disease risk. To get 0.9 g a day you can eat one of the following:

- 32 g mackerel
- 45 g (half a small tin) tuna in oil (0.45 g) plus 1 small (120 g) chicken leg portion (0.45 g)
- 2 tbsp (30 g) linseeds
- one (130 g) sweet potato
- 4 tbsp (40 g) pumpkin seeds
- 12–15 g walnuts
- 1 level tbsp linseed oil
- ι Omega-3 fortified egg* (0.7 g) plus 2 tbsp (0.2 g) spinach

*from hens fed a omega-3 rich diet

Most fish oil-based supplements supply 0.1 g omega-3 fatty acids. Taking 9 supplements a day may be unrealistic so get as close as possible to the recommended intake from food and then top up with a supplement if you need to (*see* Table 7.4 for fish sources of omega-3).

In addition, the DoH advises a minimum of 1% energy as linoleic acid. This can be met by consuming:

- 1 tbsp (15 g) sunflower seeds
- 1 tbsp (15 g) sesame seeds
- 0.5 tbsp (7.5 ml) sunflower, corn, safflower or sesame oil
- 1 tbsp (15 g) polyunsaturated margarine

How can omega-3 fatty acids help athletic performance?

Studies have shown that omega-3 fatty acids can lead to improvements in strength and endurance by enhancing aerobic metabolism (Brilla and Landerholm, 1990; Bucci, 1993) – a critical energy system for all types of activities. The benefits of omega-3 fatty acids can be summarised as follows:

- improved delivery of oxygen and nutrients to cells because of reduced blood viscosity
- more flexible red blood cell membranes and improved oxygen delivery
- enhanced aerobic metabolism
- increased energy levels and stamina
- increased exercise duration and intensity
- improved release of growth hormone in response to sleep and exercise, improving recovery and promoting anabolic (or anti-catabolic) environment
- anti-inflammatory, preventing joint, tendon, ligament strains
- reduction of inflammation caused by over-training, assisting injury healing.

Table 7.4	Omega-3 fatty acid content of some fish
Weight	Source
0.5 g or less	Cod, haddock, mullet, halibut, skipjack tuna, clams, scallops, crab, prawns
0.6–1 g	Red snapper, yellow fin tuna, turbot, swordfish, mussels, oysters
1 g or more	Rainbow trout, mackerel, herring, sardines, salmon, blue fin tuna

What are trans fatty acids?

Small amounts of trans fatty acids are found naturally in meat and dairy products, but most come from processed fats. These are produced by hydrogenation, a process which changes liquid oils into solid or spreadable fats. During this highly pressurised heat treatment, the geometrical arrangement of the atoms changes. Technically speaking, one or more of the unsaturated double bonds in the fatty acid is altered from the usual cis form to the unusual *trans* form. Hydrogenated fats and oils are used in many foods, including cakes, biscuits, margarine, low-fat spreads and pastries – check the ingredients.

The exact effect of trans fatty acids on the body is not certain, but it is thought that they may be worse than saturates: they could lower HDL and raise LDL levels. They may also increase levels of a substance that promotes blood clot formation and stops your body using essential fatty acids properly. A US study in 1993 of 85,000 nurses by researchers at Harvard Medical School linked high intakes of trans fatty acids (from processed fats, not natural fats) with a 50% increase in the risk of heart disease. Until more research has been carried out, it is probably best to regard them as similar to saturates and avoid them as far as possible. In practice, this means cutting down on hard margarine (the softer the spread, the fewer trans fatty acids it is likely to contain), fried foods from fast-food chains (many use hydrogenated oils), biscuits and other bakery products that contain hydrogenated fats (check the ingredients).

The DoH recommend that trans fatty acids make up no more than 2% of total calorie intake and that we eat no more than 5 g per day. Unfortunately, they are not normally listed on nutrition labels.

What is cholesterol?

Cholesterol is an essential part of our bodies; it makes up part of all cell membranes and helps produce several hormones. Some cholesterol comes from our diet, but most is made in the liver from saturated fats. In fact, the cholesterol we eat has only a small effect on our LDL cholesterol; if we eat more cholesterol (from meat, offal, eggs, dairy products, seafood) the liver compensates by making less, and vice versa. This keeps a steady level of cholesterol in the bloodstream.

Several factors can push up blood cholesterol levels. The major ones are obesity (especially android or central obesity), lack of exercise and the amount of saturated fatty acids we eat. Studies have shown that replacing saturated fatty acids with carbohydrates or unsaturated fatty acids can lower total and LDL cholesterol levels.

So, which are the best types of fats to eat?

In general, eat all types of fats and oils in moderation – remember, they should make up 15–30% of your total calorie intake. Most people eat considerably more than this (around 41% of calories). Use all spreading fats sparingly – there are advantages and disadvantages with butter, margarine and low-fat spreads. Butter, for example, is high in saturated fatty acids but contains no artificial additives. Most margarines and low-fat spreads contain trans fatty acids (as hydrogenated oil) and artificial additives, but are lower in saturates and higher in unsaturates. Check the label for the absence of hydrogenated or partially-hydrogenated oil. It also depends on your taste preferences. However, it is best to avoid hard margarines (those which don't spread straight from the fridge) as they have the highest content of hydrogenated fats and trans fatty acids.

For cooking and salad dressings, choose oils which are high in omega-3 fatty acids or monounsaturated fatty acids – olive, rapeseed flax and nut oils are good choices for health as well as taste. Include nuts and seeds in your regular diet; they provide many valuable nutrients apart from omega-3 fatty acids and monounsaturates. If you eat fish, include one to two portions of oily fish (e.g. mackerel, herring, salmon) per week. Vegetarians should make sure they include plant sources of omega-3 fatty acids in their daily diet.

SUMMARY OF KEY POINTS

- Excess body fat is a disadvantage in almost all sports and fitness programmes, reducing power, speed and performance.
- Very low body fat does not guarantee improved performance either. There appears to be an optimal fat range for each individual which cannot be predicted by a standard linear relationship.
- There are three main components of body-fat: essential fat (for tissue structure); sex-specific fat (for hormonal function); and storage fat (for energy).
- The minimum percentage of fat recommended for men is 5% and for women, 10%.

However, for normal health, the recommended ranges are 13–18% and 18–25% respectively. In practice, many athletes fall below these recommended ranges.
- Very low body fat levels are associated with hormonal imbalance in both sexes, and amenorrhoea, infertility, reduced bone density and increased risk of osteoporosis in women.
- Very low-fat diets can lead to deficient intakes of essential fatty acids and fat-soluble vitamins.
- A fat intake of 15–30% of energy is recommended for athletes and active people.
- Unsaturated fatty acids should make up the majority of your fat intake, with saturated fatty acids and trans fatty acids kept to a minimum.
- Greater emphasis should be placed on omega-3 fatty acids to improve the omega-3:omega-6 ratio. Include oily fish 1–2 times a week or consume 1–3 tbsp of linseed oil, pumpkin seeds, walnuts and rapeseed oil a day.
- Omega-3 fatty acids can enhance oxygen delivery to cells and therefore improve athletic performance.

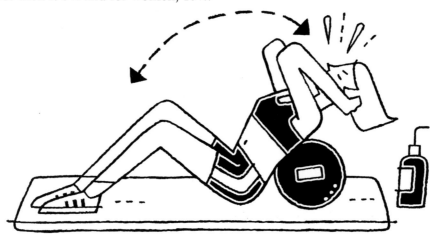

EVERYTHING YOU NEED TO KNOW ABOUT FAT LOSS

Many athletes and fitness participants wish to lose weight, either for health or performance reasons, or in order to make a competitive weight category. However, rapid weight loss can have serious health consequences leading to a marked reduction in performance. A knowledge of safe weight loss methods is, therefore, essential. Since 95% of dieters fail to maintain their weight loss within a five-year period, lifestyle management is the key to long-term weight management.

This chapter examines the effects of weight loss on performance and health, and highlights the dangers of rapid weight loss methods. It presents a simple step-by-step guide to calculating your calorie, carbohydrate, protein and fat intake on a fat-loss programme. Both nutritional and exercise strategies are given, including a detailed fat-loss exercise plan designed to minimise muscle loss and maximise fat burning. It examines the reasons why many people find it hard to lose and maintain weight, and the barriers to long-term success. Up-to-date research on appetite control and metabolism is presented, along with the dangers of 'yo-yo' dieting (repeated dieting and weight gain, also known as 'weight cycling'). It explodes many of the myths and fallacies about metabolic rates and, finally, gives safe and simple step-by-step strategies for successful weight loss.

How will losing weight affect my performance?

Unfortunately, many athletes use weight loss methods that have an adverse effect on their performance and their health. The two most common are crash dieting and dehydration. Clearly, an athlete may achieve a desirable appearance, but to the detriment of his or her performance. There is actually little evidence that attaining a very low body fat/weight automatically improves an athlete's performance; genetic endowment, strenuous training and good nutrition appear to be the main reasons for success.

Rapid weight loss results in a diminished aerobic capacity (Fogelholm, 1994). A drop of up to 5% has been measured in athletes who had lost just 2–3% of body weight through dehydration. A loss of 10% can occur in those who lose weight through strict dieting. Anaerobic performance, strength and muscular endurance are also decreased, although researchers have found that strength (expressed against body weight) can actually improve after gradual weight loss (Tiptan, 1987).

What happens to the body during rapid weight loss through crash dieting?

Strict dieting reduces vitamin and mineral status, since a lower food intake almost always means a lower intake of micro-nutrients (Steen, 1986; Colgan et al., 1991). Supplements may, therefore, be advisable if dieting for more than three weeks.

Prolonged dieting or food restriction can have more serious health consequences. In female athletes, low body weight and body fat have been linked with menstrual irregularities,

Rapid weight loss

To make weight for a competition (e.g. boxing, bodybuilding, judo), athletes may resort to rapid weight loss methods, such as fasting, dehydration, exercising in sweat suits, saunas, diet pills, laxatives, diuretics or self-induced vomiting. Weight losses of 4.5 kg in 3 days are not uncommon. In a study of 180 female athletes (Rosen et al., 1986), 32% admitted they used more than one of these methods. In another (Drummer et al., 1987), 15% of young female swimmers said they had tried one of these methods.

amenorrhoea and stress fractures; in male athletes, with reduced testosterone production. It has also been suggested that the combination of intense training, food restriction and the psychological pressure for extreme leanness may precipitate disordered eating and clinical eating disorders in some athletes. Scientists say that those who attempt to lose body fat for appearance are more likely to develop an eating disorder than those who control it only for performance purposes.

There is a fine line between dieting and obsessive eating behaviour, and many female athletes, in particular, are under pressure to be thin and improve their performance. The warning signs and health consequences of eating disorders are discussed in Chapter 10.

What happens to the body during rapid weight loss by dehydration?

Dehydration results in a reduced cardiac output and stroke volume, reduced plasma volume, slower nutrient exchange and slower waste removal, all of which have an impact on health and performance (Fogelholm, 1994; Fleck and Reimers, 1994). In moderate-intensity exercise lasting more than 30 seconds, even dehydration of less than 5% body weight will diminish strength or performance, although it does not appear to affect exercise lasting less than 30 seconds. So, for athletes relying on pure strength (e.g. weight lifting), rapid weight loss may not be as detrimental.

Will I still be able to train hard whilst losing weight?

The problem with most weight-loss diets is they do not provide enough calories or carbohydrate to support intense training. They can leave you feeling weak and lacking in energy. Instead reduce your normal calories by 10–20% (ACSM, ADA, DC, 2000). This modest change should produce weight loss in the region of 0.5 kg per week without you feeling deprived, tired or overly hungry. One consistent finding from studies is that an adequate carbohydrate intake (50–60% of energy) is critical for preserving muscular strength, endurance, and both aerobic and anaerobic capacity. A lower than optimal intake results in glycogen depletion and increased protein oxidation (muscle loss). Retaining lean mass is also vital for losing fat. The less muscle you have the lower your resting metabolic rate and the harder it is to lose fat (*see* pp. 117–18).

Can carbohydrate make you fat?

Studies have shown that eating carbohydrates increases your metabolic rate: about 10–15% of the carbohydrate calories are expended as heat (*see* p. 125, 'What is thermogenesis?'). That gives you a little leeway in your carbohydrate intake by allowing you to overconsume by around 10–15% (relative to your requirements).

So what happens to the excess carbohydrate? Well, it is converted preferentially into glycogen – provided there is spare storage capacity and provided there is only a modest rise in blood glucose. A rapid rise in blood glucose produced by high GI carbohydrates (*see* Appendix 1) can lead to fat storage. This is because it provokes a rapid release of insulin. The more insulin that is present in the bloodstream in response to high GI carbohydrates, the more likely that this insulin will turn excess carbohydrates into fat and deposit it in your fat cells.

The key to keeping insulin levels low is to eat low GI meals. In practice that means you need to eat balanced amounts of some carbohydrate, protein and healthy fat at each meal. Adding a small amount of unsaturated fat (particularly essential fatty acids) will also reduce the GI of the meal.

Can protein make you fat?

When protein is overeaten, the amino part of the molecule is excreted and the remainder of the molecule provides an energy substrate. This can either be used directly for energy production or else stored – preferably as glycogen rather than fat. Furthermore, protein ingestion stimulates thermogenesis (*see* p. 125), so a significant proportion of protein calories are given off as heat.

Researchers believe that protein is the most effective nutrient for switching off hunger signals, so it helps you to stop overeating. The most likely explanation is that we have no capacity to store excess protein so the brain readily detects when you have eaten enough and switches off hunger signals.

By including adequate amounts of protein in your meals on a fat-loss programme, you can help control hunger.

Can fat make you fat?

Dietary fat is far more likely to make you fat than any other nutrient, as it is stored as adipose tissue if it is not required straight away. In contrast to

Fat makes you fat

The hypothesis that fat is more fattening, calorie for calorie, than carbohydrate, is supported by a number of studies. (Flatt, 1993, Danforth, 1985). When men were fed 150% of their calorie requirements for two 14-day periods. In one period, the excess calories came from fat; in the other, from carbohydrate. (Horton et al., 1995) Overfeeding fat caused much greater deposition of body fat than overfeeding carbohydrate. Other researchers believe that it is unimportant whether the excess calories come from carbohydrate or fat. The best way to avoid obesity is to limit your total calories, not just the fat calories (Willett & Stampfer, 2002).

carbohydrate and protein, overeating fat does not increase fat oxidation; this only occurs when total energy demands exceed total energy intake or during aerobic exercise.

Fat is very calorie-dense; it contains more than double the calories per gram (9 kcal/g) of carbohydrate and protein (both 4 kcal/g), but it is much easier to overconsume as it is less satiating for two reasons. Firstly, carbohydrate and protein produce a rise in blood glucose, which reduces the appetite. Fat, on the other hand, is digested and absorbed less rapidly, and often actually depresses blood glucose, thereby failing to satisfy the appetite as efficiently. Secondly, fatty foods usually have a high-calorie density and low bulk, again making them less satisfying, even in the short term, and easier to overeat.

The fats you do eat should comprise unsaturated fatty acids, particularly the mono-unsaturated fats omega-3 and omega-6 fatty acids (*see* pp. 108–10).

Can alcohol make you fat?

Indirectly, alcohol can encourage fat storage. Since alcohol cannot be stored in the body, it must be oxidised and converted into energy (*see* p. 96). Whilst this is happening, the oxidation of fat and carbohydrate is suppressed, and these are channelled into storage instead.

Alcohol provides 7 kcal/g, which can significantly increase your total calorie intake if you consume large quantities. Also, many alcoholic drinks contain sugars and other carbohydrates, which increase the calorie content further.

HOW CAN I LOSE BODY FAT?

To lose body fat, you have to expend more energy (calories) than you consume. In other words, you have to achieve a negative energy balance (*see* Fig. 8.1).

Research has shown that a combination of diet and activity is more likely to result in long-term success than diet or exercise alone. Unfortunately, there are no miracle solutions or short cuts. The objectives of a healthy diet and exercise programme are to:

- achieve a modest negative energy (calorie) balance
- maintain (or even increase) lean tissue
- gradually reduce body fat percentage
- avoid a significant reduction in your resting metabolic rate (see definition below)
- obtain energy requirements from a high percentage of carbohydrate (60%) and a low percentage of fat (15–20%)
- achieve an optimal intake of vitamins and minerals.

How much carbohydrate, protein and fat should I consume if I want to lose body fat?

Calorie counting does not give you the full picture. Although you need to be in a negative energy balance to lose weight, new research suggests that the relative amounts of fat, carbohydrate and protein in your diet are important in switching on and off hunger signals. Also, the calories from each of these sources are handled by the body in quite different ways. This, in turn, has an important bearing on body fat levels.

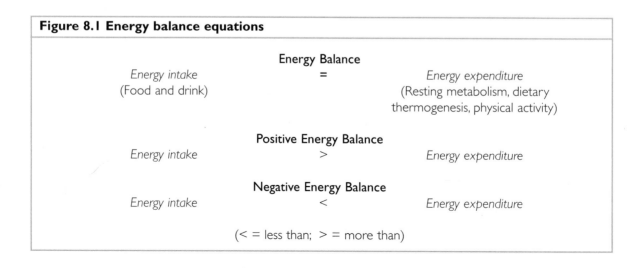

Figure 8.1 Energy balance equations

Energy Balance

| Energy intake (Food and drink) | = | Energy expenditure (Resting metabolism, dietary thermogenesis, physical activity) |

Positive Energy Balance

| Energy intake | > | Energy expenditure |

Negative Energy Balance

| Energy intake | < | Energy expenditure |

(< = less than; > = more than)

The key to successful fat loss is to cut your fat to 20–25% of total calories (Walberg-Rankin, 2000) and to reduce carbohydrates by only a modest amount. Ideally, carbohydrates should continue to contribute 50–60% of your total calories. That may not sound very different from your normal diet but remember you have now reduced your calorie intake, so your carbohydrate intake will be reduced proportionally. To convert calories to grams of carbohydrate you divide by 4. For example, if you have cut your calories from 2500 kcal (60% of calories = 375 g carbohydrate) to 2000 kcal, your new carbohydrate intake will be 60% of 2000 divided by 4 = 300 g.

If you reduce your carbohydrate intake below your daily energy requirement, glycogen stores become depleted, and not only does fat oxidation increase but protein oxidation also increases. Clearly, this is not a desirable state for athletes as it results in a loss of lean tissue. This will, of course, affect your performance and cause a reduction in your RMR. The less lean tissue you have, the lower your RMR, and the fewer calories you burn just to maintain your weight (*see* p. 126 'What makes your RMR high or low?').

A higher protein intake can offset some of the lean tissue loss. Most researchers recommend around 1.6 g/kg body weight/ day on a fat-loss programme. For example, a 75 kg athlete would need to consume 120 g protein/day. On a 2000

kcal programme, that would be equivalent to 24% total calories (i.e. 75 × 1.6 divided by 2000). This percentage is higher than the 12–15% recommended for weight maintenance but simply reflects the lower calorie intake. In other words, you maintain or slightly increase your protein intake but cut the calories from carbohydrate and fat.

Calculating calorie, carbohydrate, protein and fat requirements on a fat-loss programme

Reduce your usual calorie intake by 15%. This relatively modest reduction in calories will avoid the metabolic slowdown that is associated with more severe calorie reductions. The body will recognise and react to a smaller deficit by oxidising more fat. If you cut calories more drastically, it will not make you shed fat faster. Instead it will cause your body to lower its metabolic rate in an attempt to conserve energy stores. It will also increase protein oxidation and glycogen depletion. The end result is likely to be loss of lean muscle tissue, low energy levels, and extreme hunger.

In theory, 0.5 kg (500 g) of fat can be shed when a deficit of 4500 kcal is created since 1 g fat yields 9 kcal (9 × 500 = 4500 kcal). However, in practice, it may not work exactly like this because it depends on your initial calorie intake. For example, athlete A (male) normally eats 3000 kcal/day and athlete B (female) normally eats 2000 kcal/day. If both athletes reduced their calorie intake by 643 kcal/day (equivalent to 4500 kcal/week), athlete A now eats 2357 kcal/day and athlete B now eats 1357 kcal/day. The two athletes will, in practice, get very different results in terms of their body composition. Athlete A will almost certainly lose around 0.5 kg fat/week because his deficit is a 15% (modest) reduction. Athlete B will probably lose 0.5 kg fat/week for the first week or two, but

What is the resting metabolic rate?

Your resting metabolic rate (RMR) is the number of calories your body burns if you did *absolutely nothing* all day, i.e. lie down for 24 hours. It's basically the energy used to keep your essential body functions ticking over and accounts fo 60–75% of your total daily energy expenditure.

after that she will lose muscle tissue. That's because she has cut her calories by 32% which is too severe. In general, calorie reductions of greater than 15% will lead to a metabolic slowdown and muscle loss, making fat loss slower. Athlete B may well lose 0.5 kg of fat/week but some will come from muscle and a loss of muscle will slow her metabolism.

So, for fat loss, aim for a reduction of calories as a percentage of your maintenance calorie intake. Reducing calorie intake by 15% will lead to fat loss without slowing the metabolism. It may not allow you to lose 0.5 kg of fat/week – it may be 0.5 kg/10 days – but at least it will be fat, not muscle. Athlete B should eat 1700 kcal a day. This will produce a loss of 0.5 kg fat/11 or 12 days.

To help guide you through, calculations are shown for a 65 kg male cyclist, aged 30, who leads a mostly sedentary lifestyle and trains 10 hours on his bike (16 km/h) per week.

Step 1: Calculate your RMR (*see* Table 8.1)

Example:
RMR $= (65 \times 15.3) + 679 = 1673$ kcal

Step 2: Calculate your daily energy expenditure

Multiply your RMR by the appropriate number below:

a) If you are mostly sedentary (mostly seated or standing activities during the day):
RMR $\times 1.4$
b) If you are moderately active (regular brisk walking or equivalent during the day):
RMR $\times 1.7$

c) If you are very active (generally physically active during the day):
RMR $\times 2.0$
Example:
Daily energy expenditure $= 1673 \times 1.4 = 2342$ kcal

Step 3: Estimate the number of calories expended during exercise (*see* Table 8.2)

It's best to estimate your exercise calorie expenditure over a week (7 days) then divide by 7 to get a daily average.
Example:
Exercise calories/week $= 10 \times 385 = 3850$ kcal
Exercise calories/day $= 3850 \div 7 = 550$ kcal

Step 4: Add figures from steps 2 and 3

This is the number of calories you need to maintain your body weight. Regard this figure as your maintenance intake. If your current calorie intake is higher or lower than your maintenance intake, gradually adjust your intake until it almost matches. This may take a few weeks.
Example:
Maintenance calorie intake $= 2342 + 550 = 2892$ kcal

Step 5: Reduce your calorie intake by 15%

To do this, multiply your maintenance calories, as calculated in step 4, by 0.85 (85%) to give you your new total daily calorie intake.
Example:
New total daily calorie intake $= 2892 \times 85\% = 2458$ kcal

Table 8.1	Resting metabolic rate (RMR) in athletes	
Age	Male	Female
10–18 years	(body weight in kg × 17.5) + 651	(body weight in kg × 12.2) + 746
18–30 years	(body weight in kg × 15.3) + 679	(body weight in kg × 14.7) + 496
31–60 years	(body weight in kg × 11.6) + 879	(body weight in kg × 8.7) + 829

Table 8.2	Calories expended during exercise
Sport	**kcal/hour***
Aerobics (high intensity)	520
Aerobics (low intensity)	400
Badminton	370
Boxing (sparring)	865
Cycling (16 km/hour)	385
Cycling (9 km/hour)	250
Judo	760
Rowing machine	445
Running (3.8 min/km)	1000
Running (5.6 min/km)	750
Squash	615
Swimming (fast)	630
Tennis (singles)	415
Weight training	270–450

*Figures are based on the calorie expenditure of an athlete weighing 65 kg. Values will be greater for heavier body weights; lower for smaller body weights.

Step 6: Calculate your carbohydrate needs

Multiply the figure from step 5 by 0.6 (60%) then divide by 4 to calculate your carbohydrate intake in grams.
Example:
  Carbohydrate intake = $(2458 \times 60\%) \div 4 = 369$ g

Step 7: Calculate your protein needs

This is based on the recommended requirement of 1.6 g/kg body weight/day. Multiply your weight in kg × 1.6 to give you your daily protein intake in grams.

To calculate protein intake as a percentage of total calories, multiply the number of grams of protein by 4, divide by total calories as calculated in step 5, then multiply by 100:

% protein = (g protein × 4) ÷ (Step 5 figure) × 100.
Example:
  Protein intake = $65 \times 1.6 = 104$ g
  % protein intake = $(104 \times 4) \div 2458 = 17\%$

Step 8: Calculate your fat needs

Your fat intake as a percentage of total calories is the balance left once you have calculated the carbohydrate and protein percentages, i.e. 100% – % carbohydrate – % protein = % fat.

Then, to calculate your fat intake in grams, multiply the figure from step 5 by % fat and divide by 9.
Example:
  % fat intake = $100\% - 60\% - 17\% = 23\%$
  g fat = $(23\% \times 2458) \div 9 = 63$ g

How can I speed up my fat loss?

Increasing exercise calorie expenditure will help speed up fat loss. This can have a dual effect. Firstly, any additional aerobic exercise you perform on top of your regular training will increase fat oxidation during exercise as well as increase your metabolic rate for a while afterwards (*see* pp. 127–30 for more information on exercise and fat loss). Secondly, adding or increasing weight training exercises will offset any loss of lean tissue and maintain muscle mass.

STRATEGIES FOR PERMANENT FAT LOSS

Step 1: Set realistic goals

Before embarking on a weight loss plan, write down your goals clearly, as research has proven that by writing down your intentions, you are far more likely to turn them into actions.

These goals should be specific, positive and realistic ('I will lose 5 kg of body fat') rather than hopeful ('I would like to lose some weight'). Try to allow a suitable time frame (*see* Step 3): to lose 15 kg one month before a summer holiday is, obviously, unrealistic! Make sure, also, that you are clear about your reasons for wanting to lose weight: many normal-weight women wrongly believe that losing weight will solve their emotional or body image problems.

Step 2: Monitor body composition changes

The best way to ensure you are losing fat not muscle is to measure your body composition once a month. The simplest method is to use a combination of simple girth or circumference measurements (e.g. chest, waist, hips, arms, legs), as shown in Figure 8.2, and skinfold thickness measurements, obtained by callipers (*see* Chapter 7, pp. 102–3). Exercise physiologists

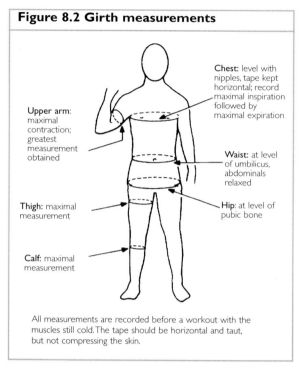

Figure 8.2 Girth measurements

Upper arm: maximal contraction; greatest measurement obtained

Chest: level with nipples, tape kept horizontal; record maximal inspiration followed by maximal expiration

Waist: at level of umbilicus, abdominals relaxed

Thigh: maximal measurement

Hip: at level of pubic bone

Calf: maximal measurement

All measurements are recorded before a workout with the muscles still cold. The tape should be horizontal and taut, but not compressing the skin.

recommend keeping a record of the skinfold thickness measurements themselves rather than converting them into body fat percentages. This is because the conversion charts are based on equations for the average, sedentary person and may not be appropriate for sportspeople or very lean or fat individuals. Monitoring changes in measurements at specific sites of the body allows you to see how your shape is changing and where most fat is being lost. This is a far better motivator than weighing scales! Alternatively, you can use one of the other methods of body composition measurement described in Chapter 7.

Step 3: Aim to lose no more than 0.5 kg/week

Weekly or fortnightly weighing can be useful for checking the speed of weight/fat loss, but do not rely exclusively on this method as it does not reflect changes in body composition! Avoid more frequent weighing as this can lead to an obsession with weight. Bear in mind that weight loss in the first week may be as much as 2 kg, but this is mostly glycogen and its accompanying fluid (1/2 kg glycogen is stored with up to 1½–2 kg water). Afterwards, aim to lose no more than 0.5 kg fat/week. Faster weight loss usually suggests a loss of lean tissue.

Step 4: Keep a food diary

A food diary is a written record of your daily food and drink intake. It is a very good way to evaluate your present eating habits and to find out exactly what, why and when you are eating. It will allow you to check whether your diet is well balanced or lacking in any important nutrients, and to take a more careful look at your usual meal patterns and lifestyle.

Weigh and write down everything you eat and drink for at least three consecutive days – ideally seven. This period should include at least one weekend day. It is important not to change your usual diet at this time and to be completely honest! Every spoonful of sugar in tea, every scrape of butter on bread should be recorded.

Use your food diary to find out about:

- the main sources of saturated fat in your diet which you need to eliminate
- the GI of your meals and snacks. Aim to consume low-GI food during the day and before exercise
- your fibre intake. Check that most meals are based on fibre-rich foods (*see* p. 22)
- the timing of your meals and snacks. Aim to eat approximately six times a day.

Step 5: Never consume fewer calories than your RMR

Calorie intake should never be less than your RMR, otherwise you risk losing excessive lean tissue, severely depleting your glycogen stores and having an inadequate nutrient intake. It is

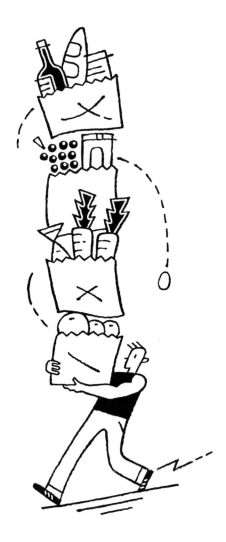

erroneous and potentially dangerous to prescribe low-calorie diets of 1000 kcal or less. Keep to the 15% rule.

Step 6: Trim saturated and hydrogenated fat

Look carefully at your food diary and identify the foods containing saturated and hydrogenated fats that you are currently eating. Fat puts on more body fat than any other nutrient. When protein or carbohydrate is eaten in excess, the body makes metabolic adjustments to promote glycogen storage and increase the use of protein or carbohydrate for fuel. You have to overeat fairly large amounts of these foods before they are converted into body fat. In contrast, excess saturated fats cause virtually no change in metabolism and are readily converted into body fat. Focus on cutting saturated rather than unsaturated fats. Table 8.3 provides suggestions on how to reduce your intake of saturated fats.

Table 8.3	Trim the fat

Eat less of the following:
- butter, hard margarine and other solid spreading fats (check label: avoid products containing animal fat, hydrogenated vegetable oil, palm oil, partially hydrogenated vegetable oil)
- deep-fried foods
- fatty meats and processed meat products (e.g. sausages, burgers, meat pies)
- pastry dishes
- cakes, biscuits, puddings
- chocolate
- cheese.

(These foods are high in saturated and/or trans fatty acids but relatively low in other essential nutrients.)

Make the following substitutions:
- semi-skimmed or skimmed milk instead of full-fat milk
- low-fat spread or peanut butter instead of butter or margarine (check label, see above)
- low-fat cheese (e.g. cottage cheese, quark) instead of ordinary cheese
- jacket or boiled potatoes instead of chips
- chicken, fish or lean meat instead of fatty meat, burgers and sausages
- crackers, rice cakes or fruit bars instead of biscuits and cakes
- fresh fruit instead of chocolate.

(These foods provide some fat together with other essential nutrients.)

Make the following changes:
- limit frying to stir frying with modest amounts of pure vegetable oil (e.g. olive oil, rapeseed oil, sunflower oil) instead of butter
- top baked potatoes with fromage frais, yoghurt or baked beans
- remove skin from chicken or turkey
- grill, bake, stir fry or boil instead of frying
- make low-fat salad dressings with flavoured vinegar (e.g. raspberry); yoghurt seasoned with fresh herbs, lemon or lime juice; fromage frais seasoned with mustard
- choose lean cuts of meat and trim off as much fat as possible.

(These will reduce your fat intake while supplying other essential nutrients.)

Step 7: Include healthy fats

Don't cut fat out of your diet completely. You need a certain amount each day to provide essential fatty acids, stimulate hormone production, keep your skin healthy, and absorb and transport fat-soluble vitamins. Dr Udo Erasmus (1996) believes that the essential fatty acids in foods such as nuts, seeds and oily fish help burn fat by assisting the transport of oxygen to the body's tissues. So, if you want to lose weight, cut down on saturated and trans fatty acids; the remainder should come from unsaturated fats. Aim for 15–20% of your total calories.

Step 8: Go for the (slow) burn

Make all of your meals low GI. This helps improve appetite regulation, increases feelings of fullness and delays hunger between meals. Remember that adding protein, fat or soluble fibre to carbohydrate always reduces the speed of absorption and produces a lower blood sugar rise. In practice, this is easy to achieve if you plan to eat a carbohydrate source (e.g. potatoes) with a high-protein source (e.g. fish) and add vegetables. Better still, choose low-GI carbohydrates, such as lentils and beans.

Step 9: Bulk up

The most filling foods are those with a high volume per calorie. Water and fibre add bulk to foods so load up on foods naturally high in these components. Fruit, vegetables, pulses and wholegrain foods give maximum fill for minimum calories. If you can eat a plate of food that is low in calories relative to its volume, you're likely to feel just as satisfied as eating smaller amounts of high-calorie food.

Step 10: Eat more fibre

Apart from reducing your risk of various cancers and heart disease, fibre slows down the emptying of food from your stomach and helps to keep you feeling full. Fibre also gives food more texture so you need to chew your food more. This slows down your eating speed, reducing the chances of overeating and gives better meal satisfaction.

Fibre also slows the digestion and absorption of carbohydrates and fats, resulting in a slow steady energy uptake and stable insulin levels (Albrink, 1978). Non-fluctuating glucose and insulin levels will encourage the use of food for energy rather than for storage as body fat; it also reduces hunger and satisfies the appetite.

Step 11: Indulge yourself

Don't cut out your favourite comfort foods. Many people find that a 'day off' from healthy eating or dieting once a week satisfies their cravings and keeps them well-motivated to eat well week after week. This means you can allow yourself to have chocolate, or your favourite ice cream or that extra large hamburger, without feeling guilty. If you know you can eat a little of your favourite food every week you'll stop thinking of it as a forbidden food and won't want to overeat on it. Studies have shown that not banning 'naughty' foods and enjoying the occasional high-fat indulgence without feeling guilty is a successful strategy for maintaining weight loss.

Step 12: Eat more frequently

Plan to eat at least 4–6 times a day, planning snacks and meals at regular intervals. This does not mean increasing the amount eaten, but eating moderate-sized meals or snacks more frequently. Some suggestions for low-fat snacks are given in Table 8.4. Research has shown that each time we eat, the metabolic rate increases by approximately 10% for a short while afterwards. This phenomenon is the *thermic* effect of food, or dietary-induced *thermogenesis* (see below). Re-searchers have also found that frequent eating keeps blood sugar and insulin levels more stable,

Table 8.4 Healthy snacks

If you feel hungry between meals, here are some suggestions on what to eat. The snacks are designed to provide balanced amounts of carbohydrate, protein and healthy fat and a low–moderate GI.

- Wholemeal sandwiches, rolls, toast, bagels with healthy fillings (e.g. cottage cheese, tuna, chicken, peanut butter)
- Wholemeal English muffins, fruit buns, scones with olive oil spread
- Smoothies (home-made or ready-made) made with crushed fruit and yoghurt
- Oat/Scotch/homemade pancakes
- Oatcakes and rice cakes with healthy toppings (e.g. peanut butter,e avocado)
- Baked beans on wholemeal toast
- Fresh fruit
- Dried fruit and nuts
- Meal replacement shake or bar
- Home-made shakes made with low-fat milk, fruit and yoghurt
- Low-fat yoghurt and fromage frais

Table 8.5 Lifestyle changes

Lifestyle	Suggestion
Not enough time to prepare healthy meals	Plan meals in advance so all ingredients and at hand. Make meals in bulk and refrigerate/freeze portions. Cook baked potatoes, pasta and rice in larger quantities and save
Work shifts	Plan regular snack breaks and take own food with you
Work involves lots of travelling	Take portable snacks (e.g. rolls, fruit, nuts, energy bars, muffins, dried fruit, diluted fruit juice)
Need to cook for rest of family	Adapt favourite family meals (e.g. spaghetti bolognese) to contain less fat, more carbohydrate and fibre (e.g. leaner mince, more vegetables, wholemeal pasta). Make meals that everyone enjoys
Overeat when stressed	Consider stress counselling or relaxation courses to learn to handle stressful situations; take up new sport/hobby/leisure interests
Eat out frequently	Choose lower fat meals in restaurants (e.g. pasta with vegetable sauces, chicken tikka with chappati, stir fried vegetables with rice)

as well as helping to control blood cholesterol levels. For regular exercisers, eating six times a day is especially beneficial for efficient glycogen replenishment between workouts, and for minimising fat deposition. A regular food intake also ensures a constant flux of nutrients for repairing body tissues.

Step 13: Make gradual lifestyle changes

Long-term weight management can be achieved with healthy eating and regular exercise. However, one of the biggest barriers to this is an unwillingness to commit to a few necessary changes in lifestyle. Table 8.5 lists some of the common reasons why many people fail to manage their weight in the long term, together with some suggestions as to how to overcome them.

TURNING UP THE HEAT

What is thermogenesis?

This technical term means heat production. Every time you consume food your RMR increases and your body temperature rises a little. If you can get your body to produce more heat by eating the right ratio of fuels, then more of the calories you consume will be burned off as heat. Some nutrients have a higher thermic effect than others. Protein exerts the strongest thermic effect, carbohydrates exerts a milder effect, but fat exerts only a tiny thermic effect. When you eat 100 kcal fat only 3 kcal will be burned off as heat. When you eat 100 kcal carbohydrate, 12–15 kcal are 'wasted' as heat. When you eat protein, approximately 20 kcal are wasted (Swaminathan et al., 1985). So eating protein and carbohydrate increases the RMR, whereas fat causes very little increase in RMR and most of the calories will be converted into body fat. That's a good reason to keep your fat intake low.

Can you lower thermogenesis?

Yes. Consuming a diet that is low in protein or carbohydrate, high in fat or simply too low in calories will cause the body to produce less heat. When you produce less heat, your body temperature falls and that means you are burning fewer calories.

How can you increase thermogenesis?

Clearly, it is advantageous to optimise thermogenesis when aiming to lose body fat. You can do this by reducing calories by a modest amount (15%), reducing fat, and keeping carbohydrate and protein at adequate levels. This way your body can tap into its fat reserves for fuel without decreasing its heat production. Cutting calories more severely (by more than 15%) will cause a drop in your metabolic rate through a loss of muscle mass and a marked decrease in heat production that is induced by foods.

If you are going to overeat, it's better to indulge on high-protein foods (low fat, of course) or high-carbohydrate foods (preferably low-GI). At least some of those extra calories will be wasted as heat rather than being turned into body fat.

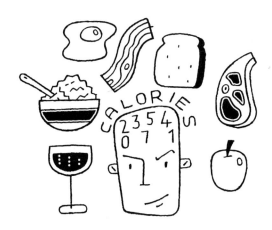

Another way to burn more calories as heat is to divide your daily calories into six meals. Every time you eat, thermogenesis increases, as extra energy is expended in digesting and absorbing food. Up to 10% of the calories you consume at a meal will be used for this purpose. So it makes sense to turn on thermogenesis as frequently as possible within your daily calorie requirements.

YOUR METABOLIC RATE

What makes your RMR high or low?

The most important factor that determines your RMR is the amount of fat-free mass you have (muscle, bone and vital organs). This is calorie-burning tissue so the more fat-free mass you have the higher your RMR will be.

Your total body weight also affects your RMR. The more you weigh the higher your RMR, because the larger your body the more calories it needs for basic maintenance.

It is a myth that overweight people have a lower RMR (except in clinical conditions such as hypothyroidism or Cushing's syndrome). Numerous studies have shown a linear relationship between total weight and metabolic rate, i.e. the RMR increases with increasing body weight. Genetics undoubtedly play a role – some people are simply born with a more 'revved-up' metabolism than others.

Can dieting slow down my RMR?

Strict dieting will sabotage long-term efforts at weight control because it sends the body into 'famine' mode. When you restrict your calories, your RMR slows down as your body becomes more energy efficient. You need fewer calories just to maintain your weight. The more severe the calorie drop the greater the decrease in your RMR. Generally the decrease is between 10–30%. However, the effect is not permanent as the RMR returns to its original level once normal eating is resumed.

Avoid a big drop in your RMR by cutting your calories as modestly as possible (15% is recommended) and always consume more calories than your RMR. For example, if your maintenance calorie intake is 2500 kcal, you should reduce this to 2125 kcal.

How can I raise my RMR?

By increasing your fat-free mass. Studies have shown that regular weight training will raise your RMR in as little as three months (Thompson et at., 1996). And a higher RMR is the key to successful weight control. Muscle tissue burns more calories than fatty tissue. Therefore, by increasing your muscle:fat ratio you will have a higher metabolic rate. Some researchers estimate that the increased lean body mass associated with exercise can increase total energy expenditure by between 8 and 14%, equivalent to 155–271 kcal/day for an average woman.

In a study conducted by Wayne Westcott, Fitness Research Director at South Shore YMCA, Massachusetts, 72 overweight adults were divided into two groups. The first followed an aerobics-only training programme for 30 minutes 3 days a week. The second did a

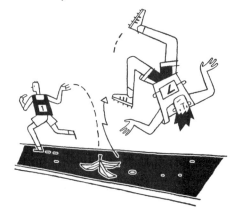

combination of weight training and aerobics for the same amount of time and frequency. After 8 weeks, those following the aerobics-only programme lost 1.4 kg body fat and 0.2 kg muscle; those following the weight training plus aerobics programme lost 4.5 kg body fat and gained 0.9 kg muscle!

How much extra muscle would it take to boost my RMR significantly?

According to Wayne Westcott's research, 0.5 kg muscle burns approximately 30–50 kcal/ day. So adding just 0.5 kg muscle would use up 350 kcal/week just for maintenance purposes. If you lose 0.5 kg fat and gain 0.5 kg muscle, that's a 1 kg improvement in your body composition.

Will exercise raise my RMR?

Your metabolic rate remains high after exercise while your body burns extra calories to pay off the oxygen debt. How high and how long depends on the type of workout, how hard and how long you exercise and how fit you are. This post-exercise increase in RMR is called the excess post-exercise oxygen consumption (EPOC). This is sometimes called the 'after-burn'. It refers to the energy needed to replenish the high-energy compounds (PC and ATP) and repair muscle tissue. This energy is obtained chiefly from the body's fat stores.

BURN FAT, NOT MUSCLE

What is the best type of exercise for fat loss?

Anyone on a calorie-reduced programme will lose both muscle and fat. On a severe calorie-reduced programme, muscle loss can account for up to 50% of weight loss. However, muscle loss can be minimised by the right choice of exercise.

When weight training exercise is added to a calorie-reduced programme, more muscle is preserved and a greater proportion of weight loss is fat loss. Intense resistence exercise should be included in your fat-loss programme for two reasons. Firstly, your RMR will be elevated for up to 15 hours post-exercise, due to the oxidation of body fat (Melby et al., 1993). Secondly, weight training acts as the stimulus to muscle retention. The more muscle you have, the faster your metabolism.

Muscle accounts for at least 60% of EPOC. So, the more muscle tissue you have, the greater the EPOC (Bosselaers et al.,1994).

Can aerobic exercise speed up fat loss?

Adding aerobic exercise to your fat-loss programme will burn more calories and offset some of the muscle wastage, but don't rely on aerobic exercise exclusively. You could still lose substantial amounts of muscle tissue with aerobic exercise – some studies have estimated as much as 40% (Aceto, 1997). This is because aerobic exercise does not act as sufficient stimulus to ensure muscle retention while you are on a calorie-reduced programme. Muscle loss will subsequentially result in a lowering of your metabolic rate.

Is high-intensity aerobics better than low-intensity?

Despite what many people believe, low-intensity, long-duration aerobic exercise is not the best method for shedding fat. Research indicates that not only does high-intensity aerobic exercise burn fat more effectively but it also speeds up your metabolism and keeps it revved-up for a while after your workout. What actually counts is the number of calories burned per unit of time. The more calories you expend, the more fat you break down. For example, walking (i.e. low-intensity aerobic exercise) for 60 minutes burns 270 kcal, of which 160 kcal (60% calories) comes from fat. Running (i.e. high-intensity aerobic exercise) for the same amount of time burns 680 kcal, of which 270 kcal (40% calories) comes from fat. Therefore, high-intensity aerobic exercise results in greater fat loss over the same time period. This principle applies to everyone no matter what your level of fitness – exercise intensity is always relative to the individual. Walking at 6 km/h may represent high-intensity exercise for an unconditioned individual; running at 10 km/h may represent low-intensity exercise for a well-conditioned athlete.

How should I construct my fat burning exercise programme?

You have two parts to your fat burning exercise programme:

1 weight training
2 high-intensity aerobic exercise.

Ideally, they should be performed on alternate days so you will have adequate time for recuperation between workouts and maximum energy for each workout. Here is a plan to achieve effective fat loss, and preservation (or building) of muscle mass and the metabolic rate:

- Perform your weight training workout 3 times a week on alternate days (e.g. Monday, Wednesday, Friday). Training sessions should be intense, causing you to reach muscular failure (maximum rating of intensity or perceived exertion on the last set of each exercise).
- Each weight training session should last 40–45 minutes.
- Alternate training the muscles of the upper and lower body (i.e. a two-way split). For example, train upper body on Monday, lower body on Wednesday, upper body on Friday, etc.
- Perform a total of 6 sets for each muscle group, choosing one or two different exercises that target that muscle group. (*See* Table 8.6 below.)

Table 8.6	Sample fat-burning exercise plan					
Monday	Tuesday	Wednesday	Thursday	Friday	Saturday	Sunday
Week 1						
UBWT: Chest, back, shoulders, arms	AT: 20–25 minutes on stationary bike	LBWT: Legs, calves, abdominals	AT: 20–25 minute run	UBWT: Chest, back, shoulders, arms	AT: 20–25 minute swim	No training
Week 2						
LBWT: Legs, calves, abdominals	AT: 20–25 minutes on stationary bike	UBWT: Chest, back shoulders, arms	AT: 20–25 minute run	LBWT: Legs, calves, abdominals	AT: 20–25 minute swim	No training

Key: UBWT = Upper body weight training
LBWT = Lower body weight training
AT = Aerobic training

Table 8.7	Sample weight training plan (upper body workout)
Muscle group/exercise	**Reps**
Chest	
Bench press (warm-up)	1 × 12–15
Bench press	3 × 8–10
Dumbbell flyes	3 × 8–10
Back	
Lat pulldown (warm-up)	1 × 12–15
Lat pulldown	3 × 8–10
Seated row	3 × 8–10
Shoulders	
Dumbell shoulder press (warm-up)	1 × 12–15
Dumbell shoulder press	3 × 8–10
Lateral raise	3 × 8–10
Arms	
Barbell curl (warm-up)	1 × 12–15
Barbell curl	3 × 8–10
Lying tricep extension (warm-up)	1 × 12–15
Lying tricep extension	3 × 8–10

Table 8.8	Sample weight training plan (lower body workout)
Muscle group/exercise	**Reps**
Legs	
Squat (warm-up)	1 × 12–15
Squat	3 × 8–10
Lunges	3 × 8–10
Calf raise (warm-up)	1 × 12–15
Calf raise	3 × 8–10
Abdominals	
Crunches	2 × 10–15
Oblique crunches	2 × 10–15
Reverse curl-ups	2 × 10–15

Note: For a full description of the exercises in Tables 8.7 and 8.8 see *The Complete Guide to Strength Training* by Anita Bean (A & C Black, 1997).

- Maintain super-strict form and focus on each repetition, keeping the weight fully in control. The importance of technique cannot be stressed enough.
- Lift and lower for a count of two on each part of the movement, and aim to hold the fully contracted position for a count of one.
- Perform your aerobic training sessions three times a week on alternate days (e.g. Tuesday, Thursday, Sunday). Each session should take approximately 20–25 minutes.
- Suitable activities include running, cycling (stationary bike or outdoor cycling), stepping, swimming, rowing or any cardiovascular apparatus. The important factor is that the activity is continuous and you are able to vary your intensity.
- Start with a 3–5 minute warm-up phase. Increase the intensity gradually over the next 4 minutes until you have reached a high-intensity effort. Maintain for 1 minute then reduce the intensity back to a moderate level for 1 minute. Repeat that pattern 4 times. Finish with a gradual reduction in intensity over 2–3 minutes.

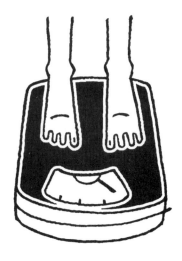

DIETING

Does 'yo-yo' dieting wreck your metabolism?

Many life-long dieters believe that repeated dieting and weight regain (known as 'yo-yo' dieting or weight cycling) makes the body so efficient at conserving energy that it permanently slows their RMR. The theory is that the body adapts to survive on fewer and fewer calories so that when the diet fails, the body stores fat more readily, making it harder to lose weight next time.

A report commissioned by the US National Institutes of Health (1994) concluded that there simply is not enough evidence to support the claims that yo-yo dieting permanently slows down your metabolism. When you restrict your food intake, your RMR falls initially, but soon returns to its original level once normal eating is resumed. A study carried out at the Dunn Clinical Nutrition Centre followed 11 overweight women over 18 weeks through three dieting cycles and found that, although their RMR decreased during the up–down cycles it returned to its original level once their weight stabilised.

Is yo-yo dieting harmful?

Repeated weight fluctuations have been linked with an increased risk of heart disease, secondary diabetes, gall bladder disease and premature death. However, researchers are divided as to the exact reason. One explanation is that fat tends to be redeposited intra-abdominally, closer to the liver, rather than in the peripheral regions of the body, such as the hips, thighs and arms, thus posing a greater heart disease risk. Another explanation is that repeated severe dieting can lead to a loss of lean tissue (including organ tissue) and nutritional deficiencies that can damage heart muscle. Yo-yo dieting can also be bad for your psychological health. Each time you regain weight, you experience a sense of failure, which can lower your confidence and self-esteem.

How effective are popular weight loss diets for athletes?

A number of quasi-scientific popular diets contradict high-carbohydrate sports diets. Here is a summary of the two most popular.

The Zone diet

The Zone diet is high in protein (30%), low in carbohydrate (40%), moderate in fat (30%) and low in calories. The two central claims are: (1) it changes the body's insulin:glucagon ratio, which in turn promotes fat oxidation rather than storage; (2) it increases eicosanoid production (a localised hormone that dilates blood vessels), thus increasing oxygen delivery to the muscles. Many eminent researchers, such as Cheuvront (1999), have disputed these claims and found absolutely no evidence that supports them. One major criticism is that the Zone diet will not cause a big enough rise in glucagon to affect fat-burning. What's more, there is no evidence that any rise in eicoanoid levels it produces affects vaso-dilation, oxygen delivery or athletic performance. In fact, researchers say the Zone diet is more likely to *reduce* athletic performance!

The Atkins Diet

The basis for Atkins' diet is that people lose weight more effectively when insulin levels are kept as low as possible. Atkins claims that a life-long high-carbohydrate diet causes a metabolic disorder called insulin resistance, which means that the body becomes unresponsive to the actions of insulin and, as a result, produces more of it. The body then goes into fat-storage mode.

The solution, according to Atkins is to cut carbohydrate intake dramatically and force the body to go into ketosis, i.e. fat is broken down in a different way to release ketones.

Again, this diet has been criticised by eminent researchers who state that it is not the insulin that makes people put on weight; the opposite is more likely to be true. In most cases, it's being fat that makes people insulin resistant. When you lose weight, resistance returns to normal.

Low-carbohydrate diets may work in the short term but only because you eat fewer calories. If you cut out virtually all sugar and starch you automatically restrict the foods you can eat and end up consuming fewer calories. In a year-long study at the University of Pennsylvania, obese people on the Atkins diet lost 10 lbs more after 6 months than volunteers on a conventional diet (Samaha, 2003). But by the end of the year, the differences between the two groups were not significant, suggesting the Atkins diet is no better at helping overweight people shed weight than traditional diets. The novelty of such a 'different' eating system appeals to certain people and that in itself is motivating. However, these diets are highly unsuitable for athletes as they provide too little carbohydrates to support athletic perform-ance. They would empty your glycogen reserves, produce fatigue and limit your endurance.

BUT WHAT IF I STILL CAN'T LOSE WEIGHT

Many people insist that they hardly eat a thing, yet cannot shift any surplus weight. Clearly, this is impossible. An alternative explanation can usually be found by delving more closely into daily eating habits, lifestyle and psychology. Keeping a detailed, honest, weighed food diary, ideally for seven days, can reveal many truths.

Why does my weight soar once I stop dieting?

There are two main explanations as to why some people gain a lot of weight after dieting. Firstly, many dieters tend to overeat or binge after 'coming off' their diet, especially on foods regarded as forbidden. You are likely, therefore, to consume a lot more calories than before. Researchers say that this is because inappropriate dieting suppresses your natural appetite control and lowers your self esteem, leading to negative moods and exaggerated appetite once you stop dieting. The second explanation is that your glycogen stores simply fill out. Since you store about 1.5 kg water for every 0.5 kg glycogen, the scales may register a larger weight gain than expected. Obviously, this is not fat weight, so don't feel disheartened!

Here are some of the most common explanations for 'resistant obesity':

Underestimating food intake

Researchers say that many 'resistant' dieters underestimate their food intake. Numerous studies have found that such people consciously or subconsciously underestimate how much they eat. In a study carried out by researchers from the University of Ulster and the Dunn Clinical Nutrition Centre (Prentice et al., 1989), 16 men and 16 women kept a 7-day, weighed-food diary, while their total energy expenditure was simultaneously measured. There was little difference in energy expenditure, but there was a wide variation in reported energy intakes.

This discrepancy between energy expenditure and apparent low intakes in some people could only be explained by under-reporting of food intake and not, according to the researchers, to any defect in energy metabolism.

Weekend splurging

Many people restrict their food intake during the week, then relax restraint at the weekend, celebrating their dieting efforts by splurging on high-fat 'treats' – often aided by alcohol. A rigid daily diet of around 1000–1200 kcal from Monday to Friday, can give way to mounting hunger by Friday night, and to a much larger consumption of food over the weekend – perhaps 3000 kcal a day. Despite weekday dieting efforts, the total weekly calorie intake ends up exactly the same as a normal, daily maintenance calorie intake (i.e. non-diet).

Guilt after the weekend splurge brings on renewed resolve to diet more strictly during the coming week. This, again, is followed by hunger, increased appetite, overeating, guilt, and so the vicious circle continues. It is easy to see how the weekday dieter becomes more and more frustrated: he or she feels constantly on a diet, yet never able to lose any weight.

Daytime starving/evening bingeing

It is common to find that many dieters eat very little during the day, skipping breakfast and surviving only on snacks. Daytime starvation leads to low energy levels, depleted glycogen stores and exaggerated hunger by the evening and consequent overeating.

If you eat in the early part of the day, you burn off more calories by a process called *dietary-induced thermogenesis* (DIT), in which energy is used up as a result of digesting and absorbing a meal. Thus, eating late at night burns off fewer calories than eating during the daytime.

Evening nibbles

A food diary may reveal that a dieter's evening meal extends to an all night sitting. It is easy to discount snacks and nibbles consumed mindlessly in front of the television. Many dieters will snack in the evening through boredom, misery, anger or other emotional reasons, without consciously realising or admitting how much they have eaten.

Eating too many low fat foods

If you're cutting fat but still not losing weight you may have simply replaced high-fat foods with greater volumes of the low-fat ones. The trouble is that feeling full is a complex mixture of physiology and psychology. A lot of people reward themselves with a double portion of low-fat ice cream because they believe it is not 'fattening'. In many cases, it's simply not true as the sugar and calorie value of low-fat foods can still be very high. Some people trade weekday low-fat eating with weekend high-fat indulgence because they think they feel virtuous. The result is their weekly fat and calorie intake stays high and they don't lose weight

Unfortunately, calories are the bottom line. To lose weight you have to eat fewer calories. Reduced-fat chocolate, for example, may temporarily satisfy the taste buds but it won't satisfy a desire for real chocolate. You can eat huge amounts of calories from reduced-fat chocolate and then go on to binge on the real thing the next day. Another problem with low-fat bars and biscuits is that they are 'energy dense'. Stripped of fibre and water, they lose their ability to make you feel full or satisfied. So it's easy to consume a lot of calories in seconds, and it's tempting to have another.

The best way to manage your weight is to concentrate on eating full-flavoured real food slowly.

Setting an unrealistic goal

Aiming for an unrealistically low body weight is a very common mistake. One theory is that we have a genetically determined 'set point' close to which the body attempts to regulate its weight and body fat. It uses a variety of adaptive

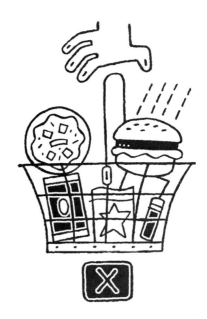

mechanisms: studies have shown that when underfed, the body reduces its spontaneous physical activity, its thermic response to food (DIT) and, temporarily, its RMR, in response to what it perceives as imminent starvation. Research by Dr Stunkard in the USA (Stunkard et al., 1986; Stunkard et al., 1990) suggests that everyone's body is programmed to be at a certain weight. So, people who are constantly striving to attain a low body weight may be fighting a losing battle with their genes, as well as putting their health at risk and creating unnecessary psychological stress.

Dieting psychology

There is evidence that a psychological difference exists between dieters and non-dieters. In dieters and weight-conscious people, the normal regulation of food intake becomes undermined as normal appetite and hunger cues are ignored. This leads to periods of restraint and semi starvation, followed by overindulgence and guilt, followed by restraint, and so on.

Psychologists have shown that habitual dieters tend to have a more emotional personality than those who are not preoccupied with weight. They also tend to be more obsessive and less able to concentrate.

The psychology of dieting

Dieters usually live by a set of rules centred around 'allowed' foods and 'banned'/'naughty' foods. For example, in one US study, dieters were given two apples (100 kcal) or two squares of chocolate (100 kcal). Those who ate the chocolate perceived themselves to be breaking their diet and went on to overindulge at the subsequent meal. Those who ate the apples continued with their diet.

At the University of Toronto, dieters and non-dieters were given a high-calorie milkshake, followed by free access to ice cream (Herman & Polivy, 1991). The dieters actually went on to eat more ice cream than the non-dieters. This is due to a phenomenon known as 'counter regulation'; having lost the inbuilt regulation system of non-dieters, they were unable to detect and thus compensate for the calorie pre-load.

Dr Barbara Rolls and colleagues at Penn State University (Rolls & Shide, 1992) demonstrated that weight worriers appear to lack the internal 'calorie counter' possessed by people who don't worry about their weight. When given a yoghurt half an hour before lunch, those who worried about their weight ate more for lunch than the free and easy people. It appears that such dieters have poor appetite control and are unable to compensate for previous food intake.

Checklist

- Keep a food diary for a week, writing down the weight of everything you normally eat and drink. This helps you become aware of your true eating pattern.
- Do not skip meals or starve yourself during the day.
- Plan regular meals and snacks throughout the day, thereby eliminating excessive hunger, satisfying appetite, facilitating efficient glycogen refuelling, improving energy levels and health.
- Set yourself a realistic weight goal that is right for your body type.
- Avoid weekday dieting and weekend splurging. Aim to eat about the same amount of food each day and don't worry if you occasionally overdo it.
- Remember, there are no banned foods; all foods are allowed.
- Do not set yourself rigid eating and exercising rules. Be flexible and never feel guilty if you overindulge or miss an exercise session.
- Examine your feelings and emotions when you eat. Food should not be used as a shield for emotional problems. Solve these with the help of a trained counsellor or eating disorder specialist.

SUMMARY OF KEY POINTS

- Rapid weight loss can result in an excessive loss of lean tissue, dehydration, and a reduction in aerobic capacity (up to 10%), strength and endurance.
- Effective fat loss can be achieved by reducing calorie intake by no more than 15%; this will minimise both lean tissue loss and resting metabolic rate (RMR) reduction.
- The recommended rate of fat loss is no more than 0.5 kg/week.
- Carbohydrate should be reduced by only a modest amount, but still contribute 60% of calories.
- Protein intake should be approx 1.6g/kg body weight/day to offset lean tissue loss.
- A reduction in saturated fat while maintaining essential fatty acids will result in an effective body-fat loss.
- Additional aerobic exercise performed for 20 minutes 3 times a week together with high intensity weight training performed on alternate days will maintain muscle mass and RMR while losing body fat.
- Your diet should be based on low GI meals, and foods with a high fibre and/or water content.
- Eating carbohydrate and protein, minimising fat and increasing meal frequency can optimise thermogenesis and, therefore, fat loss.
- The most effective way of increasing your RMR is to increase lean mass and follow a high intensity aerobic and weight training programme.
- Appetite regulation is enhanced by a high protein, high carbohydrate, low-fat eating programme.
- Yo-yo dieting can have an adverse effect on body composition, and overall physical and mental health.

- Failed attempts to lose body fat permanently may be due to inconsistent patterns of food intake, negative body image, poor motivation, unnecessary food restriction or avoidance, or a negative mental attitude.

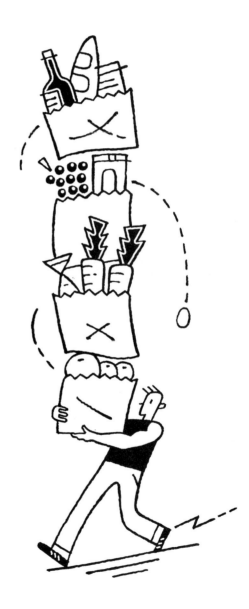

GAINING LEAN BODY WEIGHT

There are two ways to gain weight: either by increasing your lean mass or by increasing your fat mass. Both will register as weight gain on the scales but result in a very different body composition and appearance!

Lean weight gain can be achieved by combining the right type of strength training programme with a balanced diet. Strength (resistance) training provides the stimulus for muscle growth while your diet provides the right amount of energy (calories) and nutrients to enable your muscles to grow at the optimal rate. One without the other will result in minimal lean weight gain.

What type of training is best for gaining weight?

Resistance training (weight training) is the best way to stimulate muscle growth. Research shows that the fastest gains in size and strength are achieved using relatively heavy weights that can be lifted strictly for 6–10 repetitions per set. If you can do more than 10–12 repetitions at a particular weight, your size gains will be less, but you may still achieve improvements in muscular endurance, strength and power.

Concentrate on the 'compound' exercises, such as bench press, squat, shoulder press and lat pull-down, as these work the largest muscle groups of the body together with neighbouring muscles that act as 'assistors' or 'synergists'. These types of exercises stimulate the largest number of muscle fibres in one movement and are therefore the most effective and quickest way to gain muscle mass. Keep the smaller isolation exercises, such as biceps concentration curls or

tricep kickbacks, to a minimum; these produce slower mass gains and should only be added to your workout occasionally for variety.

How much weight can I expect to gain?

How much lean weight you can expect to gain depends on three main factors:

1 genetics
2 body type
3 hormonal balance.

Your genetic make up determines the proportion of different types of fibres in your muscles. The fast-twitch (type II) fibres generate power and increase in size more readily than the slow-twitch (type I or endurance) fibres. So, if you naturally have plenty of fast-twitch fibres in your muscles, you will probably respond faster to a strength training programme than someone who has a higher proportion of slow-twitch fibres. Unfortunately, you cannot convert slow-twitch into fast-twitch fibres – hence two people can follow exactly the same training programme, yet the one with lots of fast twitch muscle fibres will naturally gain weight faster than the other.

Your natural body type also affects how fast you gain lean weight. An ectomorph (naturally slim build with long lean limbs, narrow shoulders and hips) will find it harder to gain weight than a mesomorph (muscular, athletic build with wide shoulders and narrow hips) who tends to gain muscle readily. An endomorph (stocky, rounded build with wide shoulders and

Training for muscle gain

Certain compound exercises, such as dead lifts, clean and jerks, snatches and squats, not only stimulate the 'prime mover' muscles, but also have a powerful anabolic ('systemic') effect on the whole body and the central nervous system. These are the classic mass builders and should be included once a week in any serious muscle/strength training programme.

To stimulate the maximal number of muscle fibres in a muscle group, select one to three basic exercises and aim to do 4–12 total sets for that muscle group. Latest research suggests that doing fewer sets (4–8) but using heavier weights (80–90% of your one-rep maximum – i.e. the maximum weight which can be lifted through one complete repetition) results in faster size and strength gains. If you exercise that muscle group to exhaustion, you will need to allow up to 7 days for recuperation before repeating the same workout. So, aim to train each muscle group once a week (on average). In practice, divide your body parts (e.g. chest, legs, shoulders, back, arms) into three or four, and train one part per workout.

Always use strict training form and, ideally, have a partner to 'spot' for you so that you can use near-maximal weights safely. Always remember to warm up each muscle group beforehand with light aerobic training (e.g. exercise bike) and some relevant stretches. Ensure you also stretch the muscles after (and, ideally, in between each part of) the workout to help relieve soreness.

However, no matter what your genetics, natural build and hormonal balance, everyone can gain muscle and improve their shape with strength training. It is just that it takes some people longer than others.

How fast can I expect to gain weight?

Muscle and strength gains are usually faster at the start of a strength programme. Gains are often periodic as each improvement is interspersed with a plateau. As with a weight-loss programme, aim to gain weight gradually. After an initial, relatively fast gain, expect to gain no more than 0.5–1 kg per month or 0.25–1% of your body weight per week. Monitor your body composition rather than simply your weight. If you gain weight much more than 1 kg per month on an established programme, then you are likely to be gaining fat!

HOW MUCH SHOULD I EAT?

To gain lean weight and muscle strength at the optimal rate you need to be in a positive energy balance, i.e. *consuming more calories than you need for maintenance*. This cannot be stressed too much. These additional calories should come from a balanced ratio of carbohydrate, protein and fat.

hips and an even distribution of fat) gains both fat and muscle readily.

People with a higher natural level of the male (anabolic) sex hormones, such as testosterone, will also gain muscle faster. That is why women cannot achieve the muscle mass or size of men unless they take anabolic steroids.

1 Calories

Estimate your maintenance calorie intake using the formulae in Steps 1–4, Chapter 8, pp. 112–13. To gain muscle, increase your calorie intake by 20%, i.e. multiply your maintenance calories by 1.2 (120%).

Example:

If your maintenance calorie requirement is 2700 kcal, you will need to eat 2700 × 1.2 = 3240 kcal.

In practice, most athletes will need to add roughly an extra 500 kcal to their daily diet. Not all of these extra calories are converted into muscle – some will be used for digestion and absorption, given off as heat or used for physical activity. Increase your calorie intake gradually, say 200 a day for a while then after a week or two, increase it by a further 200 kcal. Slow gainers may need to increase their calorie intake as much as 1000 kcal a day.

2 Carbohydrate

In order to gain muscle, you need to train very hard, and that requires a lot of fuel. The key fuel for this type of exercise is, of course, muscle glycogen. Therefore, *you must consume enough carbohydrate to achieve high muscle glycogen levels.* If you train with low levels of muscle glycogen, you risk excessive protein (muscle) breakdown, which is just the opposite of what you are aiming for.

For muscle gain, carbohydrate should provide 60% of your calorie needs, i.e. multiply total calories by 60% then divide by 4 (because 1 g carbohydrate gives 4 kcal). Using the same example, your carbohydrate intake would be $(3240 \times 60\%) \div 4 = 486$ g/day.

3 Protein

The recommendation for strength training is 1.4–1.8 g/kg body weight/day (Tarnopolsky et al., 1992; Lemon et al., 1992). However, as your calorie requirements increase 20%, protein should increase proportionally. Thus, an intake between 1.8–2.0 g/kg body weight is recommended. For example, if you weigh 80 kg you would need between 144 g and 160 g protein a day. Studies show that increasing your intake above 2.0 g/kg body weight produces no further benefit.

To calculate protein intake as a percentage of total calories, multiply the number of grams of protein by 4, divide by total calories (as calculated above), then multiply by 100. For example, using the average value of the 144 g–160 g range (i.e. $(144 + 160) \div 2 = 152$ g):

$$\% \text{ protein} = (152 \times 4) \div 3240 = 19\%$$

4 Fat

Fat should comprise between 15–30% total calories. You can calculate your fat intake as a percentage of the total calories remaining once you have subtracted percentage of carbohydrate and the percentage of protein from 100%, i.e. % fat = 100% – % carbohydrate – % protein.

To calculate your fat intake in grams, multiply your total calorie intake by the percentage of fat and divide by 9.

Example:
$$\% \text{ fat} = 100\% - 60\% - 19\% = 21\%$$
$$\text{g fat} = (21\% \times 3240) \div 9 = 76 \text{ g}$$

What about meal timing?

Begin refuelling as soon as possible after training. You can optimise glycogen recovery after training by consuming 1 g carbohydrate/kg body weight during the 2-hour post exercise period (Ivy et al., 1988). So, for example, if you weigh 80 kg you need to consume 80 g carbohydrate within 2 hours after exercise.

However, it's not only carbohydrate that aids recovery after training: one study suggests that taking carbohydrate combined with protein after exercise, helps create the ideal hormonal environment for glycogen storage and muscle building (Zawadzki et al., 1992). Both trigger the release of insulin and growth hormone in your body. These are powerful anabolic hormones. Insulin transports amino acids into cells, reassembles them into proteins, and prevents muscle breakdown. It also transports glucose into muscle cells and stimulates glycogen storage. Growth hormone increases protein manufacture and muscle building.

In the study, nine weight trainers were given either water, a carbohydrate supplement, a protein supplement or a carbohydrate–protein supplement immediately after training and again 2 hours later. Blood levels of insulin and growth hormone were greatest during the 8 hours after exercise in those trainers who consumed the carbohydrate–protein supplement. Therefore, it seems that the combination of post-workout carbohydrate and protein promotes the best hormonal environment for muscle growth.

Suitable post-exercise snacks include carbohydrate–protein drinks (i.e. meal re-placement products (MRPs)), sports nutrition bars, pasta with tuna, and chicken or cottage cheese sandwiches.

To optimise glycogen storage and muscle growth, you should ensure a relatively steady supply of nutrients into the bloodstream by eating small meals throughout the day. In practice, divide your daily intake into at least five or six meals and snacks and avoid leaving gaps longer than 3–4 hours as this would encourage protein breakdown and slow down glycogen storage. Avoid consuming large infrequent meals or lots of high GI meals as they will produce large fluctuations in blood sugar and insulin and therefore reduce glycogen storage.

WEIGHT-GAIN SUPPLEMENTS

Should I take meal replacement products (MRPs)?

Multinutrient supplements can be useful for anyone with high nutritional requirements. They can help you achieve your weight gain goals by making up any shortfalls of calories and other nutrients in your diet. Most provide well-balanced amounts of protein (usually whey and/or casein and/or milk proteins), carbo-hydrate (usually maltodextrin and/or various sugars), vitamins and minerals. Some MRPs also contain ergogenic nutrients, such as creatine and glutamine, both of which increase muscle growth and recovery. In essence, you are getting a compact nutritious meal. MRPs, however, should be regarded as supplement meals, rather than substitutes for normal meals. One of their main advantages is that they are, of course, very convenient and quick to prepare. MRPs are portable so you have an almost instant 'meal on the go', and take much of the effort out of meal planning. For more information on MRPs, *see* Chapter 5, p. 67.

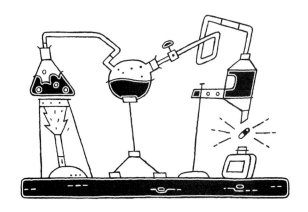

Can protein supplements help me gain weight?

Protein supplements should be regarded in the same way as MRPs, i.e. as a convenient and easy way to make up the shortfall in your diet. For example, if your requirements exceed 140 g you may find it difficult to get this amount from food alone. Vegetarians and vegans who consume mostly plant sources of protein may need to consider a protein supplement, or MRP (*see* Chapter 3 for more information).

Many brands of protein supplements contain cross micro-filtered or ion-exchanged whey protein isolates. Other protein ingredients include casein or soy protein.

The advantage of protein supplements over food include their higher BV (therefore, high bioavailability) and their high content of key amino acids such as glutamine and branched-chain amino acids. There is also evidence that whey proteins may stimulate the immune system. The high glutamine content of whey protein isolates can minimise muscle breakdown and prevent immune suppression during heavy training (*see* Chapter 5, 'Protein-based supplements, pp. 63–5).

Can creatine help me gain muscle mass?

Many studies since the mid 1990s show that both short-term and long-term creatine supplementation promotes muscle hypertrophy and *produces significant increases in lean body mass.* (*See* also Chapter 5, p. 69.)

Pooling the results from more than 40 studies, typical muscle mass gains average between 0.8 kg and 2 kg following a loading dose of 20 g/day for 5–7 days. For example, in a study carried out at Pennsylvania State University, 13 weight trainers gained an average 1.3 kg body mass after taking creatine supplements for 7 days (Volek,

1997). However, not all studies have shown a positive effect on muscle mass; some have found gains in total body weight only. Longer-term studies lasting between 14 days and 12 weeks have reported gains of up to 4 kg. The same team of researchers measured total weight gain of 1.7 kg and muscle mass gain of 1.5 kg after 1 week of creatine supplementation among 19 weight trainers (Volek, 1999). After 12 weeks, total weight gain averaged 4.8 kg and muscle gain averaged 4.3 kg.

How does creatine cause weight gain?

Weight gain is due partly to water retention in the muscle cells and partly to increased muscle growth. Researchers have found that urine volume is reduced markedly during the initial days of supplementation with creatine, which indicates the body is retaining extra water (Hultman , 1996).

Creatine draws water in to the muscle cells, thus increasing cell volume. In one study with cross-trained athletes, thigh muscle volume increased 6.6% and intra-cellular volume increased 2–3% after a creatine-loading dose (Ziegenfuss et al., 1997). It is thought that the greater cell volume caused by creatine supplementation acts as an anabolic signal for protein synthesis and therefore muscle growth (Haussinger et al., 1996). It also reduces protein breakdown during intense exercise.

The fact that studies show a substantially greater muscle mass even after long-term creatine supplementation indicates that creatine must have a direct effect on muscle growth. In studies at the University of Memphis, athletes taking creatine gained more body mass than those taking the placebo, yet both groups ended up with the same body water content (Kreider et al., 1996). If creatine allows you to train more intensely, it follows that you will gain more muscle mass. For more details on creatine supplement doses *see* Chapter 5, pp. 68–72.

Are there any other supplements that could help me gain weight?

There are literally dozens of supplements on the market that claim to enhance muscle mass, although many of the claims are not supported by scientific research. Supplements that may be worth considering include:

- multivitamin/mineral supplements
- antioxidants
- creatine
- meal replacement supplements
- protein supplements
- and possibly glutamine and HMB.

For more information on these supplements, see Chapter 5.

WEIGHT GAIN STRATEGIES

- Divide your food intake into 3 meals and 3 snacks. Eat every 2–3 hours.
- Eat larger portions.
- If you cannot eat large meals, include more snacks between meals.
- Supplement your food intake with nutritious drinks such as smoothies (blended fruit), milk shakes (fruit and milk), and yoghurt drinks.
- Use a meal replacement product or protein-based supplement as a snack.
- Snack on bananas, dried fruit, nuts, cereal or fruit bars and 'sports nutrition' bars.
- Add dried fruit, sunflower seeds, pumpkin seeds and chopped nuts to cereals and yoghurt.

SUMMARY OF KEY POINTS

- To build muscle, an intense weight-training programme must be combined with a balanced intake of calories, carbohydrate, protein and fat.
- Aim to gain 0.5–1 kg lean weight per month.
- Ultimately, the amount of lean weight you gain depends on your genetic make-up, body type and hormonal balance.
- To gain lean weight, increase your maintenance calorie intake by 20%, or about 500 kcal daily.
- A protein intake of 1.8–2.0 g/kg body weight will meet your protein needs; carbohydrates should supply about 60% of your total calories.
- Consume 1 g carbohydrate/kg body weight immediately after training, ideally combined with protein.
- Divide your food into 6 meals a day; include extra snacks if necessary.
- Meal replacement products and protein supplements can help make up for any shortfall in your diet and may provide additional benefits.
- Creatine may be worth including in a weight-gain programme.

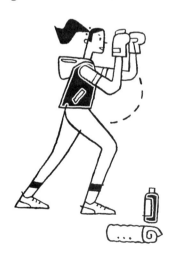

THE FEMALE ATHLETE

10

This chapter covers the issues that relate specifically to female athletes. These centre around disordered eating, amenorrhoea and bone loss, which are closely linked and relatively common among female athletes.

The emphasis placed on being lean or attaining a very low body weight in many sports is now greater than ever. To achieve this goal, many female athletes undertake an intense and excessive training programme and combine it with a restrictive diet. However, in some athletes, this can lead to an obsessive preoccupation with body weight and calorie intake, and eventually disordered eating. This chapter examines why female athletes are more prone to disordered eating and gives some of the warning signs to look out for. It considers the effects on health and how to help someone suspected of having an eating disorder.

Disordered eating is one of the risk factors for the development of amenorrhoea, a loss of normal menstrual periods. This condition is often the result of a chronic low calorie intake, low body fat and weight, high-intensity training and volume, and psychological stress. This chapter looks at the causes and treatment of amenorrhoea and explains the effect it has on health and performance. One of the most severe effects is the reduction in bone density and increased risk of bone loss, osteoporosis and stress fractures.

Female athletes are more prone than non-athletes to iron-deficiency anaemia, due to increased losses associated with training or a low dietary intake. This chapter describes the symptoms of this condition and also explains the causes of related conditions, sports anaemia and latent iron deficiency. The appropriate use of iron supplements is also covered.

Finally, details of specific nutritional considerations for female athletes during pregnancy are given, and the effect a low body fat percentage may have on the chances of conception and successful pregnancy are discussed.

DISORDERED EATING OR EATING DISORDER?

Many athletes are very careful about what they eat and often experiment with different dietary programmes in order to improve their performance. However, there is a thin line between paying attention to detail and obsessive eating behaviour. The pressure to be thin or attain higher performance makes some athletes develop eating habits that not only put their performance at risk but also endanger their health.

Eating disorders represent the extremes in a continuum of eating behaviours. An eating disorder is defined as: a *distorted pattern of thinking and behaviour about food.* In all cases, pre-occupation and obsession with food occurs and eating is out of control. It's as much about attitude and behaviour towards food as it is about consumption of food.

Clinical eating disorders such as anorexia, bulimia and compulsive eating are defined by official, specific criteria by the American Psychiatric Association (APA). *Anorexia nervosa* is the extreme of restrictive eating behaviour in which the individual continues to restrict food and feel fat in spite of being 15% or more below an ideal body weight. *Bulimia* refers to a cycle of food restriction followed by bingeing and purging. Compulsive eating is a psychological craving for food that results in uncontrollable eating.

However, many people who don't fall into these clinical categories may still have a sub-clinical eating disorder. This is often called *disordered eating*. Sufferers have an intense fear of gaining weight or becoming fat even though their weight is normal or below normal. They are preoccupied with food, their weight and body shape. Like anorexics, they have a distorted body image, imagining they are larger than they really are. They attempt to lose weight by restricting their food, usually consuming less than 1200 kcal a day, and may exercise excessively to burn more calories. The result is a chaotic eating pattern and lifestyle.

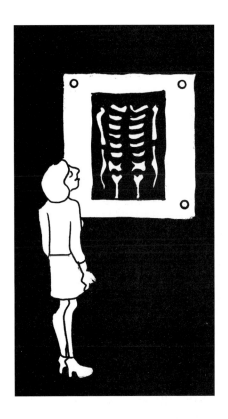

Why are athletes more likely to develop eating disorders?

Female athletes are more vulnerable to eating disorders than the general population and disordered eating may affect up to 60% of female athletes in certain sports (Sundgot-Borgon, 1994 (a) and (b); Petrie, 1993). Eating disorders are much more common in athletes in sports where a low body weight, body fat level or thin physique is perceived to be advantageous (*see* Table 10.1). The causes differ depending on the sport. Distance runners are at greater risk from eating disorders because of the close link between low body weight and performance. Those participating in aesthetic sports such as dancing, bodybuilding and gymnastics are at risk because success depends on body shape as well as physical skill. Athletes competing in weight categories sports such as judo and lightweight rowing are also more likely to develop eating disorders due to the pressures of meeting the weight criteria.

Table 10.1	Eating disorders – high risk sports
Lean sports	Distance running and cycling, horse racing
Aesthetic sports	Gymnastics, figure skating, ballet, competitive aerobics, bodybuilding,
	synchronised swimming
Weight category sports	Lightweight rowing, judo, karate, weight lifting, bodybuilding

Source: Beal & Manore, 1994.

There is no single cause of eating disorders. The demands of certain sports or training programmes or the requests made by coaches to lose weight may trigger an eating disorder in susceptible individuals. It is possible that some people with a predisposition to eating disorders are attracted to certain sports. Studies have shown that athletes in sports demanding a high degree of leanness have a more distorted body image, and are more dissatisfied with their body weight and shape compared to the general population. Researchers have found that the personality characteristics of élite athletes are very similar to those with eating disorders: obsession, competitiveness, perfectionism, compulsiveness and self-motivation. Training then becomes a way to lose weight and the positive relationship between leanness and performance further legitimises the athlete's pursuit of thinness.

Evidence is also emerging that sufferers have a disturbed body chemistry as well as a psychological predisposition to an eating disorder. For example, studies have found that more than half of those suffering from anorexia have a severe zinc deficiency and that recovery is more successful if zinc supplements are given (Bryce-Smith and Simpson, 1984). There may also be a genetic link. Around 10% of anorexics have siblings similarly affected, and it occurs more commonly than would be expected in identical twins. Researchers have identified certain genes that influence personality traits such as perfectionism and thus predispose an individual to eating disorders (Garfinkel and Garner, 1982; Davis, 1993). Scientists have recently proposed that sufferers have a defective gene that results in abnormally high levels of the brain chemical, serotonin. This causes a reduction in appetite, lowered mood and anxiety. They suggest that anorexics use starvation as a means of escaping anxiety.

What are the warning signs?

Athletes with eating disorders try to keep their disorder a secret. However, there are physical and behavioural signs you can look out for. These are detailed in Tables 10.2 and 10.3 overleaf (*see also* 'Have you got an eating problem?' p. 146).

What about the health effects of eating disorders?

The chaotic and restricted eating patterns of eating disorders often result in menstrual and fertility problems. Amenorrhoea is common among anorexics. The combination of low body fat levels, restricted calorie intake, low calcium intake, intense training and stress can result in bone thinning, stress fractures and other injuries, and, ultimately premature osteoporosis. Gastro-intestinal problems, electrolyte imbalances, kidney and bowel disorders, and depression are also common. Anorexics may develop low blood pressure and chronic low core body temperature. In bulimics, repeated vomiting and use of laxatives can lead to stomach and oesophagus pain, enamel erosion and tooth decay.

How can athletes with an eating disorder continue training?

It seems extraordinary that athletes with apparently very low calorie intake continue to exercise and compete, apparently unabated. Undoubtedly, a combination of psychological and physiological factors are involved.

On the psychological side, anorexics are able to motivate and push themselves to exercise, despite feelings of exhaustion. Sufferers are strong willed, highly driven and have a strong desire to succeed.

Some scientists believe that some athletes under-report their food intake and, in fact, eat

Table 10.2	Characteristics of anorexia nervosa		
Physical signs	**Psychological signs**	**Behavioural signs**
Severe weight loss	Obsessive about food, dieting and thinness	Eating very little
Well below average weight	Claiming to be fat when thin	Relentless exercise
Emaciated appearance	Obsessive fear of weight gain	Great interest in food and calories
Periods stop or become irregular	Low self-esteem	Anxiety and arguments about food
Growth or downy hair on face, arms and legs	Depression and anxiety	Refusing to eat in company
Feeling cold, bluish extremities	Perfectionism	Lying about eating meals
Restless, sleeping very little	High need for approval	Obsessive weighing
Dry/yellow skin	Social withdrawal	Rituals around eating

Table 10.3	Characteristics of bulimia nervosa		
Physical signs	**Psychological signs**	**Behavioural signs**
Tooth decay, enamel erosion	Low self-esteem and self-control	Out of control bingeing on large amounts of food (up to 5000 kcal)
Puffy face due to swollen salivary glands	Impulsice	Eating to numb feeling/provide comfort
Normal weight or extreme weight fluctuations	Depression, anxiety, anger	
Abrasions on knuckles from self-induced vomiting	Body dissatisfaction and distortion	Guilt, shame, withdrawal and self-deprecation after bingeing
Menstrual irregularities	Preoccupied with food, body image, appearance and weights	Purging – vomiting, laxative abuse
Muscle cramps/weakness		Frequent weighing
Frequently dehydrated		Disappearing after meals to get rid of food
		Secretive eating
		May steal food/laxatives

more than they admit. For example, a study at Indiana University on nine highly trained cross-country runners found that they were eating, on average, 2100 kcal per day but their predicted energy expenditure was 3000 kcal (Edwards, 1993). After analysing the results of a Food Attitude Questionnaire, the researchers suggested that many had a poor body image and had inaccurately reported what they ate during the study.

On the physiological side, it is likely that the body adapts by becoming more energy efficient, reducing its metabolic rate (10–30% is possible). This would allow the athlete to train and maintain energy balance on fewer calories than would be expected. Some scientists, however,

Have you got an eating problem?

This questionnaire is not intended as a diagnostic method for eating problems or as a substitute for a full diagnosis by an eating disorders specialist. If you answer yes to six or more of the following questions you could be at risk of developing an eating disorder and may benefit from further help.

- Do you count the calories of everything you eat?
- Do you think about food most of the time?
- Do you worry about gaining weight?
- Do you worry about or dislike your body shape?
- Do you diet excessively?
- Do you feel guilty during or after eating?
- Do you feel your weight is one aspect of your life you can control?
- Do your friends and family insist that you are slim while you feel fat?
- Do you exercise to compensate for eating extra calories?
- Does your weight fluctuate dramatically?
- Do you ever induce vomiting after eating?
- Have you become isolated from family and friends?
- Do you avoid certain foods even though you want to eat them?
- Do you feel stressed or guilty if your normal diet or exercise routine are interrupted?
- Do you often decline invitations to meals and social occasions involving food in case you might have to eat something fattening?

suggest that excessive exercise during dieting may augment the fall in metabolic rate.

To overcome physical and emotional fatigue, many anorexics and bulimics use caffeine-containing drinks such as strong coffee and 'diet' cola, to over-ride fatigue. However, in the long term, performance ultimately falls. As glycogen and nutrient stores become chronically depleted, the athlete's health will suffer and optimal performance cannot be sustained indefinitely. Maximal oxygen consumption decreases, chronic fatigue sets in and the athlete becomes more susceptible to injury and infection.

How should I approach someone suspected of having an eating disorder?

Approaching someone you suspect has an eating disorder requires great tact and sensitivity. Sufferers are likely to deny that have a problem; they may feel embarrassed and their self-esteem threatened so it is vital to avoid a direct confrontation about their eating behaviour or physical symptoms. Be tactful, tread very gently – do not suddenly present 'evidence' - and avoid accusations.

If the sufferer admits to having an eating problem (see box 'Have you got an eating problem'), suggest that it would be best to consult an eating disorders specialist. Various forms of specialist help are available, such as trained counsellors from a self-help organisation or private eating disorders clinic (see p. 265 for a list of useful organisations), or with a GP's referral, treatment within a multidisciplinary team of psychologists and dietitians.

AMENORRHOEA AND BONE LOSS

Are female athletes prone to amenorrhoea?

Women who are involved in regular intense exercise are more likely to have irregularities in their menstrual cycle (*oligomenorrhoea*) or even a complete loss of menstrual periods (*amenorrhoea*).

Improve your body image

This guide is not intended as a treatment for an eating disorder. Treatment should always be sought from an eating disorders specialist.

- Learn to accept your body's shape – emphasise your good points.
- Realise that reducing your body fat will not solve deep-rooted problems or an emotional crisis.
- Don't set rigid eating rules for yourself and feel guilty when you break them.
- Don't ban any foods or feel guilty about eating anything.
- Don't count calories.
- Think of foods in terms of taste and health rather than a source of calories.
- Establish a sensible healthy eating pattern rather than a strict diet.
- Listen to your natural appetite cues– learn to eat when you are hungry.
- If you do overeat, don't try to 'pay for it' later by starving yourself or exercising to burn off calories.
- Enjoy your exercise or sport for its own sake; have fun instead of enduring torture to lose body fat.
- Set positive exercise goals not related to losing weight.

A number of studies reveal that oligomenorrhoea and amenorrhoea are more common among athletes with low body weight and body fat (Sundgot-Borgon, 1994), and it has been estimated that oligomenorrhoea and amenorrhoea affect up to 62% of female endurance athletes, 60% of those involved in aesthetic sports and 50% of those involved in weight-class sports (Sundgot-Borgon and Larsen, 1993). Both of these conditions are associated with low levels of oestrogen, progesterone,

follicle-stimulating hormone (FSH) and luteinising hormone (LH).

What are the causes of amenorrhoea?

Amenorrhoea is unlikely to develop as result of exercise alone, nor does there seem to be a specific body fat percentage below which regular periods stop. A combination of factors, such as restricted calorie intake, disordered eating, intense training before menarche, high-intensity training and volume, low body-fat levels and physical and emotional stress are usually involved (see Fig. 10.1). The more of these risk factors that you have, the greater the chance of developing a menstrual disorder.

Girls who begin intense training pre-puberty usually start their periods at a later age than the average. This may be due to a combination of high-volume exercise and low body-fat levels. Some female athletes, particularly runners, may have shorter than average menstrual cycles due to anovulatory cycles, which are cycles during which an egg is not produced. This pattern is linked to lower than normal levels of oestrogen and progesterone.

Figure 10.1 Risk factors for amenorrhoea among athletes

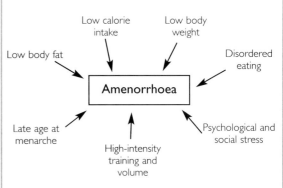

How can a low calorie intake cause amenorrhoea?

Studies show that female athletes who consistently eat fewer calories than they would seem to need for their activity (i.e. they are in chronic negative energy balance) are more likely to have menstrual disorders. It has been suggested that this is an energy-conserving adaptation by the body to a very low calorie intake. In other words, the body tries to save energy by economising on the energy costs of menstruation i.e. 'shutting down' the normal menstrual function.

The body mechanism is as follows: the combination of mental or physiological stress and a chronic negative energy balance increases cortisol production by the adrenals, which disrupts the release of gonadotrophin-releasing hormone (GnRH) from the brain. This, in turn, reduces the production of the gonadotrophin-releasing hormone, luteinising hormone (LH) and follicle-stimulating hormone (FSH), oestrogen and progesterone (Loucks et al., 1989; Edwards et al., 1993).

How does amenorrhoea cause bone loss?

It's a myth that amenorrhoea is simply a consequence of hard training; it should be regarded as a clinical state of overtraining, because of the adverse effects it has on many systems in the body.

One of the most severe effects is the reduction in bone density and increased risk of early osteoporosis and stress fractures. This is partly due to low levels of oestrogen and progesterone, both of which act directly on bone cells to maintain bone turnover (Drinkwater et al., 1984). When hormone levels drop, the natural breakdown of old bone exceeds the speed of formation of new bone. The result is loss of bone

minerals and a loss of bone density. Training, then, no longer has a positive effect on bone density: it cannot compensate for the negative effects of low oestrogen and progesterone. But high levels of cortisol and poor nutritional status – both linked to amenorrhoea – are also thought to contribute to bone loss and low bone density (Carbon, 2002).

Studies have found that the bone mineral density in the lumber spine can be as much as 20–30% lower in amenorrhoeic distance runners compared with normally menstruating runners (Cann et al., 1984; Nelson et al., 1986). Whether bone mineral density 'catches up' once menstruation resumes is not known for certain. One long-term study found that bone mass increased initially, but in the long term, it remained lower compared to active and inactive women (Drinkwater, 1986).

Does amenorrhoea affect performance?

Amenorrhoea results in many performance-hindering effects, all of which are linked to very low oestrogen levels. These include soft tissue injuries, stress fractures, prolonged healing of injuries and reduced ability to recover from hard training sessions (Lloyd et al., 1986). For example, low oestrogen levels result in a loss of

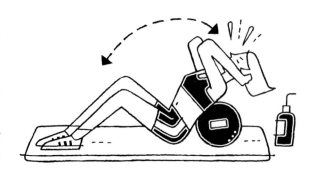

suppleness in the ligaments, which then become more susceptible to injury. Low oestrogen levels slow down bone adaptation to exercise and micro-fractures occur more readily and heal more slowly.

The good news is that performance will most likely improve once menstruation resumes. Studies show that when amenorrhoeic athletes improve their diet and restructure their training programme to improve energy balance, normal menstruation resumes within about three months and performance improves consistently (Dueck et al., 1996). This is perhaps the most persuasive reason to seek treatment if you have amenorrhoea.

How can amenorrhoea be treated?

You should definitely seek advice if you have suffered amenorrhoea for longer than six months. An initial consultation with your GP will rule out medical causes of amenorrhoea. You should then get a referral to a specialist, such as a gynaecologist, sports physician, endocrinologist or bone specialist. As part of your treatment you should consider advice from a sports nutritionist, exercise physiologist or sports psychologist. Treatment will centre on resuming 'normal' body weight and body fat, and reducing or changing your training programme. For example, you may have to reduce your training frequency, volume and intensity or change your current programme to include more cross-training. You may need to increase your food intake in order to bring your body weight and body fat within the normal range. If you have some degree of disordered eating, you will need help in overcoming this problem (*see* p. 146).

If amenorrhoea persists after this type of treatment, hormone therapy may be prescribed to prevent further loss of bone mineral density. Doses of oestrogen and progesterone, similar to those used for treating postmenopausal women, are usually used. Supplements containing calcium, magnesium and other key minerals may be advised simultaneously.

IRON DEFICIENCY

Are female athletes more likely to be iron deficient?

It has been estimated that up to 80% of élite female endurance athletes are iron deficient. However, this is based on measurements of low blood ferritin or haemoglobin, which does not give a true indication of total body iron content. In fact, iron-deficiency anaemia occurs no more frequently among athletes than in non-athletes. It is easily confused with sports anaemia, which is more common among female athletes and is simply an adaptation to endurance training. Unlike iron-deficiency anaemia, sports anaemia does not benefit from iron supplements.

So, what's the difference between iron-deficiency anaemia and sports anaemia?

Iron-deficiency anaemia occurs when there is insufficient haemoglobin to meet the body's needs. It is characterised by a low concentration of haemoglobin in the blood (the normal range is 11.5–16.5 g/100 ml) and/or a low level of ferritin in the blood, the storage form of iron (the normal level is above 12 µg/L). Sports anaemia, although associated with a low haemoglobin concentration, is not really anaemia. It arises as a consequence of regular aerobic training, which causes an increase in blood plasma volume. As a result the red blood cells are more diluted, and measures of haemoglobin and ferritin appear lower since they have effectively been 'watered down'.

What are the causes of iron-deficiency anaemia in female athletes?

Iron-deficiency anaemia may be the result of increased blood losses associated with training or a deficient dietary intake.

Training effects

Blood losses in the urine, a condition called *haematuria*, may occur in female distance runners. This is due to bruising of the bladder lining caused by repeated pounding by the abdominal contents during running. Another condition, called *haemoglobinuria* (the presence of haemoglobin in the urine), can result from repetitive foot strikes associated with poor running gait or pounding on hard surfaces. This causes some destruction of red blood cells in the soles of the feet. In haematuria, the urine has a cloudy appearance, whereas in haemoglobinuria it is clear like rosé wine. Another route of blood loss in distance runners may be via the digestive tract and may be visible with diarrhoea. This is caused by the repeated minor trauma as the abdominal contents bounce up and down with each foot strike. However, iron losses via any of these routes are relatively small.

Diet

Studies reveal that many female athletes consume less than the RDA of iron. This may be due to a low food or calorie intake, which is common among weight-conscious athletes and those involved in sports requiring a low body fat level. It is very difficult to consume enough iron on a calorie intake of less than 1500 kcal a day. Many female athletes avoid red meat (a readily absorbed source of iron) or eat very little and perhaps do not compensate by eating other sources of iron.

What are the symptoms of iron-deficiency anaemia?

The main symptoms of iron-deficiency anaemia are fatigue, headaches, light-headedness and above-normal breathlessness during exercise. Unfortunately, many of these symptoms are not specific to anaemia. Fatigue and tiredness are associated with stress and many other illnesses, making iron-deficiency anaemia difficult to diagnose without blood tests. Anaemia will affect aerobic performance so if you notice an unexplained drop in your performance and you feel excessively tired despite plenty of rest and you have no other symptoms you should consult your GP for a blood test.

What is latent iron deficiency?

Many athletes have lower concentration of ferritin in the blood than non-athletes. Values below 12 µg/L would normally indicate depleted iron stores but, in athletes this does not correlate with iron deficiency (Ashenden et al., 1998). This combination of low ferritin yet normal haemoglobin is sometimes referred to as *latent iron deficiency*. There has been considerable research investigating the possible adverse effect of low serum ferritin on sports performance. The current consensus is that a low ferritin value in the absence of symptoms of iron-deficiency anaemia does not affect your performance. This is surprising, but repeated studies have found that physical training reduces serum ferritin concentration without producing any symptoms of iron-deficiency anaemia and that iron supplementation in cases of low ferritin has no beneficial effect on performance (Cook, 1994).

Can iron supplements improve performance?

When athletes with iron-deficiency anaemia are given iron supplements, their performance will improve. The usual recommended dose is 200 mg iron sulphate 3 times a day for 1 month. However, studies have shown that iron supplementation does not increase performance in athletes with sports anaemia or latent iron deficiency (see above). In other words, the discovery of sports anaemia or latent iron deficiency should not automatically be accompanied by supplementation (Ashenden et al., 1998; Cook, 1994). Iron supplements can cause unpleasant side effects such as reduced bowel motility, constipation and dark faeces.

Which foods contain iron?

Foods rich in iron include red meat, offal, poultry (dark part of the meat), fish, pulses, wholegrains, dark green leafy vegetables, eggs, fortified foods and dried fruit (*see* Table 10.4). Iron is absorbed more efficiently when it exists in the ferrous form (as in animal sources). When it is in the ferric form (as in plant sources) it is absorbed less efficiently. However, absorption is enhanced in the presence of vitamin C or other fruit acids so it is beneficial to have vitamin C-rich fruit, vegetables, or juice, with iron-containing foods. This is especially important for vegetarians. The RDA for iron is 14.8 mg for women but the body can increase its absorption rate from the average 7–10% to 30–40% when body stores are low. This explains why people who are not consuming the RDA for iron are not necessarily anaemic.

Table 10.4	The iron content of various foods	
Food	Portion size	Mg iron
Calves liver	Average (100 g)	12.2
Bran flakes	1 bowlful (50 g)	10.0
Dried apricots (ready to eat)	5 (200 g)	7.0
Red lentils (boiled)	4 tbsp (160 g)	4.0
Prunes (ready to eat)	10 (110 g)	3.0
Baked beans	1 small tin (205 g)	2.9
Chick peas (boiled)	4 tbsp (140 g)	2.8
Lean beef fillet (grilled)	Average (105 g)	2.4
Wholemeal bread	2 large slices (80 g)	2.0
Wholemeal roll	1 (50 g)	1.8
Cashew nuts	30 (30 g)	1.8
Walnuts	12 halves (40 g)	1.2
Eggs	1 large (61 g)	1.2
Broccoli	2 spears (90 g)	1.0
Dark chicken meat	2 slices (100 g)	0.8

PREGNANCY

Female athletes share the same nutritional recommendations for pregnancy as non-athletes but there are additional issues that need to be addressed. These relate to body weight and body composiiton, which tend to differ markedly from non-athletic women. Many female athletes, particularly those in sports requiring a very lean physique, such as endurance events, aesthetic sports and weight-category sports, tend to have a lower body fat percentage than non-athletic women. In addition the physical and psychological demands of regular exercise may affect your chances of conception and of a successful pregnancy. This section highlights the sports-specific issues associated with pregnancy.

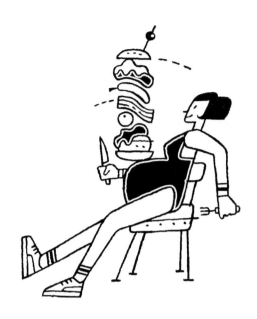

Does my body fat level affect my fertility?

A lower than average body fat level is often associated with a drop in oestrogen production which, in turn, affects normal menstrual function and can result in *oligomenorrhoea* or *amenorrhoea* (*see* pp. 146–7 'Are female athletes prone to amenorrhoea?'). Research shows that body fat is important for oestrogen production and for converting the hormone from its inactive form into its active form. However, as explained on p. 147, 'What are the causes of amenorrhoea?' loss of normal menstrual function is not simply a result of attaining a very low body fat percentage. It is often the result of a combination of factors, including a chronic low calorie intake, high training volume and intensity, and emotional and physical stress. Many female athletes are affected by one or more of these factors and, thus, fertility can be low and the chances of pregnancy small. Normal menstrual function and fertility can usually be restored within 6 months by adopting a more appropriate

training programme, increasing your food intake so that energy intake matches energy output, and reducing stress.

What are the problems with having a very low body fat percentage during pregnancy?

A low body fat level is less likely to be a problem than a small pregnancy weight gain. Provided you are in good health and are gaining weight at the recommended rate (*see* Table 10.5), low body fat levels should not present a problem. However, a small weight gain suggesting prolonged food restriction, can have an adverse effect on the baby. The baby is more likely to be underweight when born, shorter in length and have a smaller head circumference than normal. Dieting or restricting your weight gain during pregnancy is not recommended.

Short-term dietary imbalances (e.g. during the first trimester due to sickness) do not affect the baby. Hormones are produced by the mother and placenta to ensure the baby continues to receive the necessary growth factors and nutrients during occasional times of adversity. During these periods, it is the mother's health that is more likely to suffer.

How much weight should I gain during pregnancy?

The recommended average weight gain is 12.5 kg over 40 weeks although anywhere between 11.5 and 16 kg is considered healthy. The recommended weight gain guidelines are shown in Table 10.5. Distribution of weight gain (body component changes) is shown in Table 10.6. The increased level of progesterone favours body fat deposition, mainly subcutaneously (76%) in the thighs, hips and abdomen (Sohlstrom and Forsum, 1995). This extra fat deposit acts as a buffer of energy for late pregnancy when the developing baby's energy needs are highest. The hormone lactogen is produced during late pregnancy and post-pregnancy to mobilise these fat stores to provide energy for the developing baby and breast milk production should your

Table 10.5	Guidelines for weight gain during pregnancy	
Body Mass Index* category	Recommended total weight gain (kg)	Approx. rate of gain in 2nd and 3rd trimesters (kg/week)
Underweight < 19.8	12.5–18	0.5
Normal 19.8–26	11.5–16	0.4
Overweight 26–29	7.0–11.5	0.3
Obese > 29	At least 6.0	No recommended value

Source: Institute of Medicine, 1990.
*(see p. 00 'What is the BMI?')

Table 10.6	Body component changes during pregnancy
Body component	Average increase in weight (kg)
Baby	3.4
Placenta	0.65
Amniotic fluid	0.8
Uterus	0.97
Breast	0.41
Blood	1.25
Extracellular fluid	1.68
Fat	3.35
Total	12.5

Source: Hytten and Leitch, 1971

calorie intake drop. In practice, this extra fat is not necessary as there is little danger of a drop in food supply (i.e. famine). Most women have already got enough body fat to buffer against a food shortage.

Gaining extra body fat, therefore, is certainly not advantageous for female athletes as it represents surplus baggage that can potentially reduce your performance once you resume training. Thus, the 3.35 kg fat allowance in the recommended 12.5 kg pregnancy weight gain may be regarded as optional for female athletes. Provided you consume a well-balanced diet during pregnancy, you can aim to gain 9–10 kg. However, do not try to go below this level.

How many calories should I eat?

The Department of Health recommends no change in calorie intake during the first two trimesters of pregnancy for the general population. However, as an athlete, you may need to adjust your food intake if you reduce your training substantially during pregnancy. It is fine to continue exercising during pregnancy but you will almost certainly need to reduce the intensity and/or frequency of your training particularly during the third trimester (due to your increased weight and the physiological changes associated with pregnancy). Prolonged high-impact activities such as running, jumping, plyometrics and high-impact aerobics, and heavy weight training are not recommended during the second and third trimesters as they cause undue stress on the joints. During pregnancy, the ligaments, which support the joints, become softer and more lax owing to the effects of the hormone relaxin. Therefore, if you omit these activities from your routine your energy expenditure may be considerably lower than normal and you risk unnecessary fat gain unless you eat less or substitute an alternative exercise programme.

During the third trimester, there is a greater increase in your energy needs as the baby grows larger and additional pregnancy-related tissues are laid down. The DoH recommends an extra 200 kcal daily during this time. However, you may not need to eat more food because the discomfort of the growing bump may curtail your normal physical activity level. Your training may be further reduced or even stopped during the last few weeks of pregnancy so there may be no change in your net calorie intake.

General nutritional guidelines for pregnancy

- Include foods rich in omega-3 and omega-6 fatty acids in your diet. These are needed for the normal development of brain tissue, and for brain, central nervous system and eye function. *See* Chapter 7 p. 109 'What are the best food sources of essential fatty acids?'.
- A daily multivitamin and mineral supplement may be useful to help meet your increased needs. *See* Chapter 4 p. 49–50.
- The DoH recommends taking a daily folic acid supplement containing 400 µg (0.4 mg) prior to pregnancy and during the first 12 weeks to reduce the risk of neural tube defects. *See* Appendix 2, 'Glossary of Vitamins and Minerals', for food sources of folic acid.
- It is safest to avoid alcohol altogether, especially during the first trimester. After that, the Royal College of Physicians advises limiting alcohol to a maximum of two units a day (equivalent to 2 glasses of wine or 1 pint of beer).
- You should avoid vitamin A supplements (*see* Appendix 2, 'Glossary of Vitamins and Minerals'), fish liver oil supplements, liver and liver pate since very high doses (more than 10 times the RDA) may lead to birth defects

- Avoid raw or lightly cooked eggs and products made with them to reduce the risks of salmonella poisoning.
- Avoid mould-ripened soft cheeses such as camembert and brie, and also blue-veined cheeses to reduce the risk of listeria poisoning.

SUMMARY OF KEY POINTS

- Three conditions – disordered eating, amenorrhoea and bone are increasingly common among female athletes.
- Intense and excessive training programme combined with restrictive diets may lead to an obsessive preoccupation with body weight and calorie intake and eventually disordered eating.
- Eating disorders are much more common in athletes in sports where a low body weight, body fat level or thin physique is perceived to be advantageous.
- It is possible that some people with a predisposition to eating disorders are attracted to certain sports.
- It has been estimated that menstrual irregularities such as amenorrhoea affect up to 62% of endurance athletes.
- Amenorrhoea develops due to a combination of factors, such as restricted calorie intake, disordered eating, the commencement of intense training before menarche, high training intensity and volume, low body fat levels and physical and emotional stress.
- Amenorrhoea has an adverse effect on many systems in the body, including a reduction in bone density, putting you at risk of early osteoporosis and stress fractures; soft tissue injuries; prolonged healing of injuries and reduced ability to recover from hard training sessions

- Iron-deficiency anaemia is characterised by a concentration of haemoglobin in the blood below 11.5 g/dl and/or a level of ferritin below 12 µg/L, but occurs no more frequently among athletes than in non-athletes.
- Iron-deficiency anaemia may be the result of increased blood losses associated with training or a deficient dietary intake.
- Sports anaemia, although associated with a low haemoglobin concentration, arises as a consequence of regular aerobic training, which causes an increase in blood plasma volume.
- The physical and psychological demands of regular exercise, together with a very low body fat, may reduce your chances of conception.
- A low body fat level is less likely to be a problem than a small pregnancy weight gain, which may result in reduced growth of the developing baby. Dieting or restricting your weight gain during pregnancy is not recommended.
- You may need to reduce your food intake if you reduce your training substantially during pregnancy.

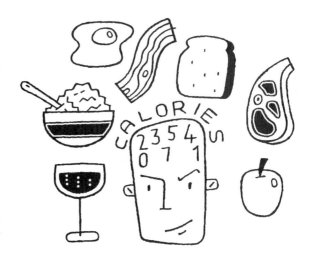

COMPETITION NUTRITION

11

Your diet before a competition will have a big impact on your performance, and could provide you with that winning edge. In addition, what you eat and drink on the day of the event can affect your ability to recover between heats and your performance in subsequent heats. This chapter covers the whole of the competition period, including the week before the event, during, and after the event. It consolidates much of the information presented in preceding chapters, in particular Chapter 2 on carbohydrate intake and Chapter 6 on fluid intake, and provides specific guidelines for arriving at your competition well-hydrated and with full glycogen stores. It gives pre-competition sample eating plans that you can use as a basis for developing your personal programme, suitable pre-competition meals and snacks that can be eaten between heats and events. For those athletes who need to make weight for their competition, this chapter gives a simple step-by-step nutrition strategy that will help you lose body fat safely and effectively.

THE WEEK BEFORE

During the week before a competition, your two main aims are:

1 to fill your muscle and liver glycogen stores so that you compete with a 'full' fuel supply.
2 to keep well hydrated.

Your preparation will be dictated by the kind of event that you are competing in, the importance of the event and how frequently you compete.

Short duration events lasing less than 4 minutes

Short duration, all-out events lasting less than 4 minutes are fuelled by ATP, PC and muscle glycogen. If you are competing in a sprint event, it is important to allow enough recovery time after your last training session, and to make sure your muscle glycogen stores are replenished. The presence of muscle damage will delay the recovery process. Training which may cause muscle fibre damage should either be scheduled earlier in the week to allow for recovery or avoided altogether. Such training includes plyometrics, heavy weight training and hard running. Reduce your training over the pre-competition week and rest during the three days prior to the competition. Aim to consume 7–8 g carbohydrate/kg body weight/day. Use Table 11.1 as a guide to the amount of carbohydrate you should be eating during the final 3 days.

Endurance events lasting more than 90 minutes

If you are competing in an endurance event lasting longer than 90 minutes you may benefit from carbohydrate loading. This is detailed in Chapter 2, 'Carbohydrate loading', p. 31–2. In summary, you should consume a moderate carbohydrate diet (5–7 g/kg body weight/day) for the first three days (this should be less than you are used to eating), followed by a high carbohydrate intake (8–10 g/kg body weight/day) for the final 3 days. Use Table 11.1 as a guide to the amount of carbohydrate you should be eating during the pre-competition week. Your last hard training session should be

Table 11.1	Recommended carbohydrate intake for athletes of different body weights	
Body weight (kg)	Daily carbohydrate intake equivalent to 7–8 g/kg body weight	Daily carbohydrate intake equivalent to 8–10 g/kg body weight
65	455–520 g	520–650 g
70	490–560 g	560–700 g
75	525–600 g	600–750 g
80	560–640 g	640–800 g
85	595–680 g	680–850 g
90	630–720 g	720–900 g

completed one week before your competition. Then taper your training during the final week so that you perform only very light exercise and rest the day prior to your competition.

Endurance events lasting less than 90 minutes; or multiple heats

If your event lasts less than 90 minutes, or if your competition schedule includes several short heats in one day, your muscle glycogen stores can become depleted. Examples of events with multiple heats include swimming, track cycling and track and field athletics. You can fill your muscle glycogen stores by tapering your training during the final week and maintaining or increasing your carbohydrate intake to about 7–8 g/kg body weight/day during the 3 days prior to your competition. This should be approximately 60–70% of your total calorie intake. Use Table 11.1 as a guide to the amount of carbohydrate you should be eating during the final 3 days.

Weekly events

If you compete weekly or even more frequently (e.g. in seasonal competitions such as football, netball and cycling), it may not be possible to rest for 3 days prior to each match or race. You would end up with virtually no training time. Perform lower intensity training or technical training during the 2 days before the match and taper only for the most important matches or races. Increase your carbohydrate intake during the final 2 days to 8–10 g/kg body weight/day. Use Table 11.1 as a guide to the amount of carbohydrate you should be eating during the final 3 days.

For all events, your total calorie intake should remain about the same as usual during the pre-competition week, but the proportions of carbohydrate, fat and protein will change. Eat larger amounts of carbohydrate-rich foods (e.g. potatoes, bread, rice, dried fruit) and carbohydrate drinks, and smaller amounts of fats and proteins. However, if you are performing a week-long taper, you may need to reduce your calories slightly to match your reduced training needs. You can do this by reducing your fat intake; otherwise you may experience fat gain.

In practice, eat at least 6 small meals a day, avoid gaps longer than 3 hours, and base all your meals on low GI foods. Use the sample eating plans in Table 11.2 as a basis for developing your own plan during the pre-competition week. While they provide the requirements for carbo-

Table 11.2	Pre-competition sample eating plans
Providing 500 g carbohydrate	Providing 700 g carbohydrate
Breakfast 1 large bowl (85 g) breakfast cereal 200 ml skimmed milk 2 tbsp (60 g) raisins 1 glass (200 ml) fruit juice	**Breakfast** 4 thick slices toast with honey 1 glass (200 ml) fruit juice 1 banana
Morning snack 1 banana sandwich (2 slices bread and 1 banana)	**Morning snack** 2 scotch pancakes 2 apples

Lunch
1 large jacket potato (300 g)
3 tbsp (90 g) sweetcorn and 1 tbsp (50 g) tuna
    or cottage cheese
2 pieces fresh fruit
1 carton low-fat fromage frais
	Lunch
	1 large bowl (125 g uncooked weight) rice
	    salad with 60 g turkey or 125 g beans and
	    vegetables
	2 slices bread
	2 pieces fruit

Pre-workout snack 1 energy bar	**Pre-workout snack** 2 bananas
Workout 1 L sports drink	**Workout** 1 L sports drink
Post-workout snack 1 serving of a meal replacement product	**Post-workout snack** 2 cereal bars 1 carton (500 ml) flavoured milk
Dinner 1 bowl (85 g uncooked weight) pasta 125 g stir-fried vegetables 60 g stir-fried chicken or tofu 2 slices bread and butter 1 large bowl (200 g) fruit salad	**Dinner** 2 large (2 × 300 g) jacket potatoes 1 carton (115 g) cottage cheese of fromage frais Broccoli or other vegetable 1 piece fresh fruit
Snack 2 slices toast with honey 1 carton low-fat yoghurt	**Snack** 1 carton (200 g) low-fat rice pudding

hydrate prior to competition, they are low in fat and protein and are not ideal for the rest of the season.

Check:
- Make sure that you rehydrate fully after training. *See* p. 87 to calculate how much

fluid you should consume before and after training. Check your hydration status by monitoring the frequency, volume and colour of your urine during the pre-competition week.

- Avoid any new, or untried foods or food combinations during the pre-competition week.
- If you will be travelling or staying away from home, be prepared to take food with you. Try to find out beforehand what type of food will be available at the event venue and predict any nutritional shortfalls.

What is the best way to make weight for my competition?

For weight-class sports such as boxing, judo, lightweight rowing and bodybuilding, it is an advantage to be as close as possible to the upper limit of your weight category. However, this should not be achieved at the expense of losing lean tissue (by rapid and severe dieting), depleting your glycogen stores (by starving) or dehydration (by fluid restriction, saunas, sweat suits, diuretics). The principles for making weight for competition are similar to those for weight loss. In summary:

- Set a realistic and achievable goal.
- Allow enough time – aim to lose 0.5 kg body fat per week. This is crucial to your strategy and *cannot be overemphasised.* You must plan to 'make weight' many weeks before your event and *not* at the last minute, as is often the case.
- Monitor your weight and body composition by skinfold thickness measurements and girth measurements (*see* Chapter 7, pp. 102–3).
- Reduce your calorie intake by 15% and never eat less than your resting metabolic rate (*see* Chapter 8, 'Calculating calorie, carbohydrate protein and fat requirements on a fat-loss programme', pp. 117–19).

- Increase the amount and frequency of aerobic training.
- Maintain carbohydrate intake at 60% of calories.
- Reduce fat intake to 15–25% of calories.
- Minimise muscle loss by consuming approximately 1.6 g/protein/kg bodyweight/day.
- Eat at frequent and regular intervals (5–6 times a day).

Avoid losing weight at the last minute by starvation or dehydration, as this can be dangerous. Starvation leads to depleted glycogen stores so you will be unable to perform at your best. Dehydration leads to electrolyte disturbances, cramp and heartbeat irregularities. It is doubtful whether you can refuel and rehydrate sufficiently between the weigh-in and your competition so aim to be at or within your weight category at least a day before the weigh-in. If you find it very difficult to make weight without resorting to these dangerous methods, consider competing in the next weight category.

A major problem with increasing the carbohydrate content of your diet in the pre-competition week is that the extra carbohydrate, stored with an amount of water equivalent to 3 times its weight, can result in weight gain. While

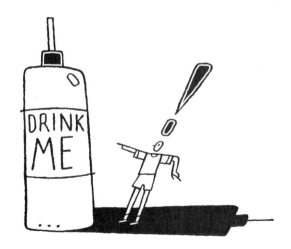

this extra glycogen is advantageous in most sports it can be a disadvantage in weight-class sports where the cut-off weight is often reached by a whisker. Ideally, you should allow for an extra weight gain of up to 1 kg during the final week. In other words, make weight in advance – aim to attain a weight at least 1 kg below your competing weight.

THE DAY BEFORE

The day before your competition your main aims are:

1 to top up muscle glycogen levels
2 to ensure you are well hydrated.

Continue eating meals high in carbohydrate that have a low GI throughout the day and drinking plenty of fluids. To maximise muscle glycogen replenishment, perform only very light exercise or rest completely. Do not skip your evening meal, even if you experience pre-competition 'nerves', as this is an important time for topping up muscle glycogen. However, stick to familiar and simple foods, avoid fatty or oily foods and avoid alcohol, as it is a diuretic.

What should I eat when I am nervous before competition?

Most athletes get pre-competition 'nerves' and this can reduce your appetite and result in problems such as nausea, diarrhoea and stomach cramps. If you find it difficult to eat solid food during this time, consume liquid meals such as meal replacement products (protein-carbo-hydrate sports supplements), sports drinks, milk shakes, yoghurt drinks and fruit smoothies. Try smooth, semi-liquid foods such as pureed fruit (e.g. apple puree, mashed banana, apple and apricot puree), yoghurt, porridge, custard and rice pudding. Bland foods such as semolina, mashed potato, or a porridge made from cornmeal or ground rice may agree with your digestive system better. To reduce problems, avoid high-fibre foods such as bran cereals, dried fruit, and pulses. You may wish to avoid vegetables that cause flatulence such as the brassica vegetables (cabbage, cauliflower, Brussel sprouts, broccoli). Caffeine can cause anxiety and problems such as diarrhoea when combined with 'nerves'. In essence, avoid anything that is new or unfamiliar. The golden rule with pre-competition eating *is stick with tried and tested foods, which you know agree with you!*

ON THE DAY

On the day of your competition, your aims are to:

1 top up liver glycogen stores following the overnight fast
2 maintain blood sugar levels
3 keep hunger at bay
4 keep well hydrated.

Plan to have your main pre-competition meal 2–4 hours before the event. This will allow enough time for your stomach to empty sufficiently and for blood sugar and insulin levels to normalise. It will also top up liver glycogen levels. Nervousness can slow down your digestion rate so if you have pre-competition nerves you may need to leave a little longer than usual between eating and competing

The actual timing of your pre-competition meal and the quantity of food eaten depends on the individual despite the fact that studies recommend consuming 200–300 g carbohydrate during the 4 hours prior to exercise. Pre-competition nerves often slow down digestion so you may find 200–300 g carbohydrate too filling.

The key is to find out what works for you and stick with it.

So, for example, if you are competing in the morning, you may need to get up a little earlier to eat your pre-competition breakfast. If your event is at 10.00 a.m., have your breakfast at 7.00 a.m. Some athletes skip breakfast, preferring to feel 'light' when they compete, however, it is not a good strategy to compete on an empty stomach, particularly if your event lasts longer than 1 hour, or you will be competing in a number of heats. Low liver glycogen and blood sugar levels may reduce your endurance and result in early fatigue. As explained in Chapter 2, liver glycogen is important for maintaining blood sugar levels and supplying fuel to the exercising muscles when muscle glycogen is depleted.

If you are competing in the afternoon, have a substantial breakfast and schedule lunch approximately 2–4 hours, before the competition. If you are competing in the evening, eat your meals at 3-hourly intervals during the day, again, scheduling your last meal approximately 2–4 hours before competition.

What should I eat on the day of my competition?

Your pre-competition meal should be:

- based on low GI carbohydrates
- low in fat
- low in protein
- low or moderate in fibre
- not too bulky or filling
- not salty or spicy
- enjoyable and familiar
- easy to digest
- include a drink – approx. 500 ml 2 hours before the event.

Suitable types of meals are given in the box, 'Pre-competition meals' on p. 158. Remember, you can reduce the GI of a meal by adding protein. If you really do not feel like eating, have a liquid meal or semi-liquid foods (*see* 'What should I eat when I am nervous before competition?' on p. 160).

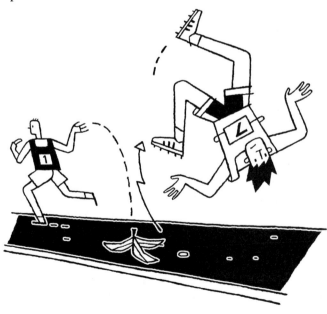

Should I eat or drink just before my competition?

Consume your pre-event meal 2–4 hours before the start of the event. This will provide a sustained supply of energy, maintain blood sugar levels during the event, particularly during the latter stages, and delay fatigue. Aim to consume about 2.5 g carbohydrate/kg body weight. (*See* p. 24, Chapter 2.) Most athletes find that low GI foods avoid any risk of hypoglycaemia at the start of the competition. However, make sure that you have rehearsed your eating programme plenty of times during training before the event. Do not try anything new on the day of competition. The timing is fairly individual, so experiment in training first!

You should also make sure that you are well hydrated before the competition (check the colour of your urine!) and aim to drink a further 125–250 ml fluid about 15–30 minutes before the event. Carry a drink bottle with you at all times.

Should I eat or drink during my competition?

If you are competing for more than about 60 minutes, you may find that extra carbohydrate will help delay fatigue and maintain your performance, particularly in the latter stages. Depending on your exercise intensity and duration, aim to take in 30–60 g carbohydrate/ hour. Start consuming the food or drink after about 30 minutes and continue at regular intervals, as it takes approximately 30 minutes for digestion and absorption.

If your glycogen stores are low at the start of the event (which hopefully they are not!), then consuming additional carbohydrate during the event will have a fairly immediate effect on your performance.

Any carbohydrate with a high or moderate GI would be suitable but you may find liquids easier

Pre-competition meals

Pre-competition breakfast (*2–4 hrs before event*)
- Breakfast cereal or porridge with low-fat milk and fresh fruit
- Toast or bread with ham/honey; low-fat yoghurt
- English muffins with honey
- Meal replacement shake

Pre-competition lunches (*2–4 hrs before event*)
- Sandwiches or rolls with tuna, cottage cheese or chicken; fresh fruit
- Pasta or rice with tomato-based sauce; fresh fruit
- Baked potato with low-fat filling; fresh fruit

Pre-competition snacks (*1 hr before event*)
- Smoothie
- Yoghurt drink
- Fruit, e.g. apples, bananas, oranges, grapes, kiwi
- Tinned fruit
- Meal replacement or energy bar
- Sports drink
- Dried apricots
- Low-fat fruit yoghurt
- Rice pudding
- Mini or Scotch pancakes

to consume than solids. Isotonic sports drinks or carbohydrate (glucose polymer) drinks are popular because they serve to replenish fluid losses and prevent dehydration as well as supplying carbohydrate. Avoid high fructose drinks, as they are not absorbed as fast as sucrose, glucose and glucose polymers. They may also cause stomach cramps or diarrhoea! Recommended quantities of isotonic drinks for different types of events are given in Table 11.3.

If you are competing in certain events such as cycling, sailing, distance canoeing, running, you may be able to take solid foods with you or

Table 11.3	Recommended quantity of a 6% isotonic drink during exercise (60 g glucose/sucrose/glucose polymer dissolved in 1 L water)		
Moderate intensity (30 g carbohydrate/h)	Moderate–high intensity (45 g carbohydrate/h)	High intensity (60 g carbohydrate/h)
500 ml/h	750 ml/h	1000 ml/h

arrange pick-up points. Suitable foods include energy bars, dried-fruit bars, cereal bars, bananas, breakfast bars, or raisins. If you are competing in matches and tournaments (e.g. football, tennis), take suitable snacks and drinks for the intervals and position them close by. Make use of every available opportunity to consume some fluid.

If you are competing for more than 60 minutes, avoid or delay dehydration by drinking *125–250 ml every 10–20 minutes* during exercise. Clearly, the more you sweat, the more you need to drink. However, do not be guided by thirst as this is not a good indicator of your hydration status. Studies have shown that you can maintain optimal performance if you can replace at least 80% of your sweat loss during exercise or keep within 1% of your body weight.

What to eat between heats or events?

If you compete in several heats or matches during the day, it's important to refuel and rehydrate as fast as possible so that you have a good chance or performing well in your next competition. Consume at least 1 g carbohydrate/kg body weight during the 2-hour post-exercise

Table 11.4	Foods suitable to eat between heats or immediately after events

- Sports drinks (home made or commercial)
- Meal replacement shake
- Bananas
- Breakfast cereal
- Meal replacement bars or energy bar
- Fruit bars
- Cereal bars or breakfast bars
- Sandwiches or rolls filled with honey, jam or bananas
- Oatmeal biscuits; fig rolls
- Dried fruit
- Home-made muffins and bars – see recipes pp. 226–8
- Rice cakes or low-fat crackers with bananas or jam
- Smoothie
- Yoghurt drink

(Accompany solid foods with sufficient water to replace fluid losses)

period (muscle glycogen replenishment is faster during the 2-hour post-exercise period). If you've only a few hours between heats, you may prefer liquid meals such as meal replacement products, sports drinks and glucose polymer drinks. These will help replace both glycogen and fluid. If you are able to eat solid food, choose carbohydrates with a high GI that you find easy to digest and are not too filling. Suitable foods are listed in Table 11.4 above. Take these with you in your kit bag. Drink at least 500 ml fluid immediately after competing and continue drinking at regular intervals to replace fluid losses.

What to eat after competition?

After your competition, your immediate aims are to replenish glycogen stores and fluid losses. If you are competing the following day or within the next few days, your post-event food intake is crucial. Again, choose foods with a moderate or high GI to ensure rapid refuelling, and aim for 1 g carbohydrate/kg body weight during the 2-hour post exercise period. Any of the foods listed in Table 11.4 above would be suitable. Drink at least 500 ml fluid immediately after competing and continue drinking at regular intervals to replace fluid losses.

Your immediate post-event food should be followed by a carbohydrate-rich meal approximately 2 hours later. Suitable post-event meals include pasta dishes, noodle dishes, thick-base pizzas (with vegetable toppings), and baked potatoes. Avoid rich or fatty meals (e.g. oily curries, chips, burgers) as these will delay refuelling and can make you feel bloated after competing. Don't forget to drink plenty of rehydrating fluid before embarking on that celebratory alcoholic drink!

SUMMARY OF KEY POINTS

Timing	Aims	Food and drink recommendations	Examples
The week before	1 Fill muscle glycogen stores 2 Maintain hydration	• Taper taining • 60–70% carbohydrate or 7–8 g/kg body weight/day • Low GI meals • Monitor fluid intake and urine	• Pasta with fish or beans • Rice with chicken or tofu • Jacket potatoes with tuna or cottage cheese
The night before	1 Top up muscle glyocen 2 Maintain hydration	• High carbohydrate meal (low GI) • Plenty of fluid • Moderate–low fibre • Low fat • Familiar foods	• Pasta dish with tomato-based sauce • Rice dishes

Summary of key points – continued

Timing	Aims	Food and drink recommendations	Examples
2–4 hours before	1 Top up liver glycogen 2 Maintain hydration 3 Prevent hunger	• Low GI meal • High carbohydrate, low fat and low protein • Easily digestible • 400–600 ml fluid	• Cereal and low-fat milk • Bread, toast, sandwiches, rolls • Potato with tuna or cottage cheese
1 hour before	1 Maintain blood sugar 2 Maintain hydration	• 1 g carbohydrate/kg body weight • Easy to digest	• Sports drink • Smoothie • Energy or meal replacement bar • Dried apricots
15–30 min before	1 Maintain hydration	• Up to 150 ml fluid	• Water • Sports drink
During events lasting more than 60 min	1 Maintain blood sugar 2 Offset fluid losses	• 30–60 g carbohydrate/hour • High or moderate GI • 150–350 ml fluid every 15–20 min	• Sports drinks • Glucose polymer drinks • Energy bars with water
Between heats or events	1 Replenish muscle and liver glycogen 2 Replace fluid	• 1 g/kg body weight within 2 hours • High GI carbohydrate • 500 ml fluid immediately after • Continue fluids	• Sports drinks • Meal replacement products • Rice cakes, energy bars, rolls • Bananas
Post-competition	1 Replenish muscle and liver glycogen 2 Replace fluid	• 1 g/kg body weight within 2 hours • High GI carbohydrate • 500 ml fluid immediately after • Continue fluids	• Sports drinks • Energy bars • Pasta dishes • Rice dishes • Pizza

DESIGNING YOUR PERSONAL NUTRITION PROGRAMME

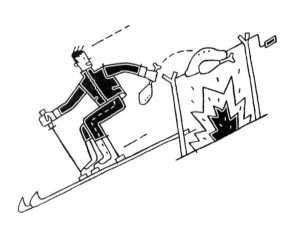

Nutrition scientists have provided general guidelines as to the proportion of nutrients athletes should consume to optimise their performance. Tailoring this information to suit your specific needs is the next critical step. Your nutritional requirements depend on many factors, including your body weight, your body composition, the energy demands of your training programme, your daily activity levels, your health status and your individual metabolism. Your diet should comprise approximately 60% calories from carbohydrate, 1.2–1.8 g/kg body weight from protein and 15–30% fat. These ratios cover your needs whether you are aiming to maintain, lose or gain weight. The main difference will be your total calorie intake.

This chapter gives a step-by-step guide to calculating your calorie, carbohydrate, protein and fat needs. The rationale for calculating your calorie requirements to lose body fat as well as the initial steps on calculating your resting metabolic rate (RMR) and your maintenance calorie needs are detailed in Chapter 8, pp. 117–19 'Calculating calorie, carbohydrate, protein and fat requirements on a fat-loss programme'. The rationale for calculating your calorie needs in a weight-gain programme is given in Chapter 9, 'How much should I eat?', pp. 137–39.

Sample daily menu plans that fit in with these nutrition recommendations are also given and can be used as a basis for developing your personal nutrition programme.

This chapter also addresses some of the most common problems faced by athletes and those leading an active lifestyle: eating on the run, in a hurry, on a budget, and adapting family meals. If you lead a busy lifestyle, it may be tempting to skip meals or rely on snacks that are high in fat or sugar. This chapter gives you plenty of practical ideas for healthy snacks that you can take with you. It also provides useful suggestions on overcoming the difficulties of putting theory into practice.

Step 1: Estimate your calorie needs

First, calculate your maintenance calorie intake by following steps 1–4 in Chapter 8, pp. 112–13. Then, if your programme aim is to:

a) lose body fat/weight: reduce your calorie intake by 15% – i.e. multiply your maintenance calories by 0.85 (85%).

b) increase lean body weight/muscle: increase your calorie intake by 20% – i.e. multiply your maintenance calories by 1.2 (120%).

Below is a sample of calculations for a 70 kg male athlete aged 18–30 years who is sedentary during the day, and performs 2 hours weight training (900 kcal) and 1 hour swimming (385 kcal) per week.

Body weight in kg: $= 70$
RMR $((70 \times 15.3) + 679)$: $= 1750$
Daily energy expenditure (1750×1.4): $= 2450$
Weekly exercise calories $(900 + 385)$: $= 1285$
Daily exercise calories $(1285 \div 7)$: $= 184$
Maintenance calorie intake
$(2450 + 184)$: $= 2634$

Calorie requirements to meet weight goal:
a) to lose fat/weight (2634×0.85) $= 2239$
b) to gain weight/muscle (2634×1.2) $= 3160$

Step 2: Calculate your carbohydrate intake

For weight maintenance fat/weight loss or muscle gain, calculate your carbohydrate needs according to your activity level and body weight,

using Table 2.1, p. 17. Carbohydrate should comprise approximately 60% of your calorie needs as calculated in Step 1.

To find the % calories from carbohydrate:
$((g\ carbohydrate \times 4) \div total\ calories) \times 100\%$

Table 12.1, below, shows a sample of calculations for weight maintenance, fat loss and muscle gain for a 70 kg male athlete aged 18–30 years who exercises for 1 hour per day.

Step 3: Calculate your protein intake

Your protein requirement is based on the following recommendations:

Endurance/aerobic athletes: 1.2–1.4 g/kg body weight/day
Power strength/cross training athletes: 1.4–1.8 g/kg body weight/day
Fat-loss programme: 1.6 g/kg body weight/day
Muscle/weight gain programme: 1.8–2.0 g body weight/day

To calculate % protein: multiply g protein by 4 (because 1 g protein gives 4 kcal), divide by total calories, then multiply by 100. Table 12.2, p. 168,

Table 12.1	Estimating carbohydrate requirements for weight maintenance, fat loss and muscle gain		
	Weight maintenance	Fat/weight loss	Muscle/weight gain
Calorie needs (calculated in Step 1)	2634	2239	3162
% calories from carbohydrate	60	60	60
Carbohydrate calories (60 × calorie needs)	1580	1343	1897
Carbohydrate needs (g) (carbohydrate calories ÷ 4)	395	336	474

Table 12.2 Estimating protein requirements	Endurance athlete (weight maintenance)	Power/strength athlete (weight maintenance)	Lose fat/ weight	Gain muscle/ weight
Body weight, kg	70	70	70	70
Protein needs, g/day	84–98	98–126	112	126–140
Calorie needs (calculated in Step 1)	2634	2634	2239	3161
% calories from protein	13–15	15–19	17	16–18

Table 12.3 Estimating fat requirements	Endurance athlete (weight maintenance)	Power/strength athlete (weight maintenance)	Lose fat/ weight	Gain muscle/ weight
Calorie needs (calculated in Step 1)	2634	2634	2239	3161
% calories from carbohydrate (calculated in Step 2)	64	64	60	60
% calories from protein (calculated in Step 3)	13–15	15–19	17	16–18
% calories from fat	21–23	17–21	23	22–24
Fat, g/day	61–67	50–61	57	77–84

shows the calculations for estimating the protein requirements for different types of athletes.

mating the fat requirements for different types of athletes based on Steps 1–3.

Step 4: Calculate your fat intake

This is the balance left once you have calculated the % carbohydrate and % protein. Therefore, % fat = 100 – % carbohydrate – % protein.

To calculate g fat: ((% fat × total calories) ÷ 100) ÷ 9 (because 1 g fat gives 9 kcal).

Table 12.3, above, shows the calculations for esti-

Step 5: Fluid intake

Researchers have found that recommended daily water intake is best calculated in relation to energy expenditure: aim to drink 1 L fluid for every 1000 kcal you consume. You will need to drink more in hot, humid weather as water loss increases due to sweating. Table 12.4 gives daily fluid intake guidelines.

Table 12.4	Daily fluid guidelines
Daily energy expenditure	Minimum daily fluid intake
2000 kcal	2 litres
2500 kcal	2½ litres
3000 kcal	3 litres
3500 kcal	3½ litres
4000 kcal	4 litres

Table 12.5	Supplements appropriate for different types of athletes			
Supplement	Endurance athlete (weight maintenance)	Power/strength athlete (weight maintenance)	Lose fat/ weight	Gain muscle/ weight
Multivitamin	✔	✔	✔	✔
Antioxidant	✔	✔	✔	✔
Creatine		✔		✔
Protein		✔		✔
Meal replacement	✔	✔	✔	✔

Follow these additional guidelines, which are based on those of the ACSM, ADA and DC (2000):

- Ensure you are fully hydrated before exercise. Consume 400–600 ml within 2 hours before exercise.
- Drink 150–350 ml every 15–20 minutes during exercise.
- For exercise lasting 1 hour or less, water is fine for replacing fluid losses.
- Do not wait until you are thirsty before you drink.
- For high-intensity exercise lasting more than 1 hour, a hypotonic or isotonic sports drink containing up to 8% carbohydrate may reduce fatigue and improve performance.

The general recommendation is to consume 30–60 g carbohydrate per hour.
- Immediately after exercise drink 250–500 ml fluid.
- Drink 1½ L for every 1 kg body weight lost during exercise.

Step 6: Supplements

Use Table 12.5, above, to choose the most beneficial supplements for your activity or sport. For more detailed information about each supplement, *see* Chapters 4 and 5.

Table 12.6	Fruit and vegetables
Food	**Amount required to equal 1 portion**
Fresh fruit	
Apple/pear/peach/orange/banana	1 fruit
Berries (strawberries, respberries, blackberries) and grapes	1 cupful (80 g)
Large fruit, e.g. mango, papaya	half a fruit
Very large fruit, e.g. melon, pineapple	1 large slice
Small fruit, e.g. apricots, plums and kiwi fruit, satsuma	2 fruit
Tinned fruit	
Any variety	⅓ of a 400 g tin (drained – the juice accounts for approx ⅓ of the weight of the tin)
Fruit juice	
100% juice	1 glass (150 ml)
Dried fruit	
Any variety	1 tbsp
Vegetables	
In general	2–3 tbsp
Carrots/courgettes	1 large
Broccoli	2 spears
Brussel sprouts	10 sprouts
Mixed salad	1 dessert bowl
Tomato	2
Cucumber	3 slices

Step 7: Timing of your meals and snacks

- Eat regular and frequent meals – 5 or 6 a day – to promote glycogen storage, lean tissue repair and growth; maintain steady blood glucose levels; regulate appetite; and discourage fat storage.
- If your calorie requirements exceed 3000 kcal or if you are aiming to gain muscle/weight, you may need to include more than 6 meals or snacks.
- Have a meal 2–4 hours before exercise. This meal should have a low GI.

- Consume a high-carbohydrate meal within 2 hours after exercise, ideally with a high or moderate GI.

Step 8: Fruit and vegetables

Both national and international targets have been set to encourage us to eat at least five 80 g portions of fruit and vegetables a day. Table 12.6 gives examples of the amount of fruit and vegetables this corresponds to in a portion.

MEAL PLANS

To help you plan your personal diet, here are some detailed sample meal plans which are in line with the nutritional recommendations outlined in the first section of this chapter. There are 3 sets of daily menu plans providing 2500 kcal, 3000 kcal and 3500 kcal. In addition, there are 3 similar sets of daily menu plans that exclude meat and fish, which are suitable for vegetarians. For each set, there are 5 daily menus designed to give you plenty of variety and plenty of ideas upon which to base your own diet. For more menu ideas, see Chapter 13 which includes more than 50 recipes for all types of diets.

The nutritional composition of each food has been listed to show its relative contribution of calories, protein, carbohydrate and fat to the daily totals. Both the total grams and the total percentage of energy contributed by protein, carbohydrate and fat are given for each daily menu. If you wish to carry out similar calculations for other foods when constructing your own menu, you may use a reputable set of food composition tables such as *McCance & Widdowson* (1991) or a dietary analysis software program, both detailed in the Further Reading section on p. 264.

Notes to menus:
Use an oil that is rich in linolenic acid, e.g. rapeseed, flax, soya, walnut.
Use a spread high in monounsaturates or polyunsaturates, containing no hydrogenated or trans fatty acids.

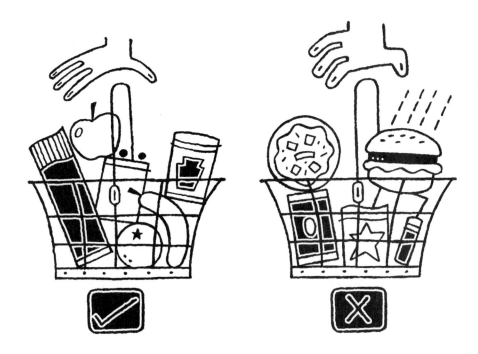

Daily menu plans providing approx 2500 kcal per day

Menu I	(2500 kcal)			
	Kcal	Protein (g)	Carbohydrate (g)	Fat (g)
Breakfast				
I average bowl (60 g) muesli	220	6	40	5
2 tbsp (80 g) low-fat yoghurt	34	3	5	0
200 ml skimmed milk	66	7	10	0
I glass (150 ml) orange juice	54	I	13	0
Mid-morning				
2 apples	94	I	24	0
I carton (150 g) low-fat fruit yoghurt	135	6	27	I
Lunch				
I large (225 g) baked potato	306	9	71	0
I tbsp (5 g) olive oil spread	85	0	0	9
I small tin (100 g) tuna in brine	99	24	0	I
I bowl (125 g) salad	15	I	2	0
I tbsp (11 g) oil/vinegar dressing	99	0	0	11
2 kiwi fruit	59	I	13	I
Mid-afternoon				
I orange	59	2	14	0
I carton (150 g) low-fat fruit yoghurt	135	6	27	I
Workout				
500 ml juice 500 ml water	180	3	44	I
Post-workout				
2 bananas	190	2	46	I
Dinner				
I portion (120 g) grilled chicken	176	36	0	4
⅓ plate (85 g uncooked weight) pasta with:	296	10	64	2
I tbsp (11 g) olive oil	99	0	0	11
I large portion (125 g) broccoli	30	4	I	I
I large portion (125 g) carrots	30	I	6	I
I tbsp (30 g) pasta sauce/tomato salsa	14	I	2	0
Evening				
I portion (85 g) red grapes	48	0	12	0
Total	2552	124	428	50
% energy		19%	63%	18%

Menu 2 (2500 kcal)

	Kcal	Protein (g)	Carbohydrate (g)	Fat (g)
Breakfast				
2 slices wholegrain toast	174	7	34	2
2 tsp (10 g) olive oil spread	57	0	0	6
2 heaped tsp (30 g) honey	86	0	23	0
1 carton (150 g) low-fat fruit yoghurt	135	6	27	1
Mid-morning				
2 apples	94	1	24	0
1 cereal or energy bar (33 g)	154	3	20	7
Lunch				
1 large (225 g) baked potato	306	9	71	0
Chopped cooked chicken (70 g)	103	21	0	2
Sweetcorn (125 g)	153	4	33	2
1 bowl (125 g) salad	15	1	2	0
1 tbsp (11 g) oil/vinegar dressing	99	0	0	11
Mid-afternoon				
2 portions (200 g) berries e.g. strawberries	54	2	12	0
Workout				
500 ml juice 500 ml water	180	3	44	1
Post-workout				
1 serving meal replacement product	174	18	26	0
Dinner				
1 average portion (175 g) grilled salmon	308	35	0	19
⅓ plate (85 g uncooked weight) brown rice	303	6	69	2
1 large portion (125 g) spinach	24	3	1	1
Evening				
1 carton (150 g) low-fat fruit yoghurt	135	6	27	1
Total	**2577**	**123**	**413**	**59**
% energy		**19%**	**60%**	**21%**

Menu 3   (2500 kcal)

	Kcal	Protein (g)	Carbohydrate (g)	Fat (g)
Breakfast				
1 cup (60 g) porridge oats	241	7	44	5
300 ml skimmed milk	99	10	15	0
1 tbsp (30 g) raisins	82	1	21	0
1 glass (200 ml) orange juice	72	1	18	0
Mid-morning				
1 cereal or fruit bar (33 g)	154	3	20	7
Lunch				
1 bagel (90 g)	241	8	46	4
spread with 2 tsp (10 g) olive oil spread	57	0	0	6
Half a carton (100 g) low-fat soft cheese	98	14	2	4
1 bowl (125 g) salad	15	1	2	0
1 tbsp (11 g) oil/vinegar dressing	99	0	0	11
Mid-afternoon				
1 large handful (60 g) dried fruit, e.g. dates, apricots	162	2	41	0
Workout				
500 ml juice 500 ml water	180	3	44	1
Post-workout				
4 rice cakes	129	2	29	1
1 carton (150 g) low-fat fruit yoghurt	135	6	27	1
Dinner				
Spicy chicken with rice (recipe p. 205)	610	58	74	11
1 portion (85 g) green cabbage	14	1	2	0
1 portion (85 g) peas	64	0	16	0
Evening				
1 pear	57	0	0	6
Total	**2509**	**123**	**409**	**53**
% energy		**20%**	**61%**	**19%**

Menu 4 (2500 kcal)

	Kcal	Protein (g)	Carbohydrate (g)	Fat (g)
Breakfast				
1 glass (150 ml) orange juice	54	1	13	0
2 slices (80 g) wholegrain toast	174	7	34	2
2 tsp (10 g) olive oil spread	57	0	0	6
2 scrambled or poached eggs	160	14	0	12
Mid-morning				
1 banana	95	1	23	0
1 portion (100 g) berries	27	1	6	0
Lunch				
Pasta salad made with:				
pasta (100 g uncooked weight)	348	12	76	2
2 tbsp (85 g) tuna in brine	84	20	0	1
1 large handful (100 g) chopped peppers	32	1	6	0
1 tbsp (11 g) oil dressing	99	0	0	11
1 orange	59	2	14	0
Mid-afternoon				
1 small cereal or protein bar (33 g)	154	3	20	7
Workout				
500 ml juice 500 ml water	180	3	44	1
Post-workout				
1 serving meal replacement product	174	18	26	0
Dinner				
1 portion (100 g) turkey breast (baked/grilled)	105	23	0	2
1 portion noodles (100 g uncooked weight)	388	12	76	6
1 portion (85 g) curly kale	20	2	1	1
1 portion (85 g) cauliflower	24	2	2	1
Evening				
½ mango (150 g)	86	1	21	0
2 Weetabix and 150 ml skimmed milk	191	9	37	1
Total	2510	133	400	53
% energy		21%	60%	19%

Menu 5 (2500 kcal)

	Kcal	Protein (g)	Carbohydrate (g)	Fat (g)
Breakfast				
3 Shredded Wheat (70 g)	228	7	48	2
200 ml skimmed milk	66	7	10	0
2 tbsp (60 g) raisins	163	1	42	0
1 glass (150 ml) orange juice	54	1	13	0
Mid-morning				
Peanut butter sandwich with:				
2 slices (80 g) wholegrain bread	174	7	34	2
and 1 tbsp (40 g) peanut butter	242	10	3	21
Lunch				
1 wholewheat pitta bread (80 g)	174	7	34	2
2 tsp (14 g) olive oil spread	80	0	0	9
2 slices (70 g) turkey	74	17	0	1
1 bowl (125 g) salad	15	1	2	0
Mid-afternoon				
125 g berries	27	1	6	0
1 carton (150 g) low-fat fruit yoghurt	135	6	27	1
Workout				
500 ml juice 500 ml water	180	3	44	1
Post-workout				
2 cereal or energy bars	308	6	40	14
Dinner				
1 portion (175 g) grilled white fish	168	37	0	2
1 large (300 g) sweet potato	345	5	84	1
1 portion (85 g) carrots	20	1	4	0
1 portion (85 g) courgettes	16	2	2	0
Evening				
2 oranges	118	4	28	0
Total	**2509**	**121**	**399**	**58**
% energy		**19%**	**60%**	**21%**

Daily menu plans providing approx 3000 kcal per day

Menu 1	(3000 kcal)	Kcal	Protein (g)	Carbohydrate (g)	Fat (g)
Breakfast					
1 average bowl (60 g) muesli		220	6	40	5
2 tbsp (80 g) low-fat yoghurt		34	3	5	0
200 ml skimmed milk		66	7	10	0
1 glass (150 ml) orange juice		54	1	13	0
1 slice (40 g) wholegrain toast		87	4	17	1
1 heaped tsp (7 g) olive oil spread		40	0	0	4
Mid-morning					
2 apples		94	1	24	0
1 carton (150 g) low-fat fruit yoghurt		135	6	27	1
Lunch					
1 large (225 g) baked potato		306	9	71	0
1 tbsp (5 g) olive oil spread		85	0	0	9
1 small tin (100 g) tuna in brine		99	24	0	1
1 bowl (125 g) salad		15	1	2	0
1 tbsp (11 g) oil/vinegar dressing		99	0	0	11
2 kiwi fruit		59	1	13	1
Mid-afternoon					
1 orange		59	2	14	0
1 carton (150 g) low-fat fruit yoghurt		135	6	27	1
Workout					
500 ml juice 500 ml water		180	3	44	1
Post-workout					
2 bananas		190	2	46	1
Dinner					
1 portion (120 g) grilled chicken		176	36	0	4
½ plate (125 g uncooked weight) pasta with:		435	15	95	2
1 tbsp (11 g) olive oil		99	0	0	11
1 large portion (125 g) broccoli		30	4	1	1
1 large portion (125 g) carrots		30	1	6	1
1 tbsp (30 g) pasta sauce/tomato salsa		14	1	2	0
Evening					
1 portion (85 g) red grapes		48	0	12	0
1 slice (40 g) wholegrain toast		87	4	17	1
1 heaped tsp (7 g) olive oil spread		40	0	0	4
Total		**3018**	**138**	**505**	**63**
% energy			**18%**	**63%**	**19%**

Menu 2	(3000 kcal)			
	Kcal	Protein (g)	Carbohydrate (g)	Fat (g)
Breakfast				
4 slices wholegrain toast	347	14	67	4
4 tsp (20 g) olive oil spread	114	0	0	13
4 heaped tsp (60 g) honey	173	0	46	0
1 carton (150 g) low-fat fruit yoghurt	135	6	27	1
Mid-morning				
2 apples	94	1	24	0
1 cereal or energy bar (33 g)	154	3	20	7
Lunch				
1 large (225 g) baked potato	306	9	71	0
Chopped cooked chicken (70 g)	103	21	0	2
Sweetcorn (125 g)	153	4	33	2
1 bowl (125 g) salad	15	1	2	0
1 tbsp (11 g) oil/vinegar dressing	99	0	0	11
Mid-afternoon				
2 portions (200 g) berries e.g. strawberries	54	2	12	0
Workout				
500 ml juice 500 ml water	180	3	44	1
Post-workout				
1 serving meal replacement product	174	18	26	0
Dinner				
1 average portion (175 g) grilled salmon	308	35	0	19
½ plate (115 g uncooked weight) boiled brown rice	411	8	93	3
1 large portion (125 g) spinach	24	3	1	1
Evening				
1 carton (150 g) low-fat fruit yoghurt	135	6	27	1
Total	3023	133	494	71
% energy		18%	61%	21%

Menu 3	(3000 kcal)	Kcal	Protein (g)	Carbohydrate (g)	Fat (g)
Breakfast					
1½ cups (100 g) porridge oats		401	12	73	9
500 ml skimmed milk		165	16	25	1
2 tbsp (60 g) raisins		163	1	42	0
1 glass (200 ml) orange juice		72	1	18	0
Mid-morning					
1 cereal or fruit bar (33 g)		154	3	20	7
Lunch					
1 bagel (90 g)		241	8	46	4
with 2 tsp (10 g) olive oil spread		57	0	0	6
Half a carton (100 g) low-fat soft cheese		98	14	2	4
1 bowl (125 g) salad		15	1	2	0
1 tbsp (11 g) oil/vinegar dressing		99	0	0	11
Mid-afternoon					
2 large handfuls (120 g) dried fruit, e.g. dates, apricots		162	2	41	0
Workout					
500 ml juice 500 ml water		180	3	44	1
Post-workout					
4 rice cakes		129	2	29	1
1 carton (150 g) low-fat fruit yoghurt		135	6	27	1
Dinner					
Spicy chicken with rice (recipe p. 205)		610	58	74	11
1 portion (85 g) green cabbage		14	1	2	0
1 portion (85 g) peas		64	0	16	0
Evening					
1 pear		57	0	0	6
Total		**2979**	**138**	**510**	**57**
% energy			**18%**	**64%**	**17%**

Menu 4 (3000 kcal)

	Kcal	Protein (g)	Carbohydrate (g)	Fat (g)
Breakfast				
1 glass (150 ml) orange juice	54	1	13	0
3 slices (120 g) wholegrain toast	260	11	50	3
3 tsp (15 g) olive oil spread	85	0	0	9
2 scrambled or poached eggs	160	14	0	12
Mid-morning				
2 bananas	190	2	46	1
1 portion (100 g) berries	27	1	6	0
Lunch				
Pasta salad made with:				
(150 g uncooked weight) pasta	522	18	114	3
2 tbsp (85 g) tuna in brine	84	20	0	1
1 large handful (100 g) chopped peppers	32	1	6	0
1 tbsp (11 g) oil dressing	99	0	0	11
1 orange	59	2	14	0
Mid-afternoon				
1 small cereal or protein bar (33 g)	154	3	20	7
Workout				
500 ml juice 500 ml water	180	3	44	1
Post-workout				
1 serving meal replacement product	174	18	26	0
Dinner				
1 portion (100 g) turkey breast (baked/grilled)	105	23	0	2
1 large portion (125 g uncooked weight) noodles	485	15	95	8
1 portion (85 g) curly kale	20	2	1	1
1 portion (85 g) cauliflower	24	2	2	1
Evening				
½ mango (150 g)	86	1	21	0
2 Weetabix and 150 ml skimmed milk	191	9	37	1
Total	**2991**	**147**	**497**	**60**
% energy		**20%**	**62%**	**18%**

Menu 5   (3000 kcal)

	Kcal	Protein (g)	Carbohydrate (g)	Fat (g)
Breakfast				
4 Shredded Wheat (100 g)	325	11	68	3
300 ml skimmed milk	99	10	15	0
2 tbsp (60 g) raisins	163	1	42	0
1 glass (150 ml) orange juice	54	1	13	0
Mid-morning				
Peanut butter sandwich with:				
2 slices (80 g) wholegrain bread	174	7	34	2
and 1 tbsp (40 g) peanut butter	242	10	3	21
Lunch				
2 wholewheat pitta bread (160 g)	348	14	68	4
2 heaped tsp (14 g) olive oil spread	80	0	0	9
3 slices (100 g) turkey	105	24	0	1
1 bowl (125 g) salad	15	1	2	0
Mid-afternoon				
125 g berries	27	1	6	0
1 carton (150 g) low-fat fruit yoghurt	135	6	27	1
Workout				
500 ml juice 500 ml water	180	3	44	1
Post-workout				
2 cereal or energy bars	308	6	40	14
Dinner				
1 portion (175 g) grilled white fish	168	37	0	2
2 large (450 g total weight) sweet potato	518	7	126	2
1 portion (85 g) carrots	20	1	4	0
1 portion (85 g) courgettes	16	2	2	0
Evening				
2 oranges	118	4	28	0
Total	3017	144	500	62
% energy		19%	62%	19%

Daily menu plans providing approx 3500 kcal per day

Menu I	(3500 kcal)				
		Kcal	Protein (g)	Carbohydrate (g)	Fat (g)
Breakfast					
I average bowl (60 g) muesli		220	6	40	5
2 tbsp (80 g) low-fat yoghurt		34	3	5	0
200 ml skimmed milk		66	7	10	0
I glass (150 ml) orange juice		54	1	13	0
2 slices (80 g) wholegrain toast		174	7	34	2
2 heaped tsp (14 g) olive oil spread		80	0	0	9
Mid-morning					
2 apples		94	1	24	0
I carton (150 g) low-fat fruit yoghurt		135	6	27	1
Lunch					
2 average (350 g total weight) baked potatoes		476	14	111	1
2 tbsp (10 g) olive oil spread		170	0	0	18
I small tin (100 g) tuna in brine		99	24	0	1
I bowl (125 g) mixed salad		15	1	2	0
I tbsp (11 g) oil/vinegar dressing		99	0	0	11
2 kiwi fruit		59	1	13	1
Mid-afternoon					
I orange		59	2	14	0
I carton (150 g) low-fat fruit yoghurt		135	6	27	1
Workout					
500 ml juice 500 ml water		180	3	44	1
Post-workout					
2 bananas		190	2	46	1
Dinner					
I large portion (150 g) grilled chicken		221	45	0	5
½ plate (125 g uncooked weight) pasta with:		435	15	95	2
I tbsp (11 g) olive oil		99	0	0	11
I large portion (125 g) broccoli		30	4	1	1
I large portion (125 g) carrots		30	1	6	1
I tbsp (30 g) pasta sauce/tomato salsa		14	1	2	0
Evening					
I portion (85 g) red grapes		48	0	12	0
2 slices (80 g) wholegrain toast		174	7	34	2
2 heaped tsp (14 g) olive oil spread		80	0	0	9
Total		3571	159	579	85
% energy			18%	61%	21%

Menu 2 (3500 kcal)

	Kcal	Protein (g)	Carbohydrate (g)	Fat (g)
Breakfast				
4 slices wholegrain toast	347	14	67	4
4 tsp (20 g) olive oil spread	114	0	0	13
4 heaped tsp (60 g) honey	173	0	46	0
1 carton (150 g) low-fat fruit yoghurt	135	6	27	1
Mid-morning				
2 apples	94	1	24	0
1 cereal or energy bar (33 g)	154	3	20	7
Lunch				
1 very large (300 g) baked potato	408	12	95	1
Chopped cooked chicken (100 g)	147	30	0	3
Sweetcorn (150 g)	183	4	40	2
1 bowl (125 g) salad	15	1	2	0
1 tbsp (11 g) oil/vinegar dressing	99	0	0	11
Mid-afternoon				
1 wholegrain roll	121	5	24	1
2 tsp (10 g) oilive oil spread	57	0	0	6
2 portions (200 g) berries e.g. strawberries	54	2	12	0
Workout				
500 ml juice 500 ml water	180	3	44	1
Post-workout				
1 serving meal replacement product	174	18	26	0
Dinner				
1 average portion (175 g) grilled salmon	308	35	0	19
½ plate (150 g uncooked weight) boiled brown rice	536	10	122	4
1 large portion (125 g) spinach	24	3	1	1
Evening				
1 carton (150 g) low-fat fruit yoghurt	135	6	27	1
Total	3502	152	577	81
% energy		17%	62%	21%

Menu 3 (3500 kcal)	Kcal	Protein (g)	Carbohydrate (g)	Fat (g)
Breakfast				
1½ cups (100 g) porridge oats	401	12	73	9
500 ml skimmed milk	165	16	25	1
2 tbsp (60 g) raisins	163	1	42	0
1 glass (200 ml) orange juice	72	1	18	0
Mid-morning				
2 energy or cereal bars (66 g)	309	7	40	15
Lunch				
2 bagels (180 g) with:	482	17	93	8
4 tsp (20 g) olive oil spread	114	0	0	13
1 carton (200 g) low-fat soft cheese	196	28	4	8
1 bowl (125 g) salad	15	1	2	0
1 tbsp (11 g) oil/vinegar dressing	99	0	0	11
Mid-afternoon				
2 large handful (120 g) dried fruit, e.g. dates, apricots	162	2	41	0
Workout				
500 ml juice 500 ml water	180	3	44	1
Post-workout				
4 rice cakes	129	2	29	1
1 carton (150 g) low-fat fruit yoghurt	135	6	27	1
Dinner				
Spicy chicken with rice (recipe p. 205)	610	58	74	11
1 portion (85 g) green cabbage	14	1	2	0
1 portion (85 g) peas	64	0	16	0
Evening				
1 pear	57	0	0	6
Total	**3530**	**163**	**578**	**79**
% energy		**18%**	**61%**	**20%**

Menu 4 (3500 kcal)

	Kcal	Protein (g)	Carbohydrate (g)	Fat (g)
Breakfast				
1 glass (150 ml) orange juice	54	1	13	0
4 slices (160 g) wholegrain toast	347	14	67	4
4 tsp (20 g) olive oil spread	114	0	0	13
2 scrambled or poached eggs	160	14	0	12
Mid-morning				
2 banana	190	2	46	1
1 portion (100 g) berries	27	1	6	0
Lunch				
Pasta salad made with:				
pasta (175 g uncooked weight)	609	21	133	3
2 tbsp (85 g) tuna in brine	84	20	0	1
1 large handful (100 g) chopped peppers	32	1	6	0
1½ tbsp (16 g) oil dressing	144	0	0	16
1 orange	59	2	14	0
Mid-afternoon				
2 energy or cereal bars	309	7	40	15
Workout				
500 ml juice 500 ml water	180	3	44	1
Post-workout				
1 serving meal replacement product	174	18	26	0
Dinner				
1 large portion (125 g) turkey breast (baked/grilled)	131	28	0	2
1 large portion noodles (150 g uncooked weight)	582	18	114	9
1 portion (85 g) curly kale	20	2	1	1
1 portion (85 g) cauliflower	24	2	2	1
Evening				
½ mango (150 g)	86	1	21	0
2 Weetabix and 150 ml skimmed milk	191	9	37	1
Total	**3516**	**166**	**572**	**78**
% energy		**19%**	**61%**	**20%**

Menu 5 (3500 kcal)

	Kcal	Protein (g)	Carbohydrate (g)	Fat (g)
Breakfast				
4 Shredded Wheat (100 g)	325	11	68	3
300 ml skimmed milk	99	10	15	0
4 tbsp (120 g) raisins	326	3	83	0
1 glass (150 ml) orange juice	54	1	13	0
Mid-morning				
Peanut butter sandwich with:				
2 slices (80 g) wholegrain bread	174	7	34	2
and 1 tbsp (40 g) peanut butter	242	10	3	21
Lunch				
2 wholewheat pitta bread (160 g)	348	14	68	4
2 heaped tsp (14 g) olive oil spread	80	0	0	9
3 slices (100 g) turkey	105	24	0	1
1 bowl (125 g) salad	15	1	2	0
Mid-afternoon				
125 g berries	27	1	6	0
1 carton (150 g) low-fat fruit yoghurt	135	6	27	1
Workout				
500 ml juice 500 ml water	180	3	44	1
Post-workout				
2 cereal or energy bars	308	6	40	14
Dinner				
1 portion (175 g) grilled white fish	168	37	0	2
2 large (450 g total weight) sweet potato	518	7	126	2
1 portion (85 g) carrots	20	1	4	0
1 portion (85 g) courgettes	16	2	2	0
Evening				
3 small (scotch) pancakes (90 g)	263	5	39	11
2 oranges	118	4	28	0
Total	3435	167	560	73
% energy		20%	61%	19%

VEGETARIAN MEAL PLANS

Notes:

Use an oil that is rich in linolenic acid, e.g. rapeseed, flax, soya, walnut.

Use a spread high in monounsaturates on poly-unsaturates, containing no hydrogenated or trans fatty acids.

Daily menu plans providing approx 2500 kcal per day

V **Menu 1** Vegetarian – (2500 kcal)	Kcal	Protein (g)	Carbohydrate (g)	Fat (g)
Breakfast				
1 average bowl (60 g) muesli	220	6	40	5
2 tbsp (80 g) low-fat yoghurt	34	3	5	0
200 ml skimmed milk	66	7	10	0
1 glass (150 ml) orange juice	54	1	13	0
Mid-morning				
2 apples	94	1	24	0
1 carton (150 g) low-fat fruit yoghurt	135	6	27	1
Lunch				
1 large (225 g) baked potato	306	9	71	0
1 tbsp (5 g) olive oil spread	85	0	0	9
½ carton (125 g) cottage cheese	123	17	3	5
1 bowl (125 g) salad	15	1	2	0
1 tbsp (11 g) oil/vinegar dressing	99	0	0	11
2 kiwi fruit	59	1	13	1
Mid-afternoon				
1 orange	59	2	14	0
1 carton (150 g) low-fat fruit yoghurt	135	6	27	1
Workout				
500 ml juice 500 ml water	180	3	44	1
Post-workout				
2 bananas	190	2	46	1
Dinner				
Mixed bean hotpot (without potatoes) (recipe p. 219)	234	16	41	1
¼ plate (65 g uncooked weight) pasta with:	226	8	49	1
1 tbsp (11 g) olive oil	99	0	0	11
1 large portion (125 g) broccoli	30	4	1	1
1 large portion (125 g) carrots	30	1	6	1
1 tbsp (30 g) pasta sauce/tomato salsa	14	1	2	0
Evening				
1 portion (85 g) red grapes	48	0	12	0
Total	**2564**	**96**	**457**	**52**
% energy		**15%**	**67%**	**18%**

V Menu 2   Vegetarian – (2500 kcal)

	Kcal	Protein (g)	Carbohydrate (g)	Fat (g)
Breakfast				
2 slices wholegrain toast	174	7	34	2
2 tsp (10 g) olive oil spread	57	0	0	6
2 heaped tsp (30 g) honey	86	0	23	0
1 carton (150 g) low-fat fruit yoghurt	135	6	27	1
Mid-morning				
2 apples	94	1	24	0
1 cereal or energy bar (33 g)	154	3	20	7
Lunch				
1 large (225 g) baked potato	306	9	71	0
2 tbsp (60 g) hummus	112	5	7	8
Sweetcorn (125 g)	153	4	33	2
1 bowl (125 g) salad	15	1	2	0
1 tbsp (11 g) oil/vinegar dressing	99	0	0	11
Mid-afternoon				
2 portions (200 g) berries e.g. strawberries	54	2	12	0
Workout				
500 ml juice 500 ml water	180	3	44	1
Post-workout				
1 serving meal replacement product	174	18	26	0
Dinner				
1 wheat tortilla filled with:	144	4	33	1
¾ pack (150 g) marinated tofu	110	12	1	6
Shredded mixed vegetables (90 g)	38	3	6	0
⅓ plate (85 g uncooked weight) boiled brown rice	303	6	69	2
1 large portion (125 g) spinach	24	3	1	1
Evening				
1 carton (150 g) low-fat fruit yoghurt	135	6	27	1
Total	**2569**	**91**	**460**	**53**
% energy		14%	67%	19%

V Menu 3 — Vegetarian – (2500 kcal)

	Kcal	Protein (g)	Carbohydrate (g)	Fat (g)
Breakfast				
1 cup (60 g) porridge oats	241	7	44	5
300 ml skimmed milk	99	10	15	0
1 tbsp (30 g) raisins	82	1	21	0
1 glass (200 ml) orange juice	72	1	18	0
Mid-morning				
1 cereal or fruit bar (33 g)	154	3	20	7
Lunch				
1 bagel (90 g) with:	241	8	46	4
2 tsp (10 g) olive oil spread	57	0	0	6
Half a carton (100 g) low-fat soft cheese	98	14	2	4
1 bowl (125 g) salad	15	1	2	0
1 tbsp (11 g) oil/vinegar dressing	99	0	0	11
Mid-afternoon				
1 large handful (60 g) dried fruit, e.g. dates, apricots	162	2	41	0
Workout				
500 ml juice 500 ml water	180	3	44	1
Post-workout				
4 rice cakes	129	2	29	1
1 carton (150 g) low-fat fruit yoghurt	135	6	27	1
Dinner				
Rice, bean and vegetable stir-fry (recipe p. 205)	526	18	94	11
1 portion (85 g) green cabbage	14	1	2	0
1 portion (85 g) peas	64	0	16	0
Evening				
1 pear	57	0	0	6
Total	**2509**	**88**	**450**	**52**
% energy		**14%**	**67%**	**19%**

V Menu 4 Vegetarian – (2500 kcal)

	Kcal	Protein (g)	Carbohydrate (g)	Fat (g)
Breakfast				
1 glass (150 ml) orange juice	54	1	13	0
2 slices (80 g) wholegrain toast	174	7	34	2
2 tsp (10 g) olive oil spread	57	0	0	6
2 scrambled or poached eggs	160	14	0	12
Mid-morning				
1 banana	95	1	23	0
1 portion (100 g) berries	27	1	6	0
Lunch				
Pasta salad made with:				
pasta (100 g uncooked weight)	348	12	76	2
2 tbsp (85 g) kidney beans	85	6	15	1
1 large handful (100 g) chopped peppers	32	1	6	0
1 tbsp (11 g) oil dressing	99	0	0	11
1 orange	59	2	14	0
Mid-afternoon				
1 small cereal or protein bar (33 g)	154	3	20	7
Workout				
500 ml juice 500 ml water	180	3	44	1
Post-workout				
1 serving meal replacement product	174	18	26	0
Dinner				
Tofu with noodles (recipe p. 213)	533	21	75	19
1 portion (85 g) curly kale	20	2	1	1
1 portion (85 g) cauliflower	24	2	2	1
Evening				
½ mango (150 g)	86	1	21	0
2 Weetabix and 150 ml skimmed milk	191	9	37	1
Total	**2581**	**107**	**415**	**64**
% energy		**17%**	**60%**	**23%**

V Menu 5 — Vegetarian – (2500 kcal)

	Kcal	Protein (g)	Carbohydrate (g)	Fat (g)
Breakfast				
3 Shredded Wheat (70 g)	228	7	48	2
200 ml skimmed milk	66	7	10	0
2 tbsp (60 g) raisins	163	1	42	0
1 glass (150 ml) orange juice	54	1	13	0
Mid-morning				
Peanut butter sandwich with:				
2 slices (80 g) wholegrain bread	174	7	34	2
and 1 tbsp (40 g) peanut butter	242	10	3	21
Lunch				
1 wholewheat pitta bread (80 g)	174	7	34	2
2 heaped tsp (14 g) olive oil spread	80	0	0	9
2 heaped tbsp (85 g) cottage cheese	83	12	2	3
1 bowl (125 g) salad	15	1	2	0
Mid-afternoon				
125 g berries	27	1	6	0
1 carton (150 g) low-fat fruit yoghurt	135	6	27	1
Workout				
500 ml juice 500 ml water	180	3	44	1
Post-workout				
2 cereal or energy bars (66 g)	308	6	40	14
Dinner				
1 beanburger (100 g)	193	11	14	11
1 large (300 g) sweet potato	345	5	84	1
1 portion (85 g) carrots	20	1	4	0
1 portion (85 g) courgettes	16	2	2	0
Evening				
2 oranges	118	4	28	0
Total	**2547**	**90**	**415**	**70**
% energy		**14%**	**61%**	**25%**

Daily menu plans providing approx 3000 kcal per day

V Menu I — Vegetarian – (3000 kcal)

	Kcal	Protein (g)	Carbohydrate (g)	Fat (g)
Breakfast				
I average bowl (60 g) muesli	220	6	40	5
2 tbsp (80 g) low-fat yoghurt	34	3	5	0
200 ml skimmed milk	66	7	10	0
I glass (150 ml) orange juice	54	1	13	0
I slice (40 g) wholegrain toast	87	4	17	1
I heaped tsp (7 g) olive oil spread	40	0	0	4
Mid-morning				
2 apples	94	1	24	0
I carton (150 g) low-fat fruit yoghurt	135	6	27	1
Lunch				
I large (225 g) baked potato	306	9	71	0
I tbsp (15 g) olive oil spread	85	0	0	9
½ carton (125 g) cottage cheese	123	17	3	5
I bowl (125 g) mixed salad	15	1	2	0
I tbsp (11 g) oil/vinegar dressing	99	0	0	11
2 kiwi fruit	59	1	13	1
Mid-afternoon				
I orange	.3759	2	14	0
I carton (150 g) low-fat fruit yoghurt	135	6	27	1
Workout				
500 ml juice 500 ml water	180	3	44	1
Post-workout				
2 bananas	190	2	46	1
Dinner				
Mixed bean hotpot (without potatoes) (recipe p.219)	234	16	41	1
½ plate (100 g uncooked weight) pasta with:	348	12	76	2
I tbsp (11 g) olive oil	99	0	0	11
I large portion (125 g) broccoli	30	4	1	1
I large portion (125 g) carrots	30	1	6	1
I tbsp (30 g) pasta sauce/tomato salsa	14	1	2	0
Evening				
I portion (85 g) red grapes	48	0	12	0
I slice (40 g) wholegrain toast	87	4	17	1
I heaped tsp (7 g) olive oil spread	40	0	0	4
Total	**3012**	**109**	**530**	**65**
% energy		**14%**	**66%**	**19%**

V Menu 2   Vegetarian – (3000 kcal)

	Kcal	Protein (g)	Carbohydrate (g)	Fat (g)
Breakfast				
4 slices wholegrain toast	347	14	67	4
4 tsp (20 g) olive oil spread	114	0	0	13
4 heaped tsp (60 g) honey	173	0	46	0
1 carton (150 g) low-fat fruit yoghurt	135	6	27	1
Mid-morning				
2 apples	94	1	24	0
1 cereal or energy bar (33 g)	154	3	20	7
Lunch				
1 large (225 g) baked potato	306	9	71	0
2 tbsp (60 g) hummus	112	5	7	8
Sweetcorn (125 g)	153	4	33	2
1 bowl (125 g) salad	15	1	2	0
1 tbsp (11 g) oil/vinegar dressing	99	0	0	11
Mid-afternoon				
2 portions (200 g) berries, e.g. strawberries	54	2	12	0
Workout				
500 ml juice 500 ml water	180	3	44	1
Post-workout				
1 serving meal replacement product	174	18	26	0
Dinner				
1 wheat tortilla filled with:	144	4	33	1
¾ pack (150 g) marinated tofu	110	12	1	6
Shredded mixed vegetables (90 g)	38	3	6	0
½ plate (115 g uncooked weight) boiled brown rice	411	8	93	3
1 large portion (125 g) spinach	24	3	1	1
Evening				
1 carton (150 g) low-fat fruit yoghurt	135	6	27	1
Total	**3016**	**101**	**541**	**65**
% energy		**13%**	**67%**	**19%**

V Menu 3 — Vegetarian – (3000 kcal)

	Kcal	Protein (g)	Carbohydrate (g)	Fat (g)
Breakfast				
1½ cup (100 g) porridge oats	401	12	73	9
500 ml skimmed milk	165	16	25	1
2 tbsp (60 g) raisins	163	1	42	0
1 glass (200 ml) orange juice	72	1	18	0
Mid-morning				
1 cereal or fruit bar (33 g)	154	3	20	7
Lunch				
1 bagel (90 g) with:	241	8	46	4
2 tsp (10 g) olive oil spread	57	0	0	6
Half a carton (100 g) low-fat soft cheese	98	14	2	4
1 bowl (125 g) salad	15	1	2	0
1 tbsp (11 g) oil/vinegar dressing	99	0	0	11
Mid-afternoon				
2 large handfuls (120 g) dried fruit, e.g. dates, apricots	162	2	41	0
Workout				
500 ml juice 500 ml water	180	3	44	1
Post-workout				
4 rice cakes	129	2	29	1
1 carton (150 g) low-fat fruit yoghurt	135	6	27	1
Dinner				
Rice, bean and vegetable stir-fry (recipe p. 205)	526	18	94	11
1 portion (85 g) green cabbage	14	1	2	0
1 portion (85 g) peas	64	0	16	0
Evening				
1 pear	57	0	0	6
Total	3023	102	550	61
% energy		14%	68%	18%

V Menu 4 — Vegetarian – (3000 kcal)

	Kcal	Protein (g)	Carbohydrate (g)	Fat (g)
Breakfast				
1 glass (150 ml) orange juice	54	1	13	0
3 slices (120 g) wholegrain toast	260	11	50	3
3 tsp (15 g) olive oil spread	85	0	0	9
2 scrambled or poached eggs	160	14	0	12
Mid-morning				
2 banana	190	2	46	1
1 portion (100 g) berries	27	1	6	0
Lunch				
Pasta salad made with pasta (150 g uncooked weight)	522	18	114	3
2 tbsp (85 g) kidney beans	85	6	15	1
1 large handful (100 g) chopped peppers	32	1	6	0
1 tbsp (11 g) oil dressing	99	0	0	11
1 orange	59	2	14	0
Mid-afternoon				
1 small cereal or protein bar (33 g)	154	3	20	7
Workout				
500 ml juice 500 ml water	180	3	44	1
Post-workout				
1 serving meal replacement product	174	18	26	0
Dinner				
1 large portion Tofu with noodles (recipe p. 213) (use 100 g noodles)	591	23	86	20
1 portion (85 g) curly kale	20	2	1	1
1 portion (85 g) cauliflower	24	2	2	1
Evening				
½ mango (150 g)	86	1	21	0
2 Weetabix and 150 ml skimmed milk	191	9	37	1
Total	**3008**	**119**	**501**	**70**
% energy		**16%**	**63%**	**21%**

V Menu 5 — Vegetarian – (3000 kcal)

	Kcal	Protein (g)	Carbohydrate (g)	Fat (g)
Breakfast				
4 Shredded Wheat (100 g)	325	11	68	3
300 ml skimmed milk	99	10	15	0
2 tbsp (60 g) raisins	163	1	42	0
1 glass (150 ml) orange juice	54	1	13	0
Mid-morning				
Peanut butter sandwich with:				
2 slices (80 g) wholegrain bread	174	7	34	2
and 1 tbsp (40 g) peanut butter	242	10	3	21
Lunch				
2 wholewheat pitta bread (160 g)	348	14	68	4
2 heaped tsp (14 g) olive oil spread	80	0	0	9
½ carton (100 g) cottage cheese	98	14	2	4
1 bowl (125 g) salad	15	1	2	0
Mid-afternoon				
125 g berries	27	1	6	0
1 carton (150 g) low-fat fruit yoghurt	135	6	27	1
Workout				
500 ml juice 500 ml water	180	3	44	1
Post-workout				
2 cereal or energy bars (66 g)	308	6	40	14
Dinner				
1 beanburger (100 g)	193	11	14	11
2 large (450 g total weight) sweet potato	518	7	126	2
1 portion (85 g) carrots	20	1	4	0
1 portion (85 g) courgettes	16	2	2	0
Evening				
2 oranges	118	4	28	0
Total	3039	108	516	74
% energy		14%	64%	22%

Daily menu plans providing approx 3500 kcal per day

V Menu I	Vegetarian – (3500 kcal)			
	Kcal	Protein (g)	Carbohydrate (g)	Fat (g)
Breakfast				
1 average bowl (60 g) muesli	220	6	40	5
2 tbsp (80 g) low-fat yoghurt	34	3	5	0
200 ml skimmed milk	66	7	10	0
1 glass (150 ml) orange juice	54	1	13	0
2 slices (80 g) wholegrain toast	174	7	34	2
2 heaped tsp (14 g) olive oil spread	80	0	0	9
Mid-morning				
2 apples	94	1	24	0
1 carton (150 g) low-fat fruit yoghurt	135	6	27	1
Lunch				
2 average (350 g total weight) baked potatoes	476	14	111	1
2 tbsp (30 g) olive oil spread	170	0	0	18
¾ carton (150 g) cottage cheese	147	21	3	6
1 bowl (125 g) mixed salad	15	1	2	0
1 tbsp (11 g) oil/vinegar dressing	99	0	0	11
2 kiwi fruit	59	1	13	1
Mid-afternoon				
1 orange	59	2	14	0
1 carton (150 g) low-fat fruit yoghurt	135	6	27	1
Workout				
500 ml juice 500 ml water	180	3	44	1
Post-workout				
2 bananas	190	2	46	1
Dinner				
Mixed bean hotpot (without potatoes) (recipe p. 219)	234	16	41	1
3 tbsp (50 g) soya mince added to hotpot	132	22	6	3
½ plate (100 g uncooked weight) pasta with:	348	12	76	2
1 tbsp (11 g) olive oil	99	0	0	11
1 large portion (125 g) broccoli	30	4	1	1
1 large portion (125 g) carrots	30	1	6	1
1 tbsp (30 g) pasta sauce/tomato salsa	14	1	2	0
Evening				
1 portion (85 g) red grapes	48	0	12	0
2 slices (80 g) wholegrain toast	174	7	34	2
1 heaped tsp (7 g) olive oil spread	80	0	0	9
Total	**3529**	**126**	**607**	**83**
% energy		**14%**	**64%**	**21%**

V Menu 2 — Vegetarian – (3500 kcal)

	Kcal	Protein (g)	Carbohydrate (g)	Fat (g)
Breakfast				
4 slices wholegrain toast	347	14	67	4
4 tsp (20 g) olive oil spread	114	0	0	13
4 heaped tsp (60 g) honey	173	0	46	0
1 carton (150 g) low-fat fruit yoghurt	135	6	27	1
Mid-morning				
2 apples	94	1	24	0
1 cereal or energy bar (33 g)	154	3	20	7
Lunch				
1 very large (300 g) baked potato	408	12	95	1
2 heaped tbsp (100 g) hummus	187	8	12	13
Sweetcorn (150 g)	183	4	40	2
1 bowl (125 g) salad	15	1	2	0
1 tbsp (11 g) oil/vinegar dressing	99	0	0	11
Mid-afternoon				
1 wholegrain roll	121	5	24	1
2 tsp (10 g) olive oil spread	57	0	0	6
2 portions (200 g) berries e.g. strawberries	54	2	12	0
Workout				
500 ml juice 500 ml water	180	3	44	1
Post-workout				
1 serving meal replacement product	174	18	26	0
Dinner				
1 wheat tortilla filled with:	144	4	33	1
1 pack (175 g) marinated tofu	128	14	1	7
Shredded mixed vegetables (90 g)	38	3	6	0
½ plate (125 g uncooked weight) boiled brown rice	446	8	102	3
1 large portion (125 g) spinach	24	3	1	1
Evening				
1 carton (150 g) low-fat fruit yoghurt	135	6	27	1
Total	3501	117	612	82
% energy		13%	65%	21%

V **Menu 3**	**Vegetarian – (3500 kcal)**			
	Kcal	Protein (g)	Carbohydrate (g)	Fat (g)
Breakfast				
1½ cups (100 g) porridge oats	401	12	73	9
500 ml skimmed milk	165	16	25	1
2 tbsp (60 g) raisins	163	1	42	0
1 glass (200 ml) orange juice	72	1	18	0
Mid-morning				
2 energy or cereal bars (66 g)	309	7	40	15
Lunch				
2 bagels (180 g) with:	482	17	93	8
4 tsp (20 g) olive oil spread	114	0	0	13
1 carton (200 g) low-fat soft cheese	196	28	4	8
1 bowl (125 g) salad	15	1	2	0
1 tbsp (11 g) oil/vinegar dressing	99	0	0	11
Mid-afternoon				
2 large handfuls (120 g) dried fruit, e.g. dates, apricots	162	2	41	0
Workout				
500 ml juice 500 ml water	180	3	44	1
Post-workout				
4 rice cakes	129	2	29	1
1 carton (150 g) low-fat fruit yoghurt	135	6	27	1
Dinner				
Rice, bean and vegetable stir-fry (recipe p. 205)	526	18	94	11
1 portion (85 g) green cabbage	14	1	2	0
1 portion (85 g) peas	64	0	16	0
Evening				
1 pear	57	0	0	6
Total	3548	128	619	79
% energy		14%	65%	20%

V Menu 4 — Vegetarian – (3500 kcal)

	Kcal	Protein (g)	Carbohydrate (g)	Fat (g)
Breakfast				
1 glass (150 ml) orange juice	54	1	13	0
4 slices (160 g) wholegrain toast	347	14	67	4
4 tsp (20 g) olive oil spread	114	0	0	13
2 scrambled or poached eggs	160	14	0	12
Mid-morning				
2 bananas	190	2	46	1
1 portion (100 g) berries	27	1	6	0
Lunch				
Pasta salad made with:				
Pasta (175 g uncooked weight)	609	21	133	3
4 tbsp (150 g) red kidney beans	150	10	27	1
1 large handful (100 g) chopped peppers	32	1	6	0
1½ tbsp (16 g) oil dressing	144	0	0	16
1 orange	59	2	14	0
Mid-afternoon				
2 energy or cereal bars (66 g)	309	7	40	15
Workout				
500 ml juice 500 ml water	180	3	44	1
Post-workout				
1 serving meal replacement product	174	18	26	0
Dinner				
Large portion tofu with noodles (recipe p. 213) (use 100 g noodles)	725	30	105	24
1 portion (85 g) curly kale	20	2	1	1
1 portion (85 g) cauliflower	24	2	2	1
Evening				
½ mango (150 g)	86	1	21	0
2 Weetabix and 150 ml skimmed milk	191	9	37	1
Total	**3434**	**134**	**550**	**91**
% energy		16%	60%	24%

V Menu 5 — Vegetarian – (3500 kcal)

	Kcal	Protein (g)	Carbohydrate (g)	Fat (g)
Breakfast				
4 Shredded Wheat (100 g)	325	11	68	3
300 ml skimmed milk	99	10	15	0
4 tbsp (120 g) raisins	326	3	83	0
1 glass (150 ml) orange juice	54	1	13	0
Mid-morning				
Peanut butter sandwich with 2 slices (80 g) wholegrain bread with:	174	7	34	2
1 tbsp (40 g) peanut butter	242	10	3	21
Lunch				
2 wholewheat pitta bread (160 g)	348	14	68	4
2 heaped tsp (14 g) olive oil spread	80	0	0	9
3/4 carton (175 g) cottage cheese	172	24	4	7
1 bowl (125 g) salad	15	1	2	0
Mid-afternoon				
125 g berries	27	1	6	0
1 carton (150 g) low-fat fruit yoghurt	135	6	27	1
Workout				
500 ml juice 500 ml water	180	3	44	1
Post-workout				
2 cereal or energy bars (66 g)	308	6	40	14
Dinner				
1 beanburger (100 g)	193	11	14	11
1 portion (175 g) grilled white fish	168	37	0	2
2 large (450 g total weight) sweet potato	518	7	126	2
1 portion (85 g) carrots	20	1	4	0
1 portion (85 g) courgettes	16	2	2	0
Evening				
3 small (scotch) pancakes (90 g)	263	5	39	11
2 oranges	118	4	28	0
Total	**3456**	**124**	**578**	**88**
% energy		14%	63%	23%

EATING ON THE RUN

I often have to eat on the run. What can I do?

Try to organise your food in advance. If you don't have time for proper meals, take a supply of healthy snacks with you. This way you can keep up your energy levels, refuel after training and ensure you are getting a good intake of nutrients. Plan to eat a small snack every two or three hours – *see* Table 12.7 for ideas on high carbohydrate, low fat, portable foods.

If you have to buy takeaways and ready-made snacks, choose sandwiches with low-fat fillings, jacket potatoes (with baked beans/cottage cheese/chicken/fish), pizza slices (with vegetable based topping), pasta and rice salads.

Always make time to relax while eating. If you are rushed or tense, you may develop indigestion, heartburn and trapped air, all of which can be very uncomfortable, especially if you will be training later on! So, reserve at least 5–10 minutes to sit down, unwind and eat slowly.

Never skip meals altogether or leave long gaps without food. This will result in low blood sugar levels, poor glycogen replenishment, a lower nutrient intake and greater lethargy. So,

the key is to be prepared and plan your eating around your daily schedule.

How can I eat cheaply but healthily?

A healthy diet need not be expensive if you make just a few simple changes to your shopping and eating habits. In fact, many of the most nutritious foods are inexpensive and readily available: potatoes, pasta, oats, rice and other cereal grains (e.g. bulgar wheat, couscous, millet), pulses (dried or tinned) and milk. These foods can be used to form the basis of your diet, for example: jacket potatoes with fillings; pasta, rice and grain dishes with a simple sauce; grain based salads; curries, salads, stews and soups based on pulses and vegetables in season; milk drinks and puddings (e.g. custard, rice pudding).

- Buy fruit and vegetables in season; look out for special offers in the shops or buy from market stalls, if possible.
- Avoid ready prepared meals and 'convenience' products – they may seem to save you time, but it's cheaper and just as easy to make large amounts of the same dish yourself and freeze the remainder.

Table 12.7	Snacks for eating on the run

- Sandwiches/rolls/pitta/bagels (filled with cottage cheese/peanut butter/banana/salad/honey/marmite/tuna/chicken/turkey/ham)
- Low fat yoghurt and fromage frais
- Fresh fruit (e.g. apples, bananas, nectarines, grapes)
- English muffins/scones/crumpets/potato cakes
- Scotch pancakes
- Dried fruit and cereal bars
- Fruit juice or cordial (diluted)
- Nuts and dried fruit mixtures
- Rice cakes/crackers/breakfast cereal

- High protein foods from plants (pulses, cereals, nuts, soya products) are less expensive than those from animals (meat, poultry, fish, eggs), so make greater use of these in your diet, e.g. risotto with beans instead of chicken.
- If you feel hungry, fill up on inexpensive, nutritious foods like bread, toast and fruit instead of other less nutritious snacks, such as confectionery bars, crisps and cakes.
- Buy the largest packs of breakfast cereals, frozen fish and poultry, pasta, rice, and dairy products as these are usually cheaper. Organise your storage space well or share the pack with a friend!

I don't have much time to cook and prepare healthy meals. What can I do?

Healthy meals can be very quick and easy to prepare. Many require no or very little cooking. Here are a few tips:

- Make larger quantities than you need of soups, casseroles, potatoes, pasta, rice, etc., then cover and keep the remainder in the fridge or freezer. Before eating, add extra ingredients (e.g. beans, poultry, vegetables or sauce) as toppings or fillings.

- Make a large bowl of vegetables or fruit salad, enough to last 2–3 days, and keep in the fridge so you have an instant supply.
- The following speedy meals can be made in less than 10 minutes: baked beans or spaghetti on toast: pizza made with ready made base, tinned tomatoes and cheese; sandwiches and pitta; pasta with tomato/ vegetable sauce; eggs or cheese on toast; baked potato with beans/cheese/tuna.

In fact, there's no need even to cook! Make substantial sandwiches using the ideas in the Sandwich box (Table 12.8).

I often have to eat late in the evening. What are my best choices?

If you train in the evening and do not arrive home until late, you should plan to have most of your food during the morning and afternoon. Have a substantial breakfast and make lunch your main meal of the day. Include frequent high carbohydrate snacks in between, with a snack about 1–2 hours before your evening training sessions. That way you will feel less hungry before and after training.

It is still important to eat after training to refuel your glycogen stores, but avoid a large or fatty

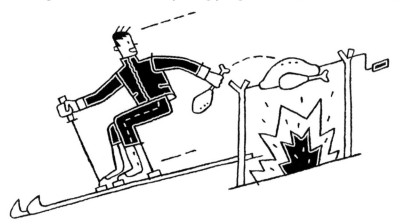

Table 12.8	Sandwich box

Bread

Cut thick slices from any of the following breads:

Multi grain, rye, sourdough, herb, Italian bread with olives, sun dried tomatoes or onions, Spanish bread with sunflower seeds, baguettes, ciabatta, country style bread

Fillings

Any combination of the following:

- Low fat soft cheese, dates and walnuts
- Hummous, lettuce and onion slices
- Peanut butter and banana
- Turkey and cranberry sauce
- Cottage cheese and dried/fresh apricots
- Salmon, watercress and low calorie dressing
- Ham, pears and lettuce
- Sun dried tomatoes, mozzarella and green salad leaves
- Tuna, red kidney beans and tabasco
- Chopped chicken, sweetcorn, onion and fromage frais
- Reduced fat hard cheese and pineapple
- Egg, lettuce, red pepper and low calorie salad dressing
- Grated carrot, raisins and cashews

meal which takes a long time to digest. Good late evening choices include pasta with a tomato based sauce, breakfast cereal, fruit and milk, beans on toast and thick sandwiches. Try to leave at least one or two hours before retiring to bed, as a full stomach can make you feel uncomfortable and disrupt your sleep.

I have to eat the same meals as the rest of my family!

The whole family can benefit from eating healthy meals – there is no need to prepare separate dishes. Simply fill up on larger portions of high carbohydrate foods, such as bread, pasta and potatoes, avoid large helpings of rich sauces and trim off any fat from meat.

Most traditional family meals can be easily adapted to contain less fat and more carbohydrate without affecting the taste or enjoyment. *For example:*

- Replace full-fat milk with low-fat milk in sauces, custard and puddings.
- Sauté onions or meat in minimal amounts of oil.
- Omit the butter or oil in sauces and thicken with cornflour.
- Add extra vegetables or pulses to stews, bolognese, soups or curries.
- Reduce the amount of fat in puddings, cakes and desserts and serve with extra fruit or yoghurt.

I like eating out. What are the best choices from the menu?

You can still enioy eating out and eating healthily provided you make the right menu choices. Check below.

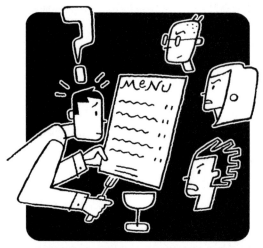

Table 12.9	Restaurant guide	
	Good choices	**Unhealthy choices**
Pizzeria	Tomato, vegetable, ham, spicy chicken, or seafood pizza toppings	Salami, mince, beef, pepperoni, extra cheese toppings
Hamburger joint	Plain, grilled hamburger, flame grilled chicken	Large burgers, fries, doughnuts, apple pies
Steak house	Grilled steak, salads, jacket potatoes, fruit	Fried/battered fish, garlic mushrooms, garlic bread, scampi, steak with creamy sauces, puddings
Indian	Chicken tikka, tandoori chicken, dahl, channa dahl, rice, naan bread, chappati, dry vegetable curries	Meat curries, meat dansak/ korma/madras, samosa, bhajis, puri, paratha
Chinese	Chicken, vegetable or prawn chop suey, stir fried vegetables, seafood or chicken, rice, noodles	Duck dishes, sweet and sour pork balls, fried noodles
French	Grilled fish, meat (e.g. steak au poivre), boeuf bourguignonne, poultry dishes without creamy sauces, ratatouille, salads (e.g. niçoise), bouillabaisse (fish stew), vegetables, consommé, sorbet	Cream or butter sauces (e.g. à la normandie, béarnaise), buttered vegetables, pastry dishes, profiteroles

Table 12.9	Restaurante guide – continued	
	Good choices	Unhealthy choices
Greek	Greek salad, tomato or cucumber salad, tzatzika, hummus, pitta, dolmadhes, stuffed tomatoes, souvlakia, grilled or barbecued fish, fresh fruit, Greek yoghurt	Taramasalata, moussaka, lamb dishes, pastitsio, keftethakia (meatballs), spicy sausages, baklava
Spanish/Portugese	Paella, grilled fish, shellfish dishes, salads, gazpacho, tortillas	Buttery/oily sauces, fried fish, pies, fried chicken
Japanese	Sushi, sashmi, sukiyaki, teryaki chicken	Tempura dishes
Mexican	Bean burrito, tortillas or tostadas with beans/vegetable chilli, fajitas with vegetables/chicken, gaucamole	Tortilla chips, potato skins, beef chilli, tortillas/burritos with beef, chimichangas
Thai	Steamed fish, rice and vegetable dishes, seafood salad	Prawn crackers, fried noodles or rice
Italian	Grissini, ciabatta, pasta with tomato/vegetable or seafood sauces (e.g. neopolitan, primavera, spinach), risotto, gnocchi, grilled chicken/fish, pasta filled with spinach/ricotta	Pasta with creamy/buttery/meat based sauce (e.g. carbonara, alfredo, bolognese), lasagne, cannelloni

THE RECIPES

The following recipes are quick, simple and fun to make. They are specially designed for sports-people who need to eat a diet high in carbo-hydrate, low in fat and rich in essential nutrients. Each recipe provides a nutritional analysis to help you put together numerous healthy menus.

The main meal recipes are divided into sections based on high carbohydrate foods to enable you to plan your meals according to the recommended nutritional guidelines. Recipes suitable for vegetarians contain no meat, poultry or fish and are marked with a 'V' symbol.

Rice and other grains

Rice is high in complex carbohydrates and makes a tasty and versatile base for main meals. Brown rice is a little higher in fibre and B vitamins than white, although it is not as high as other wholegrain cereals. Experiment with different types of rice: American, Italian, Basmati or wild. Try different types of grains, too: bulgar wheat, couscous, millet and barley. Most are available in supermarkets.

V Beans 'n' Rice

This healthy combination appears in many American and West Indian cuisines. The beans can be black, red or white, and the dish can be spicy or mild – adapt it to taste.

Serves 2

1 tbsp (15 ml) oil
1 onion, chopped
1 green chilli, chopped finely
175 g (6 oz) rice
1 large tomato, chopped
450 ml (¾ pint) stock
400 g (15 oz) beans or cooked dried beans (e.g. red kidney beans, borlotti beans or blackbeans)
25 g (1 oz) creamed coconut
1 tbsp chopped coriander or parsley

- Heat oil in a pan.
- Add onion and cook for 5 minutes.
- Add chilli and rice, stir well for 2 minutes.
- Add tomato and stock.
- Bring to the boil, cover and simmer for 15 mins.
- Add cooked beans and cook for a further 5 mins.
- Gradually stir in creamed coconut until melted, followed by coriander or parsley.

Nutritional information (per serving):

Calories = 637; protein = 23 g; carbohydrate = 112 g; fat = 13.9 g; fibre = 12.8 g

Spicy Chicken with Rice

Serves 2

2 tsp (10 ml) sunflower oil
2 chicken breasts (approx. 175 g (6 oz) each)
175 g (6 oz) brown rice
1 onion, chopped
2 cloves garlic, crushed
1–2 tsp (5–10 ml) curry powder (to taste)
1 tbsp tomato puree
3 tbsp (45 ml) water

- Cook the chicken breasts under a hot grill for 10–15 mins, turning a few times.
- Boil rice for 20–25 mins.
- Meanwhile, heat oil in a large non-stick pan and cook onion for 5 mins, until golden.
- Add garlic and curry powder and cook for a further 2 mins.
- Cut chicken into chunks and add to pan with tomato puree and water.
- Cover and cook for a further 5–10 mins.
- Serve with rice and green vegetables.

V Rice, Bean and Vegetable Stir Fry

Serves 2

175 g (6 oz) brown rice
1 tbsp (15 ml) olive oil
1 onion, chopped
2 cloves garlic, crushed
1 piece fresh root ginger, chopped
100 g (4 oz) large mushrooms, sliced
2 stalks celery, chopped
100 g (4 oz) peas
½ a 400 g (14 oz) can red kidney beans

- Cover rice with plenty of boiling water.
- Bring to the boil and simmer for 25–30 mins.
- Meanwhile, heat oil in a wok over a high heat.
- Add the onion, and stir fry for 1 min.
- Add garlic, ginger, mushrooms, celery and peas, and stir fry for 3 mins.
- Tip in red kidney beans and cooked rice.
- Cook for a further 2 mins, until all ingredients are thoroughly heated through.

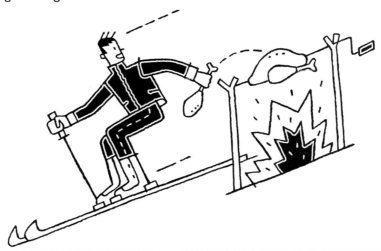

Nutritional information (per serving):

Calories = 657; protein = 58 g;
carbohydrate = 74 g; fat = 16.1 g;
fibre = 2.2 g

Nutritional information (per serving):

Calories = 526; protein = 18.3 g;
carbohydrate = 94.2 g; fat = 11.3 g;
fibre = 11.1 g

V Vegetarian Chilli Con Carne

Serves 2

1 clove garlic, crushed
1 onion, chopped
1 green or red pepper, chopped
½ tsp chilli powder (or to taste)
225 g (8 oz) can tomatoes
50 g (2 oz) red lentils
300 ml (½ pint) water
175 g (6 oz) rice
½ a 400 g (14 oz) can red kidney beans

- Place garlic, onion, pepper, chilli, tomatoes, lentils, water and rice in a large pan.
- Bring to the boil and simmer for 20 mins.
- Add drained kidney beans and cook for a further 5 mins.
- Season to taste.
- Serve with broccoli or green salad.

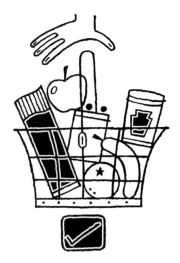

Rice Salad

This salad can be served as a main course. The vegetables can be varied according to what is in season.

Serves 2

175 g (6 oz) rice
2 spring onions, chopped
50 g (2 oz) raisins or chopped
½ red pepper and ½ green pepper, chopped
100 g (4 oz) can tuna (in brine or water), drained, *or*
2 hard boiled eggs, chopped, *or*
½ a 400 g (14 oz) can red kidney beans *or*
100 g (4 oz) cooked chicken or turkey, chopped, *or*
50 g (2 oz) peanuts

For the dressing: 2 tbsp (30 ml) olive oil
1 tsp (5 ml) wine vinegar
1 tsp (5 ml) orange juice

- Cook rice, and mix with vegetables, raisins or dates and tuna.
- Shake ingredients for dressing together.
- Combine with salad.

Nutritional information (per serving):

Calories = 550; protein = 21 g;
carbohydrate = 119 g; fat = 2.3 g;
fibre = 10.4 g

Nutritional information (per serving):

Calories = 598; protein = 20 g;
carbohydrate = 97 g; fat = 16.7 g;
fibre = 2.2 g

V Bulgar Wheat and Lentil Pilaff

Bulgar wheat has a slightly nutty flavour and can be used instead of rice for most dishes. It is very easy to cook, and is available from most health food shops and supermarkets.

Serves 2

175 g (6 oz) bulgar wheat
450 ml (¾ pint) boiling water
1 small onion, chopped
1 small green pepper, chopped
2 carrots, sliced
1 tbsp (15 ml) concentrated vegetable stock (e.g. Vecon) *or*
1 vegetable stock cube
100 g (4 oz) green lentils, pre-soaked in water

- Cover the bulgar wheat with the boiling water and leave to stand for 20 mins.
- Meanwhile, place the remaining ingredients in a large pan.
- Bring to the boil, cover and simmer for 30 mins, until the lentils are soft. (In a pressure cooker, reduce cooking time to 7 mins, and release steam slowly.)
- Spoon bulgar wheat onto a serving plate and top with lentil mixture.

Nutritional information (per serving):

Calories = 489; protein = 22 g;
carbohydrate = 98 g; fat = 2.8 g;
fibre = 6.2 g

Pilaff with Plaice

Serves 2

175 g (6 oz) brown rice
600 ml (1 pint) water
1 small onion, chopped
Pinch of turmeric (or mild curry powder)
1 courgette
1 small red pepper
350 g (12 oz) plaice fillets, cut into strips
Salt and freshly ground black pepper
1 tbsp sunflower seeds (optional)

- Place rice, water, onion and turmeric in a large saucepan.
- Bring to the boil, cover and simmer for 20 mins.
- Add courgette, red pepper, plaice and seasoning.
- Cook for a further 5 mins or until fish is cooked and water absorbed.
- Scatter sunflower seeds over before serving.

Nutritional information (per serving):

Calories = 530; protein = 40 g;
carbohydrate = 76 g; fat = 9.5 g;
fibre = 3.1 g

Couscous with Fish Stew

Couscous is available from supermarkets partly cooked, and requires very little further cooking. It fluffs up to produce a huge amount – a little certainly goes a long way. It is excellent with a little dried fruit, such as raisins or dates, and can also be used to accompany a hearty stew.

Serves 2

175 g (6 oz) couscous
½ a 400 g (14 oz) tin chick peas
25 g (1 oz) raisins
350 g (12 oz) white fish (e.g. haddock, sea bass or cod)
1 large onion, roughly chopped
450 ml (¾ pint) water
225 g (8 oz) vegetables (e.g. carrots or celery)
1 tsp mixed herbs

* Place couscous in a bowl and cover with boiling water.
* Leave to stand for 20 mins, to absorb water.
* Then, mix in chick peas and raisins.
* Meanwhile, place all ingredients for fish stew in a large saucepan.
* Bring to the boil, cover and simmer for 15 mins.
* Place couscous on a plate and top with fish stew.

Nutritional information (per serving):

Calories = 548; protein = 49 g;
carbohydrate = 78 g; fat = 6 g;
fibre = 7.1 g

V Couscous aux Sept Legumes

For an authentic Moroccan dish, make a vegetable stew with couscous, as follows.

Serves 2

450 g (1 lb) mixed vegetables (choose 7 varieties, e.g. carrots, aubergines, potatoes, broad beans, French beans, courgettes, mushrooms)
150 ml (¼ pint) water
1 tbsp (15 ml) concentrated vegetable stock (e.g. Vecon) *or*
1 vegetable stock cube

* Leave couscous to stand in a bowl of boiling water, in which the stock is dissolved, for 20 mins.
* Then bring vegetables to the boil, cover and simmer for 15 mins.
* Serve with couscous.

Nutritional information (per serving):

Calories = 435; protein = 14.9 g;
carbohydrate = 89 g; fat = 4.6 g;
fibre = 9.3 g

PASTA AND NOODLES

Pasta is made from durum wheat flour and water or egg. It is an excellent source of carbohydrate and has a lower glycaemic index than other cereals. Pasta is also very quick to cook: usually 10 mins for dried types and 2–4 mins for fresh. It can form the basis of many healthy, low-fat meals. Wholemeal varieties are higher in fibre and are therefore more filling. Top pasta shapes with one of the following sauces for a quick, nourishing meal.

V Lentil Sauce

Serves 2

1 onion, chopped
1 clove garlic, crushed
225 g (8 oz) tin tomatoes
100 g (4 oz) red lentils
600 ml (1 pint) water
1 tsp oregano

- Place all ingredients in a large pan.
- Bring to the boil, cover and simmer for 20 mins. (Alternatively, cook in a pressure cooker for 3 mins.)

V Easy Tomato Sauce

Serves 2

1 onion, chopped
1 clove garlic, crushed
400 g (14 oz) tin tomatoes
1 tsp oregano
1 tbsp tomato puree
Dash of tabasco

Topping:
2 tsp parmesan cheese
Freshly ground black pepper and salt to taste

- Place all ingredients in a large pan, bring to the boil and simmer for 5–10 mins. (Liquidise for a smoother sauce.)
- Top with parmesan cheese, and serve with salad.

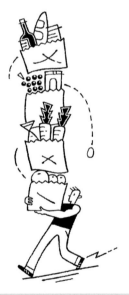

Nutritional information (per serving):

Calories = 177; protein = 13 g; carbohydrate = 31.5 g; fat = 0.8 g; fibre = 3.2 g

Nutritional information (per serving):

Calories = 37; protein = 2.3 g; carbohydrate = 7 g; fat = 0.2 g; fibre = 1.6 g

Salmon and Broccoli Sauce

Serves 2

175 g (6 oz) broccoli florets
300 ml (½ pint) skimmed or semi-skimmed milk
1 tbsp cornflour
200 g (7 0z) tin salmon, drained and flaked

Topping:
2 tsp parmesan cheese
Freshly ground black pepper

- Cook broccoli in a small amount of boiling water for 7 mins, and drain.
- Mix together milk and cornflour.
- Heat gently until thickened (can be done in a microwave oven).
- Stir in broccoli and salmon.
- Serve topped with parmesan cheese and black pepper.

Nutritional information (per serving):

Calories = 283; protein = 31.1 g;
carbohydrate = 16 g; fat = 10.8 g;
fibre = 2.3 g

'Cream' Chicken Sauce

Serves 2

225 g (8 oz) cooked chicken, chopped
225 g (8 oz) fromage frais (8% fat)
1 tbsp (15 ml) lemon juice
Freshly ground black pepper
Fresh parsley, chopped

- Combine chicken, fromage frais, lemon juice and black pepper.
- Heat gently, not quite to boiling point (otherwise the sauce will curdle). Sprinkle with parsley, and serve with green salad.

Nutritional information (per serving):

Calories = 311; protein = 14.1 g;
carbohydrate = 6.4 g; fat = 13.5 g;
fibre = 0 g

V Tomato and Aubergine Sauce

Serves 2

2 tsp (10 ml) olive oil
1 quantity easy tomato sauce (see p. 209)
1 small aubergine, cubed
2 tsp parmesan or cottage cheese

- Cook the aubergine in the oil for 10 mins.
- Stir in the tomato sauce, and serve with a little parmesan *or* cottage cheese.

Noodles with Prawns and Green Beans

Serves 2

225 g (8 oz) frozen or fresh whole green beans
175 g (6 oz) egg noodles
1 tsp (5 ml) oil
175 g (6 oz) peeled prawns
1 tbsp (15 ml) soy sauce

- Cook green beans in a little boiling water for 5 mins, then drain.
- Cook noodles in a large pan for 10 mins.
- Meanwhile, heat oil in a wok or frying pan and stir fry prawns for 2 mins.
- Add beans, noodles and soy sauce, and heat through.

Nutritional information (per serving):

Calories = 102; protein = 3.5 g;
carbohydrate = 9.8 g; fat = 5.7 g;
fibre = 4.2 g

Nutritional information (per serving):

Calories = 483; protein = 32.4 g;
carbohydrate = 66 g; fat = 11.8 g;
fibre = 5.2 g

V Mushroom Pasta

Serves 2

100 g (4 oz) mushrooms
2 tsp (10 ml) olive oil
1 onion, sliced
½ green pepper, sliced
2 tbsp (30 ml) fromage frais (8% fat)
175 g (6 oz) pasta shapes

- Either leave mushrooms whole or, if quite large, roughly slice.
- Heat oil in a pan and cook onion and pepper for 5 mins.
- Add mushrooms and continue cooking for 5 mins.
- Remove from heat and stir in fromage frais. Do not boil.
- Meanwhile, cook pasta for about 10 mins in boiling water.
- Drain and combine with the mushroom sauce.
- Serve with green salad.

Seafood Tagliatelle

Serves 2

1 tsp (5 ml) oil
1 small onion, sliced
15 g (½ oz) flour
150 ml (¼ pint) low-fat milk
3 tbsp (45 ml) water or white wine
Freshly ground black pepper
50 g (2 oz) mushrooms, sliced
225 g (8 oz) haddock fillet, cubed
50 g (2 oz) peeled prawns
175 g (5 oz) tagliatelle

- Heat oil in a pan and cook onion until soft.
- Stir in flour and cook for 1 min.
- Remove from heat and gradually stir in milk.
- Return to heat and cook, stirring all the time, until thickened and smooth.
- Add water or white wine, black pepper, mushrooms and haddock fillet.
- Simmer for about 5 mins.
- Stir in prawns and cook for a further 1–2 mins until the prawns are hot.
- Meanwhile, cook and drain tagliatelle, then combine with seafood sauce.

Nutritional information (per serving):

Calories = 438; protein = 13.6 g; carbohydrate = 71 g; fat = 13 g; fibre = 3.7 g

Nutritional information (per serving):

Calories = 507; protein = 45.2 g; carbohydrate = 73 g; fat = 5.7 g; fibre = 3.2 g

V Tofu with Noodles

Serves 2

For the marinade:
2 tbsp (30 ml) soy sauce
2 tbsp (30 ml) dry sherry
1 tbsp (15 ml) wine vinegar

For the dish:
225 g (8 oz) tofu (bean curd), cubed
1 tbsp (15 ml) olive oil
1 clove garlic, crushed
1 piece fresh root ginger, chopped
1 red pepper, sliced
100 g (4 oz) mange tout
1 tsp cornflour
175 g (6 oz) noodles, cooked in water

- Mix ingredients for marinade together.
- Add tofu and leave for at least 30 mins in fridge (or overnight).
- Heat oil in a wok and stir fry the garlic, ginger and vegetables for 4 mins.
- Remove tofu from marinade.
- Blend marinade with cornflour, and pour over the vegetables.
- Stir until sauce has thickened.
- Place vegetables and sauce in a serving dish.
- Stir fry tofu for 2 mins, and add to vegetables.
- Serve with noodles.

Nutritional information (per serving):

Calories = 533; protein = 21 g;
carbohydrate = 75 g; fat = 18.5 g;
fibre = 3.8 g

POTATOES

Potatoes are excellent sources of complex carbohydrate. They also provide vitamin C and fibre, and are a good basis for all meals.

Baked potatoes

Baked potatoes are quick to cook if you have a microwave – about 10 mins is enough for one large potato. If you are cooking with a conventional oven, save time by cooking several potatoes at once. Wrap in foil, and bake for about one hour. Allow them to cool and keep them in the fridge. They will last for up to a week.

Here are some recipes for quick and nutritious toppings. Simply cut the potato in half and spoon the topping over. Serve with a salad or vegetables.

Mexican Tuna Filling

Serves 1

100 g (4 oz) tin tuna, drained
2 tbsp tinned red kidney beans
2 tbsp sweetcorn
Dash of tabasco (or chilli) sauce

- Combine all ingredients in a saucepan.
- Heat through.

Nutritional information (per serving):

Calories = 247; protein = 34 g;
carbohydrate = 22 g; fat = 2.8 g;
fibre = 5 g

V Chick Pea Filling

Serves 1

Half an onion
½ tsp coriander and cumin, or curry powder
¼ of 400 g (14 oz) can chick peas, drained
2 tbsp plain yoghurt

- Scoop out flesh from potato, keeping skin intact.
- Blend flesh and ingredients in food processor until almost smooth, or mash with a fork.
- Pile filling back in potato skin.
- Heat through again.

V Peanut and Yoghurt Filling

Serves 1

1 tbsp crunchy peanut butter
2 tbsp (30 ml) plain yoghurt

- Scoop out some of potato flesh and mash with peanut butter and yoghurt.
- Pile back into skin.
- Heat through.

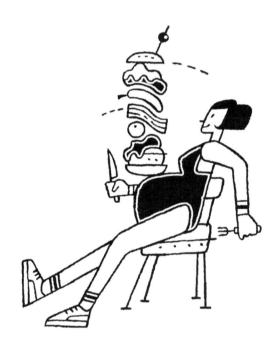

Nutritional information (per serving):

Calories = 149; protein = 10.3 g;
carbohydrate = 21 g; fat = 3.4 g;
fibre = 4.1 g

Nutritional information (per serving):

Calories = 183; protein = 8.5 g;
carbohydrate = 7.6 g; fat = 13.4 g;
fibre = 1.3 g

Chicken and Sweetcorn Filling

Serves 1

100 g (4 oz) cooked chicken,
3 tbsp sweetcorn chopped
2 tbsp cottage cheese

- Simply combine chicken, sweetcorn and cottage cheese, and serve hot or cold.

Potato and Fish Pie

Serves 2

450 g (1 lb) potatoes
200 g (7 oz) white fish fillets (e.g. cod or plaice)
3 tbsp (45 ml) skimmed milk
2 eggs
1 tbsp parsley
1 tbsp (15 ml) lemon juice

- Cut potatoes into chunks and boil until tender.
- Drain, then mash with flaked fish, milk, eggs, parsley and lemon juice.
- Place in a dish, then cook either in microwave at full power for 5 mins, or in oven at 200°C/400°F/gas mark 6 for 20 mins.
- Serve with green vegetables.

Nutritional information (per serving):

Calories = 322; protein = 42 g; carbohydrate = 18.9 g; fat = 9.3 g; fibre = 2 g

Nutritional information (per serving):

Calories = 352; protein = 33.3 g; carbohydrate = 39.4 g; fat = 7.9 g; fibre = 2.8 g

V Cheese and Potato Layer

Serves 2

450 g (1 lb) potatoes, thinly sliced
1 large onion, cut into thin rings
100 g (4oz) half-fat Cheddar cheese, grated
1 tsp herbs (e.g. sage or thyme)
150 ml (¼ pint) skimmed milk
Freshly ground black pepper

- In a dish, layer potatoes, onion, cheese, black pepper and herbs, finishing with a layer of cheese.
- Pour milk over the dish and cover.
- Cook either in microwave at full power for 15 mins or in oven at 200°C/400°F/gas mark 6 for 1 hour.
- Serve with vegetables or salad.

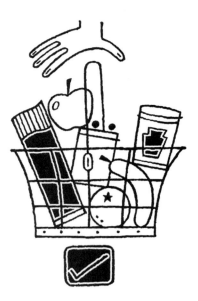

Nutritional information (per serving):

Calories = 479; protein = 27.6 g;
carbohydrate = 79 g; fat = 8.1 g;
fibre = 6.8 g

V Spicy Potatoes with Courgettes

Serves 2

450 g (1 lb) small new potatoes
100 g (4 oz) cauliflower, broken into florets
1 tbsp (15 ml) oil
1 onion, sliced
2 tsp mild curry powder
Pinch chilli powder
3 courgettes, sliced

- Boil potatoes in their skins and cauliflower for 10 mins, then drain.
- Meanwhile, heat oil in a wok or heavy based pan, and stir fry onion and spices for 3 mins.
- Add courgettes and stir fry for a further 2 mins.
- Add potatoes and cauliflower and cook for a further 3 mins or until heated through.

Follow this dish with a high protein dessert, such as cheesecake or yoghurt (*see* pp. 228; 230).

Nutritional information (per serving):

Calories = 278; protein = 7.1 g;
carbohydrate = 45 g; fat = 9 g;
fibre = 4.5 g

V Spanish Potato Omelette

Serves 2

450 g (1 lb) potatoes
1 tsp (5 ml) oil
1 onion, chopped
6 eggs
Salt and black pepper
Paprika

- Boil potatoes in their skins.
- Cool and cut into thick slices.
- Cook onion in oil for 5 mins, then add potatoes.
- Beat eggs with salt and pepper and pour into the pan with vegetables.
- Sprinkle with paprika. Lower heat and cook for about 5 mins until nearly set.
- Finish off under a hot grill for 1–2 mins or until top sets.
- Serve with tomato salad.

Nutritional information (per serving):

Calories = 458; protein = 27 g;
carbohydrate = 40 g; fat = 22 g;
fibre = 3.1 g

BEANS AND LENTILS

Beans and lentils supply protein, fibre and a wide range of important vitamins and minerals. You can buy them ready-cooked in tins – simply drain them, and use them in these recipes. Dried beans need soaking for several hours, although you can reduce the soaking time to just one hour if you use boiling water. Using a pressure cooker is quicker – follow the recommended times. Alternatively, boil them in a saucepan (times are given in the recipes). It is worth making a larger quantity than you need and freezing or keeping some in the fridge for a few days to save time.

Beans and lentils can be rather bland on their own, but they readily absorb the flavour of other ingredients. These recipes should give you lots of ideas for using them in exciting ways.

V Soya Bean Curry

Soya beans are best cooked in a pressure cooker, since they require a long cooking time. The addition of sultanas gives a subtle, sweet flavour that complements the beans well.

Serves 2

175 g (6 oz) soya beans, soaked for several hours
1 tbsp curry powder
1 onion, chopped
1 clove garlic, crushed
2 carrots, sliced
2 courgettes, sliced
2 tbsp sultanas
1 tbsp tomato puree

- Drain beans and place in pressure cooker with about 300 ml (½ pint) water.
- Add curry powder and bring to the boil.
- Cook for 15 mins.
- Release steam slowly, then add remaining ingredients.
- Bring to the boil and cook for a further 3 mins, before releasing steam slowly.
- Serve with baked potatoes.

Chicken with Chick Peas and Apricots

Chicken with apricots sounds an unusual combination, but it tastes delicious and supplies lots of valuable nutrients. Apricots are high in beta-carotene (vitamin A).

Serves 2

1 tsp (5 ml) oil
1 onion, chopped
1 piece fresh root ginger, finely chopped
2 chicken breasts, cut into large pieces
2 cloves garlic, crushed
75 g (3 oz) dried, ready-to-eat apricots
150 ml (¼ pint) water
400 g (14 oz) tin chick peas

- Heat oil in a wok or a heavy based pan.
- Stir fry onion, garlic, ginger and chicken for about 4 mins.
- Add apricots, water and chick peas.
- Simmer for 15 mins.
- Serve with boiled rice and green vegetables.

Nutritional information (per serving):

Calories = 396; protein = 33 g;
carbohydrate = 31 g; fat = 16.6 g;
fibre = 16.2 g

Nutritional information (per serving):

Calories = 502; protein = 47 g;
carbohydrate = 52 g; fat = 13.3 g;
fibre = 11.6 g

V Mixed Bean Hotpot

Serves 2

400 g (14 oz) can of beans (e.g. red kidney beans, chick peas or haricot beans)
100 g (4 oz) green beans
225 g (8 oz) can tomatoes
1 tbsp tomato puree
1 tsp mixed herbs
450 g (1 lb) potatoes, boiled and cooled

* Place drained can of beans in large casserole dish and mix in green beans, tomatoes, puree and herbs.
* Thinly slice potatoes and arrange on top.
* Bake at 170°C/325°F/gas mark 3 for 30 mins until the potatoes are cooked, or microwave on full for 8 mins.
* Serve with green vegetables or salad.

Nutritional information (per serving):

Calories = 346; protein = 16.8 g;
carbohydrate = 71 g; fat = 1.5 g;
fibre = 14.2 g

V Pasta and Chick Pea Salad

The combination of chick peas and pasta is wonderful. This dish is simple to make, using mostly store cupboard ingredients. Vary the vegetables according to what is at hand.

Serves 2

175 g (6 oz) pasta twists
100 g (4 oz) cooked peas
100 g (4 oz) sweetcorn
100 g (4 oz) canned pineapple
½ red pepper, diced
225 g (8 oz) cooked chick peas
100 g (4 oz) fromage frais

* Cook pasta for 10 mins.
* Drain and combine with remaining ingredients.

Nutritional information (per serving):

Calories = 576; protein = 28 g;
carbohydrate = 109 g; fat = 6.5 g;
fibre = 11.6 g

V Lentil and Vegetable Lasagne

This lasagne has a fluffy, light topping and is lower in fat than the traditional version. It is also an impressive dish when entertaining. If you are in a hurry, simply top with fromage frais.

Serves 2

6 sheets ready-cooked lasagne

For the lentil and vegetable sauce:
100 g (4 oz) red lentils
1 onion, chopped
400 g (14 oz) tin of tomatoes
2 carrots, chopped
1 tsp oregano
150 ml (¼ pint) water

For the topping:
100 g (4 oz) fromage frais
2 eggs
1 tbsp parmesan cheese

- Place all ingredients for lentil and vegetable sauce in a saucepan and bring to the boil.
- Simmer for 20 mins or cook in pressure cooker for 3 mins (release steam slowly).
- Place half of the sauce in a dish, with several lasagne sheets on top. Then add rest of sauce, followed by remaining lasagne sheets. For topping, beat eggs with fromage frais, then spoon them on top of lasagne. Sprinkle with parmesan cheese. Bake at 200°C/400°F/gas mark 6 for 40 mins, until the topping is golden. Serve with large mixed salad.

V Lentil and Vegetable Stew

Cooking this dish in a pressure cooker saves a lot of time. You can substitute red lentils or beans for green lentils.

Serves 2

100 g (4 oz) green lentils, soaked for a few hours
1 tbsp (15 ml) concentrated vegetable stock (e.g. Vecon), or
1 vegetable stock cube
300 ml (½ pint) water
1 onion, chopped
2 carrots
1 red or green pepper, sliced
1 potato, chopped
2 courgettes

- Drain lentils and place in a large saucepan with vegetable stock and water.
- Bring to the boil, reduce the heat and simmer for 30 mins.
- Release steam, then add vegetables.
- Bring back to the boil and cook for a further 3 mins, then release steam slowly.
- Serve with boiled or baked potatoes.

Nutritional information (per serving):

Calories = 513; protein = 33 g; carbohydrate = 75 g; fat = 10.9 g; fibre = 6 g

Nutritional information (per serving):

Calories = 232; protein = 15.2 g; carbohydrate = 42 g; fat = 1.7 g; fibre = 8.2 g

V Lentil Loaf

This loaf is surprisingly easy to make and looks impressive. It is also extremely low in fat, cut any leftovers into slices and use as a sandwich filling.

Serves 4

100 g (4 oz) red lentils
1 onion, chopped
1 tbsp (15 ml) concentrated vegetable stock (e.g. Vecon), *or*
1 vegetable stock cube
300 ml (½ pint) water
50 g (2 oz) oats or fresh breadcrumbs
1 egg, beaten

- Place lentils, onion, stock concentrate and water in a large pan.
- Bring to the boil and simmer for 20 mins, or cook in pressure cooker for 3 mins and release steam slowly.
- Stir in oats or breadcrumbs, and egg.
- Spoon into 450 g (1 lb) non-stick loaf tin.
- Cover with foil and bake at 190°C/375°F/gas mark 5 for 30 mins.
- Leave in the tin for 2 mins, then loosen and turn out.
- Serve with rice and vegetables.

V Bean Burgers

These are much lower in fat than beef burgers. Make a large batch, so that you can keep some in the freezer for when you are in a hurry.

Serves 2

400 g (14 oz) tin red kidney beans, drained
2 tsp (10 ml) oil
1 small onion, finely chopped
1 clove garlic, crushed
1 tbsp parsley
1 tbsp (15 ml) lemon juice
Oats for coating

- Cook the onion and garlic in the oil for 5 mins.
- Mash with a fork or blend in food processor with other ingredients, except the oats, till a coarse puree.
- Add a little flour if necessary for a firmer texture.
- Place oats in a dish.
- In your hands, form mixture into 4 large burgers, coating them with oats.
- Grill for about 2 mins on each side, fry in a small amount of hot oil, or barbecue.
- Serve in a wholemeal bap or pitta bread with lots of salad.

Nutritional information (per serving):

Calories = 321; protein = 19.4 g; carbohydrate = 50 g; fat = 6.1 g; fibre = 4.9 g

Nutritional information (per serving):

Calories = 234; protein = 11.6 g; carbohydrate = 34 g; fat = 6.6 g; fibre = 10.2 g

PUDDINGS AND DESSERTS

Puddings and desserts can make a substantial nutritional contribution to diet. They need not be full of sugar or dripping in cream. They can, in fact, be very healthy if based on fruit and low-fat ingredients like yoghurt and fromage frais.

These desserts and puddings are all easy to make. If you really are pressed for time, fresh fruit and yoghurt are always a good choice. If you have a little longer or are entertaining, these recipes will help to add a new dimension to your diet!

Apricot and Lemon Mousse

You can use other dried fruits such as peaches or prunes in this recipe instead of apricots, if you wish.

Serves 2

100 g (4 oz) dried apricots
300 ml (½ pint) orange juice
Juice and rind of 1 lemon
225 g (8 oz) plain fromage frais

- Soak apricots in orange juice in a bowl over-night.
- In a liquidiser or food processor, blend them into a puree.
- Add remaining ingredients and blend until smooth.
- Spoon into glasses.
- Chill in the fridge before serving.

Banana and Oat Pudding

Serves 2

2 ripe bananas
25 g (1 oz) porridge oats
300 ml (½ pint) plain yoghurt

- Mash one banana with oats and yoghurt.
- Put the mixture into individual bowls.
- Decorate with remaining banana, cut into slices.

Nutritional information (per serving):

Calories = 221; protein = 12.9 g; carbohydrate = 44.3 g; fat = 0.3 g; fibre = 3.8 g

Nutritional information (per serving):

Calories = 213; protein = 10.3 g; carbohydrate = 40 g; fat = 2.6 g; fibre = 2 g

Banana Pancakes

Makes 8 pancakes

100 g (4 oz) wholemeal flour, or fine oatmeal
300 ml (½ pint) skimmed or semi-skimmed milk
2 eggs
1 tsp (5 ml) oil
3 ripe bananas

- Blend all ingredients, except bananas, in a liquidiser for 30 secs.
- Then heat a non-stick frying pan and add oil.
- Pour in 1 tbsp of batter, tilting the pan to coat evenly.
- Cook until underside of pancake is brown.
- Turn, and cook for a further 10 secs until other side is brown.
- Repeat till batter used up.
- Stack pancakes on an oven proof plate and keep warm in the oven on a very low heat.
- Then, mix one mashed banana with two sliced bananas.
- Place spoonful on each pancake and fold into quarters.
- Serve with low-fat yoghurt.

Baked Apples

Make this pudding in the autumn, when apples are cheap.

Serves 1

1 large cooking apple
1 tbsp raisins or sultanas
1 tsp honey
1 tsp toasted, chopped hazelnuts (optional)

- Remove core from apple.
- Score skin lightly around middle. Place in small dish. Mix together raisins or sultanas, honey and nuts and fill centre of apple.
- Cover loosely with foil and bake at 180°C/350°F/gas mark 4 for 45–60 mins or cover with another dish and microwave on medium power for 5–7 mins (depending on the size of apple).
- Serve with yoghurt, low-fat custard or fromage frais.

Nutritional information (per serving):

Calories = 103; protein = 5.1 g;
carbohydrate = 17.1 g; fat = 2 g;
fibre = 1.5 g

Nutritional information (per serving):

Calories = 144; protein = 1.2 g;
carbohydrate = 33 g; fat = 1.8 g;
fibre = 0.6 g

Chocolate and Banana Cheesecake

Makes 8 slices

For the base:
25 g (1 oz) margarine or butter
2 tbsp honey
50 g (2 oz) milk chocolate
100 g (4 oz) oatmeal

For the cheesecake:
2 ripe bananas, chopped
225 g (8 oz) fromage frais
2 tbsp (30 ml) honey
4 tbsp (60 ml) plain yoghurt
2 eggs

- For base, melt margarine, honey and chocolate in small bowl in microwave or saucepan.
- Do not allow to boil.
- Stir in the oatmeal.
- Press into base of 20 cm (8") microwave cake dish or loose-bottomed cake tin.
- Blend cheesecake ingredients in liquidiser for 1 min.
- Pour onto the base.
- Cook, either in the microwave on medium power for 20 mins, or in conventional oven at 325°F/160°C/gas mark 3 for 1–1½ hours.
- Cool and decorate with grated chocolate, if you wish.

Tropical Fruit Salad

Exotic fruits are available all year round now in supermarkets. They are packed with vitamins A and C.

Serves 2

1 mango (or paw paw)
1 orange
1 banana
1 kiwi fruit
4 rings fresh or tinned pineapple
150 ml (¼ pint) orange juice

- Simply peel and chop mango, orange, banana and kiwi fruit.
- Mix with pineapple and orange juice.
- Keep in fridge before serving to preserve vitamins.

Nutritional information (per serving):

Calories = 194; protein = 7.2 g; carbohydrate = 26 g; fat = 7.4 g; fibre = 1.1 g

Nutritional information (per serving):

Calories = 220; protein = 2.7 g; carbohydrate = 56 g; fat = 0.2 g; fibre = 7 g

Wholemeal Bread and Butter Pudding

This pudding is great for athletes, as it is high in complex carbohydrates from the bread, and has lots of protein, calcium and B vitamins from the milk. It is worth making a larger quantity that you need, as it will keep in the fridge for several days.

Serves 4

8 slices wholemeal bread
40 g (1 1/2 oz) low-fat spread
75 g (3 oz) sultanas
1 tbsp brown sugar
3 eggs
600 ml (1 pint) skimmed milk
Nutmeg

- Spread bread with low fat spread.
- Cut each slice into 4 squares and put in 1 litre (2 pint) dish.
- Scatter sultanas between each slice.
- Beat together sugar, eggs, and milk and pour over bread.
- Sprinkle with a little grated nutmeg.
- Leave to soak for 30 mins, if time allows.
- Bake at 350°F/180°C/gas mark 4 for 1 hour, until the top is golden.

Raisin and Lemon Ice Cream

This ice cream is easy to make, low in fat and absolutely delicious!

Makes 4 servings

50 g (2 oz) raisins
Juice of 1 lemon
250 ml (8 fl oz) evaporated milk
50 g (2 oz) castor sugar

- Soak raisins in lemon juice for 2 hours.
- Whisk evaporated milk until foamy and holding its shape.
- Whisk in sugar.
- Stir in raisins and lemon juice.
- Freeze in ice cream maker or shallow container, whisking once or twice.

Nutritional information (per serving):

Calories = 345; protein = 17 g;
carbohydrate = 49 g; fat = 10.5 g;
fibre = 3.9 g

Nutritional information (per serving):

Calories = 178; protein = 5.5 g;
carbohydrate = 27 g; fat = 5.9 g;
fibre = 0.3 g

Banana Yoghurt Ice Cream

Makes 4 servings

2 ripe bananas
2 tbsp honey
250 ml (8 fl oz) plain yoghurt
1 tbsp (15 ml) lemon juice

- Blend ingredients in liquidiser until smooth.
- Freeze in ice cream maker or shallow container, whisking once or twice.

Nutritional information (per serving):

Calories = 139; protein = 7.0 g;
carbohydrate = 27 g; fat = 1.2 g;
fibre = 0.6 g

SNACKS – MUFFINS, BREADS AND COOKIES

These recipes for homemade, high energy snacks are not only low in fat and highly nutritious, but they are simple and quick to make (even if you have never baked before!). It's worth investing in bun tins for these recipes. Make a large batch, wrap in foil and take in your kit bag so you'll never be stuck for snacks before or after training again.

Oatbran and Raisin Muffins

High in carbohydrate and soluble fibre but very low in fat, these muffins are delicious and simple to make. Try some of the numerous variations below!

Makes 12 muffins

225 g (8 oz) oatbran
1 tbsp baking powder
1 tsp cinnamon
50 g (2 oz) brown sugar or honey
1 tbsp (15 ml) oil
2 egg whites
50 g (2 oz) raisins
350 ml (12 fl oz) skimmed milk

- Combine oatbran, baking powder and sugar.
- Stir in remaining ingredients.
- Leave to stand for a few mins to allow some of liquid to absorb.
- Spoon into 12 non-stick bun tins (or paper cases).
- Bake at 220°C/425°F/gas mark 7 for 12–15 mins.

Variations:

- Substitute 1 grated apple for the raisins.
- Add 50 g (2 oz) dates and 50 g (2 oz) walnuts instead of the raisins and omit the cinnamon.
- Substitute 100 g (4 oz) tinned black cherries (pitted) for the raisins and omit the cinnamon.
- Substitute 225 g (8 oz) tinned crushed pineapple in juice (drained) for the raisins and omit the cinnamon.
- Substitute 2 mashed bananas for the raisins and omit the cinnamon.

Nutritional information (per muffin):

Calories = 123; protein = 4.6 g;
carbohydrate = 20 g; fat = 2.8 g;
fibre = 3.6 g

Banana Muffins

These heavenly muffins can be varied according to the fruit available.

Makes 10 muffins

50 g (2 oz) butter
75 g (3 oz) brown sugar
1 egg
225 g (8 oz) flour (wholemeal or half wholemeal, half white)
2 mashed bananas
Pinch salt
1 tsp baking powder
1 tsp (5 ml) vanilla essence
5 tbsp (75 ml) skimmed milk

- Combine all ingredients in a large bowl.
- Spoon into 10 non stick bun tins (or paper cases).
- Bake at 190°C/375°F/gas mark 5 for approx 20 mins.

Variations:

– Add 50 g (2 oz) chocolate chips to the mixture (recommended!).
– Substitute 225 g (8 oz) fresh blueberries or 75 g (3 oz) dried blueberries for the bananas.
– Substitute 225 g (8 oz) fresh cranberries or 75 g (3 oz) dried cranberries for the bananas. Add 50 g (2 oz) chopped walnuts.
– Substitute 100 g (4 oz) chopped dried apricots for the bananas. Add the grated rind of 1 lemon instead of the vanilla essence.

Peanut Butter Muffins

Peanut butter is simply ground peanuts with a little salt and is therefore an excellent source of unsaturated fatty acids, zinc, protein and fibre. If you have a weakness for peanut butter, these muffins won't last long!

Makes 10 muffins

100 g (4 oz) crunchy peanut butter
100 g (4 oz) honey
2 eggs
1 tsp (5 ml) vanilla essence
225 g (8 oz) half wholemeal, half white self-raising flour
3–4 tbsp (45–60 ml) milk
25 g (1 oz) plain peanuts

- Combine peanut butter and honey.
- Add eggs, vanilla essence, flour and milk.
- Spoon into 10 non stick bun tins.
- Press a few peanuts on top of each muffin.
- Bake at 190°C/375°F/gas mark 5 for 25 mins.

Nutritional information (per muffin):

Calories = 164; protein = 4.1 g; carbohydrate = 27 g; fat = 5.3 g; fibre = 2.2 g

Nutritional information (per muffin):

Calories = 192; protein = 7.1 g; carbohydrate = 24g; fat = 8.2 g; fibre = 2.2 g

Polenta/Cornmeal Muffins

Yellow cornmeal or polenta, gives a moreish, soft texture to these unusual muffins. A little lower in fibre than wholemeal flour but higher than white flour, cornmeal is good for iron, B vitamins and carbohydrate.

Makes 12 muffins

175 g (6 oz) cornmeal
50 g (2 oz) self raising white flour
1 tbsp baking powder
2 tbsp honey
50 g (2 oz) sultanas
1 tsp (5 ml) vanilla essence
2 egg whites
300 ml (10 fl oz) skimmed milk
2 tbsp (30 ml) oil or melted butter

- Mix all ingredients together in a bowl. (Batter should be fairly runny as cornmeal absorbs a lot of liquid during cooking.)
- Spoon into 12 non stick bun tins (or paper cases).
- Bake at 400°C/200°F/gas mark 6 for 15 mins.

Variations:

- Substitute 225 g (8 oz) fresh or 75 g (3 oz) dried cranberries for the sultanas.
- Substitute 50 g (2 oz) chopped dates for the sultanas.
- Add 1 tbsp carob powder or cocoa powder to the mixture.
- Substitute 50 g (2 oz) glace cherries for the sultanas.

Oatmeal Biscuits

Makes 24

75 g (3 oz) wholemeal flour
150 g (5 oz) oatmeal
1 tsp (5 ml) vanilla essence
2 tbsp (30 ml) oil
50 g (2 oz) brown sugar
50 g (2 oz) chopped walnuts or raisins
1 egg

- Mix all ingredients together in a bowl.
- Place heaped tablespoonfuls on a non stick baking tray about 5 cm (2") apart (they will spread while cooking).
- Bake at 180°C/350°F/gas mark 4 for 10 mins.

Nutritional information (per muffin):

Calories = 126; protein = 3.2 g; carbohydrate = 22 g; fat = 3.1 g; fibre = 0.5 g

Nutritional information (per biscuit):

Calories = 71; protein = 1.8 g; carbohydrate = 9 g; fat = 3.6 g; fibre = 0.8 g

Raisin Bread

Makes one loaf (10 slices)

225 g (8 oz) strong flour (half wholemeal, half white)
½ tsp salt
1½ tbsp sugar
1 sachet easy-blend yeast
1 tbsp melted butter
180 ml (6 fl oz) warm water
100 g (4 oz) raisins

- Mix together flour, salt, sugar, yeast and butter.
- Add warm water to form a dough.
- Turn out onto floured surface and knead for 5–10 mins.
- Knead in the raisins.
- Place in bowl, cover and leave in warm place or at room temperature to rise until doubled in size (approximately 1 hour).
- Knead for a few mins then shape into a loaf.
- Place on oiled baking tray and bake at 220°C/425°F/gas mark 7 for 20 mins or until it sounds hollow when tapped underneath.

Variations:

– Add 2 tsp cinnamon to the flour mixture.
– Substitute 100 g (4 oz) chopped dried apricots for the raisins.
– Substitute 100 g (4 oz) sultanas for the raisins.
– Add 1 tsp grated orange rind.
– Add 50 g (2 oz) toasted chopped hazelnuts with the raisins.

Blueberry Bread

A cross between cake and bread, this recipe is a firm favourite with my family and friends!

Makes 1 large loaf (12 slices)

225 g (8 oz) strong white flour
100 g (4 oz) yellow cornmeal
1 sachet easy blend yeast
1 tsp salt
2 tbsp sugar
1 tbsp butter
100 g (4 oz) cottage cheese
5 tbsp (75 ml) water
225 g (8 oz) fresh or 75 g (3 oz) dried blueberries

- Mix all ingredients, except water and blueberries, in a bowl or combine in a food processor.
- Add water and mix until a dough forms.
- Turn out onto a floured surface and knead for 5–10 mins.
- Knead in blueberries carefully.
- Cover and leave to rise until doubled in size.
- Knead briefly, then shape into oblong or round loaf.
- Place on oiled baking tray and bake at 220°C/425°F/gas mark 7 for approx. 20 mins until it sounds hollow when tapped underneath.

Nutritional information (per slice):

Calories = 120; protein = 3.0 g; carbohydrate = 25 g; fat = 1.7 g; fibre = 1.6 g

Nutritional information (per slice):

Calories = 131; protein = 4.3 g; carbohydrate = 24 g; fat = 2.4 g; fibre = 1.4 g

Apple and Cinnamon Oat Bars

Makes 12 bars

2 apples, sliced and cooked, or 175 g (6 oz) apple puree
175 g (6 oz) oats
2 tsp cinnamon
4 egg whites
1 tbsp honey
50 g (2 oz) raisins
6 tbsp (90 ml) skimmed milk

- Mix all ingredients together in a bowl.
- Transfer to non-stick baking tin 23 cm × 15 cm (approx. 9" × 6").
- Bake at 200°C/400°F/gas mark 6 for 15 mins.
- When cool, cut into squares.

Nutritional information (per bar):

Calories = 87; protein = 3.1 g;
carbohydrate = 17 g; fat = 1.3 g;
fibre = 1.3 g

Peanut Bars

Makes 8 bars

4 tbsp crunchy peanut butter
4 tbsp honey
225 g (8 oz) oats
50 g (2 oz) raisins
1 tbsp wholemeal flour

- Melt peanut butter and honey in a saucepan.
- Add remaining ingredients.
- Press into non stick baking tin 23 cm × 15 cm (approximately 9" × 6").
- Bake at 190°C/375°F/gas mark 5 for 15 mins.
- Cut into 8 bars.

Nutritional information (per bar):

Calories = 203; protein = 5.8 g;
carbohydrate = 32 g; fat = 6.5 g;
fibre = 2.7 g

Muesli Bars

Makes 16 bars

50 g (2 oz) butter or margarine
3 tbsp honey
75 g (3 oz) muesli
75 g (3 oz) wholemeal flour (self raising)
2 eggs
225 g (8 fl oz) low-fat natural yoghurt
225 g (8 oz) low-fat soft cheese
100 g (4 oz) mixed dried fruit

- Combine butter and honey.
- Mix in yoghurt, soft cheese and eggs, followed by remaining ingredients.
- Spoon into non-stick baking tin (approximately 30 cm × 18 cm (12" × 7")).
- Bake for 20–25 mins or until firm and golden.
- Slice into 16 bars.

Real Fruit Cake

Makes 10 large slices

2 apples or pears, grated
1 banana, mashed
100 g (4 oz) sultanas
50 g (2 oz) chopped dates
50 g (2 oz) dried ready-to-eat apricots
150 ml (¼ pint) orange juice
3 eggs
1 tbsp honey
100 g (4 oz) wholemeal flour
100 g (4 oz) cornmeal or white flour
1 tbsp baking powder
150 ml (1/4 pint) skimmed milk

- Mix all ingredients together.
- Spoon mixture into non-stick, 20 cm (8") round cake tin.
- Bake at 160°C/350°F/gas mark 4 for approx. 1 hour or until firm to the touch.

Variations:

Substitute any of the following for the equivalent weight in the recipe: dried mango slices; dried tropical fruit mixture; tinned pineapple/mango/apricots/cherries; fresh or dried blueberries or cranberries; dried pineapple/papaya pieces; figs; ready-to-eat prunes; plums; fresh, tinned or dried peaches.

Nutritional information (per bar):

Calories = 112; protein = 4.8 g; carbohydrate = 14 g; fat = 4.5 g; fibre = 0.9 g

Nutritional information (per slice):

Calories = 176; protein = 5.6 g; carbohydrate = 34 g; fat = 2.7 g; fibre = 2.3 g

APPENDIX ONE

The Glycaemic Index and Carbohydrate Content of Foods

Appendix 1 lists the carbohydrate and calorie content of standard portions of various foods. Included in the appendix is the GI value of the foods. Although the values form a continuum, they have been divided into three categories – high, moderate and low – to help you select appropriate foods for different times. For example, during and after exercise, you will need to select high GI foods. Pre-exercise, you will need to select foods with a low GI. When constructing your daily diet, you can combine high GI and low GI foods to produce a meal combination with a moderate GI. Remember, adding foods high in protein, fat or soluble fibre will reduce the GI of the food combination. For example, combining a high GI food, such as white bread with a high-fat food, such as butter will result in a lower GI.

Table 1A	High GI foods (60–100)			
Food	Portion size	GI	Carbohydrate (g) per portion	Kcal per portion
Breakfast cereals				
Corn flakes	1 small bowl (30 g)	84	26	108
Rice crispies	1 small bowl (30 g)	82	27	111
Sustain	1 small bowl (30 g)	68	25	
Cheerios	1 small bowl (30 g)	74	23	111
Shredded wheat	2 (45 g)	67	31	146
Weetabix	2 (40 g)	69	30	141
Grains/pasta				
Couscous	5 tbsp (150 g)	65	77	341
Brown rice	6 tbsp (180 g)	76	58	254
White rice	6 tbsp (180 g)	87	56	248
Bread				
Bagel	1 (90 g)	72	46	241
Croissant	1 (60 g)	67	23	216
Baguette	3 inches (40 g)	95	22	108
White bread	1 large slice (38 g)	70	18	85
Wholemeal bread	1 large slice (38 g)	69	16	82
Pizza	1 large slice (115 g)	60	38	288

Table 1A	High GI foods (60–100) – continued			
Food	Portion size	GI	Carbohydrate (g) per portion	Kcal per portion
Crackers/crispbreads				
Puffed crispbread	1 (10 g)	81	7	32
Ryvita	1 (10 g)	69	7	32
Water biscuit	1 (8 g)	78	6	35
Rice cakes	1 (8 g)	85	6	28
Biscuits				
Shortbread	1 (13 g)	64	8	65
Vegetables				
Parsnip	2 tbsp (65 g)	97	8	43
Baked potato	1 medium (180 g)	85	22	94
Boiled potato, new	7 small (175 g)	62	27	116
Mashed potato	4 tbsp (180 g)	70	28	188
Chips	average portion (165 g)	75	59	450
Swede	2 tbsp (60 g)	72	1	7
Broad beans	2 tbsp (120 g)	79	7	58
Fruit				
Cantaloupe melon	1 slice (200 g)	65	6	26
Pineapple	1 slice (80 g)	66	8	33
Raisins	1 tbsp (30 g)	64	21	82
Watermelon	1 slice (200 g)	72	14	62
Dairy products				
Ice cream	1 scoop (60 g)	61	14	62
Drinks				
Fanta	375 ml can	68	51	191
Lucozade	250 ml bottle	95	40	150
Isostar	250 ml can	70	18	68
Gatorade	250 ml bottle	78	15	56
Squash (diluted, made up from 50 ml concentrate)	250 ml glass	66	14	54
Snacks				
Tortillas/corn chips	1 bag (50 g)	72	30	230
Confectionery				
Mars Bar	1 standard (65 g)	68	43	287
Museli bar	1 (33 g)	61	20	154

Table 1A	High GI foods (60–100) – continued			
Food	Portion size	GI	Carbohydrate (g) per portion	Kcal per portion
Sugars				
Glucose	1 tsp (5 g)	100	5	19
Sucrose	1 tsp (5 g)	65	5	19

Table 1B	Moderate GI foods (40–60)			
Food	Portion size	GI	Carbohydrate (g) per portion	Kcal per portion
Breakfast cereals				
All Bran	1 small bowl (40 g)	42	19	104
Sultana bran	1 small bowl (30 g)	52	20	91
Porridge (made with water)	1 small bowl (160 g)	42	14	78
Muesli	1 small bowl (50 g)	56	34	183
Grains/pasta				
Buckwheat	4 tbsp (80 g)	54	68	292
Bulgar wheat	4 tbsp (56 g)	48	44	196
Basmati rice	4 tbsp (60 g)	58	48	215
Instant noodles	4 tbsp (230 g cooked)	46	30	143
Macaroni	4 tbsp (230 g cooked)	45	43	198
Spaghetti	4 tbsp (220 g cooked)	41	49	229
Bread				
Pitta bread	1 large (75 g)	57	43	199
Rye bread	1 slice (25 g)	41	11	55
Biscuits				
Digestive	1 (15 g)	59	10	71
Oatmeal	1 (13 g)	55	8	57
Rich Tea	1 (10 g)	55	8	40
Cakes				
Muffin	1 (68 g)	44	34	192
Sponge cake	1 slice (60 g)	46	39	181

Table 1B	Moderate GI foods (40–60) – continued			
Food	Portion size	GI	Carbohydrate (g) per portion	Kcal per portion
Vegetables				
Carrots	2 tbsp (60 g)	49	3	14
Boiled potato	2 medium (175 g)	56	30	126
Peas	2 tbsp (70 g)	48	7	48
Sweetcorn	2 tbsp (85 g)	55	17	94
Sweet potato	1 medium (130 g)	54	27	109
Yam	1 medium (130 g)	51	43	173
Pulses				
Baked beans	1 small tin (205 g)	48	31	166
Fruit				
Apricots	1 (40 g)	57	3	12
Banana	1 (100 g)	55	23	95
Grapes	1 small bunch (100 g)	46	15	57
Kiwi fruit	1 (68 g)	52	6	29
Mango	½ (75 g)	55	11	43
Orange	1 (208 g)	44	12	54
Papaya	½ (175 g)	58	12	47
Peach (fresh)	1 (121 g)	42	8	36
Plum	1 (58 g)	39	5	20
Sultanas	1 tbsp (18 g)	56	12	50
Dairy products				
Custard	2 tbsp (120 g)	43	20	140
Drinks				
Apple juice	1 glass (160 ml)	40	16	61
Orange juice	1 glass (160 ml)	46	14	58
Snacks				
Crisps	1 pkt (30 g)	54	16	159
Confectionery				
Milk Chocolate	1 bar (54 g)	49	31	281
Sugars				
Honey	1 heaped tsp (17 g)	58	13	49

Table 1C	Low GI foods (0–40)			
Food	Portion size	GI	Carbohydrate (g) per portion	Kcal per portion
Pulses				
Butter beans	4 tbsp (120 g)	31	22	124
Chick peas	4 tbsp (140 g)	33	24	168
Red kidney beans	4 tbsp (120 g)	27	20	124
Green/brown lentils	4 tbsp (160 g)	30	28	164
Red lentils	4 tbsp (160 g)	26	28	160
Soya beans	4 tbsp (120 g)	18	6	169
Fruit				
Apples	1 (100 g)	38	12	47
Dried apricots	5 (40 g)	31	15	63
Cherries	1 small handful (100 g)	22	10	39
Grapefruit	½ (80 g)	25	5	24
Tinned peaches	½ tin (120 g)	30	12	47
Pear	1 (160 g)	38	16	64
Plum	1 (55 g)	39	5	20
Dairy products				
Full cream milk	½ pint (300 ml)	27	14	198
Skimmed milk	½ pint (300 ml)	32	15	99
Yoghurt, fruit (low-fat)	1 carton (150 g)	33	27	135
Snacks				
Peanuts	1 small handful (50 g)	14	4	301
Sugars				
Fructose	1 tsp (5 g)	23	5	19

Sources:
1. Leeds et al., 2000.
2. McCance and Widdowson's, 1991.
3. CompEat 5 software.

APPENDIX TWO

Glossary of Vitamins and Minerals

Vitamin	Function(s)	Sources	RNI and SUL*
A	Essential for normal colour vision and for the cells in the eye that enable us to see in dim light; promotes healthy skin and mucous membranes lining the mouth, nose, digestive system, etc.	Liver, meat, eggs, whole milk, cheese, oily fish, butter and margarine	Men: 700 µg/day Women: 600 µg/day *SUL*: 1500 µg/day (800 µg for pregnant women)
Beta-carotene	Converted into vitamin A (6 µg produces 1 µg vitamin A): a powerful antioxidant and free radical scavenger	Brightly coloured fruit and vegetables (e.g. carrots, spinach, apricots, tomatoes)	No official RNI. 15 mg is suggested intake *SUL*: 7 mg
B_1 (Thiamin)	Forms a co-enzyme essential for the conversion of carbohydrates into energy; used for the normal functioning of nerves, brain and muscles	Wholemeal bread and cereals, liver, kidneys, red meat, pulses (beans, lentils and peas)	Men: 0.4 mg/ 1000 calories Women: 0.4 mg/ 1000 calories No *SUL*. FSA recommends 100 mg
B_2 (Riboflavin)	Required for the conversion of carbohydrates to energy; promotes healthy skin and eyes and normal nerve functions	Liver, kidneys, red meat, chicken, milk, yoghurt cheese, eggs	Men: 1.3 mg/day Women: 1.1 mg/ day No *SUL*. FSA recommends 40 mg

Claim(s) of supplements	The evidence	Possible dangers of high doses
Maintains normal vision, healthy skin, hair and mucous membranes; may help to treat skin problems such as acne and boils; may affect protein manufacture	Not involved in energy production; little evidence to suggest it can improve sporting performance	Liver toxicity from taking supplements: symptoms include liver and bone damage; abdominal pain; dry skin; double vision; vomiting; hair loss; headaches. May also cause birth defects. Pregnant women should avoid liver. Never exceed 9000 µg/day (men), 7500 µg/day (women)
Reduces risk of heart disease, cancer and muscle soreness	As an antioxidant, may help prevent certain cancers. Other carotenoids in food may also be important	Orange tinge to the skin – probably harmless and reversible
May optimise energy production and performance; is usually present with a B-complex of multivitamin	Involved in energy (ATP) production, so the higher the thiamin requirement; increased needs can normally be met in the diet (cereals and other foods high in complex carbohydrates); there is no evidence to suggest that high intakes enhance performance; supplements are probably unnecessary	Cannot be stored – excess is excreted therefore unlikely to be toxic; toxic symptoms (rare) may include insomnia, rapid pulse, weakness and headaches. Avoid taking more than 3 g/day
Sportspeople may need more B_2 because they have higher energy needs – supplements may optimise energy production; usually present within a B-complex or multivitamin	Forms part of the enzymes involved in energy production, so exercise may increase the body's requirements; however, these can usually be met by a balanced diet; there is no evidence that supplements improve performance; if you take the contraceptive pill you may need extra B_2	Rarely toxic as it cannot be stored; any excess is excreted in the urine (a bright yellow colour)

Vitamin	Function(s)	Sources	RNI and SUL*
Niacin	Helps to convert carbohydrates into energy; promotes healthy skin, normal nerve functions and digestion	Liver, kidneys, red meat, chicken, turkey, nuts, milk, yoghurt and cheese, eggs, bread and cereals	Men: 6.6 mg/ 1000 calories Women: 6.6 mg/ 1000 calories *SUL:* 17 mg
B$_6$ (Pyridoxine)	Involved in the metabolism of fats, proteins and carbohydrates; promotes healthy skin, hair and normal red blood cell formation; is actively used in many chemical reactions of amino acids and proteins	Liver, nuts, pulses, eggs, bread, cereals, fish, bananas	Men: 1.4 mg/day Women: 1.2 mg/day *SUL:* 80 mg
Pantothenic acid (B vitamin)	Involved in the metabolism of fats, proteins and carbohydrates; promotes healthy skin, hair and normal growth; helps in the manufacture of hormones and antibodies, which fight infection; helps energy release from food	Liver, wholemeal bread, brown rice, nuts, pulses eggs, vegetables	No RNI in the UK No *SUL*
Folic acid (B vitamin)	Essential in the formation of DNA; necessary for red blood cell manufacture	Liver and offal, green vegetables, yeast extract, wheatgerm, pulses	Men: 200 µg/day Women: 200 µg/ day *SUL:* 1000 µg (1 mg)

Claim(s) of supplements	The evidence	Possible dangers of high doses
Sportspeople need more niacin since it is involved in metabolism; higher doses may help to reduce blood cholesterol levels	**Not enough evidence to** prove that high doses can help to improve performance; requirements can be met by a balanced diet	**Excess is excreted in the** urine; doses of more than 200 mg of nicotinic acid may cause dilation of the blood vessels near the skin's surface (hot flushes)
Sportspeople may need higher doses to meet their increased energy requirements	Requirements are related to protein intake, so sportspeople on high-protein diets may need extra B_6; endurance work may cause greater-than-normal losses; there is no evidence to suggest that high doses improve performance; extra doses may help to alleviate PMS (the premenstrual syndrome)	Excess is excreted in the urine; very high doses (over 2 g/day) over months or years may cause numbness and unsteadiness
Since it is involved in protein, fat and carbohydrate metabolism, sportspeople may need higher doses; usually present in a B-complex or multivitamin – for overall wellbeing	No evidence to suggest that high doses improve performance	Excess is excreted in the urine
Supplements help overall wellbeing, and also prevent folic acid deficiency and anaemia; these would, in theory, hinder aerobic performance	No studies have been carried out on athletic performance and folic acid	Dangers of toxicity are very small, though high doses may reduce zinc absorption and disguise a deficiency of vitamin B_{12}

Vitamin	Function(s)	Sources	RNI and SUL*
B12	Needed for red blood cell manufacture and to prevent some forms of anaemia; used in fat, protein and carbohydrate metabolism; promotes cell growth and development; needed for normal nerve functions	Meat, fish, offal, milk, cheese, yoghurt; vegan sources (fortified foods) are soya protein and milk, yeast extract, breakfast cereals	Men: 1.5 µg/day Women: 1.5 µg/day *SUL:* 2 mg
Biotin	Involved in the manufacture of fatty acids and glycogen, and in protein metabolism; needed for normal growth and development	Egg yolk, liver and offal, nuts, wholegrain and oats	No RNI in the UK; 10–200 µg/day is thought to be a safe and adequate range *SUL:* 900 µg
C	Growth and repair of body cells; collagen formation (in connective tissue) and tissue repair; promotes healthy blood vessels, gums and teeth; haemoglobin and red blood cell production; manufacture of adrenalin; powerful antioxidant	Fresh fruit (especially citrus), berries and currants, vegetables (especially dark green, leafy vegetables, tomatoes and peppers)	Men: 40 mg day Women: 40 mg/day *SUL:* 1000 mg

Claim(s) of supplements	The evidence	Possible dangers of high doses
Since it is involved in the development of red blood cells, the implication is that B_{12} can improve the body's oxygen carrying capacity (and therefore its aerobic performance); athletes have been known to use injections of vitamin B_{12} before competition in the hope that it will improve their endurance; usually present within a B-complex or multivitamin	Extra vitamin B12 has no effect on endurance or strength; there is no benefit to be gained from taking supplements (deficiencies are very rare)	Excess is excreted in the urine
Although biotin was once known amongst body builders as the 'dynamite vitamin', no specific role for this vitamin in sporting performance has been claimed; it is usually present within a B-complex or multivitamin	The body can make its own biotin, so supplements are unnecessary	There are no known cases of biotin toxicity
Vitamin C may help to increase oxygen uptake and aerobic energy production; exercise causes an increased loss so extra may be needed; intense exercise tends to cause greater free radical damage, so sportspeople need higher doses	A deficiency reduces physical performance; exercise may increase requirements to approximately 80 mg/day – these can be met by including 5 portions of fresh fruit and vegetables in the diet each day; intakes of 100–150 mg may help prevent heart disease and cancer	Excess is excreted, so toxic symptoms are unlikely; high doses nay lead to diarrhoea and increase the risk of kidney stones in people who are prone to them

Vitamin	Function(s)	Sources	RNI and SUL*
D	Controls absorption of calcium from the intestine and helps to regulate calcium metabolism; prevents rickets in children and osteomalacia in adults; helps to regulate bone formation	Sunlight (UV light striking the skin), fresh oils and oily fish, eggs, vitamin-D-fortified cereals, margarines and some yoghurts	No RNI in the UK (5 µg in EU) *SUL:* 25 µg
E	As an antioxidant, it protects tissues against free radical damage; promotes normal growth and development; helps in normal red blood cell formation	Pure vegetable oils, wheatgerm, wholemeal bread and cereals, egg yolk, nuts, sunflower seeds, avocado	No RNI in the UK; FSA suggests 4 mg (men) 3 mg (women) (10 mg in EU) *SUL:* 540 mg

Mineral	Function(s)	Sources	RNI and SUL*
Calcium	Important for bone and teeth structure; helps with blood clotting; acts to transmit nerve impulses; helps with muscle contraction	Milk, cheese, yoghurt, soft bones of small fish, seafood, green leafy vegetables, fortified white flour and bread, pulses	700 mg *SUL:* 1500 mg

Claim(s) of supplements	The evidence	Possible dangers of high doses
No specific claims for athletic performance	So far not shown to be beneficial to performance	Fat-soluble and can be stored in the body; toxicity is rare but symptoms may include high blood pressure, nausea, and irregular heart beat and thirst
Since it is an antioxidant, it may improve oxygen utilisation in the muscle cells; it may also helo to protect the cells from the damaging effects of intense exercise; may help to protect against heart disease and cancer	Supplements may have a beneficial effect on performance at high altitudes, and may help reduce heart disease, cancer risk, and post-exercise muscle soreness; requirements are related to intake of polyunsaturated fatty acids	Although it cannot be excreted, toxicity is extremely rare
Claim(s) of supplements	**The evidence**	**Possible dangers of high doses**
May help to prevent calcium deficiency and, in some cases, osteoporosis (brittle bone disease)	There is no evidence that extra calcium prevents osteoporosis; exercise (with adequate calcium intake) prevents bone loss, so supplements would seem to be unnecessary; sportspeople who eat few or no dairy products may find calcium supplements useful for meeting basic dietary require-ments; extra calcium may help to reduce the risk of stress fractures in sportswomen with menstrual irregularities	The balance of calcium in the bones and blood is finely controlled by hormones – calcium toxicity is thus virtually unknown. Very high intakes may interfere with the absorption of iron and with kidney function

Mineral	Function(s)	Sources	RNI and SUL*
Sodium	Helps to control body fluid balance; involved in muscle and nerve functions	Table salt, tinned vegetables, fish, meat, ready-made sauces and condiments, processed meats, bread, cheese	Men: 1.6 g/day (= 4 g salt) Women: 1.6 g/ day (= 4 g salt) FSA recommends a maximum daily intake of 2.5 g (= 6 g salt)
Potassium	Works with sodium to control fluid balance and muscle and nerve functions	Vegetables, fruit and fruit juices, unprocessed cereals	Men: 3.5 g/day Women: 3.5 g/day SUL: 3.7 g
Iron	Involved in red blood cell formation and oxygen transport and utilisation	Red meat, liver, offal, fortified breakfast cereals, shellfish, wholegrain bread, pasta and cereals, pulses, green leafy vegetables	Men: 6.7 mg/day Women: 16.4 mg/ day SUL: 17 mg

Claim(s) of supplements	The evidence	Possible dangers of high doses
It has been claimed that extra salt is needed if you sweat a lot or exercise in hot, humid conditions; advocated for treating cramp	Excessive sweating during exercise may cause a marked loss of sodium, but as salt is present in most foods, supplements are usually unnecessary; extra salt is more likely to cause, rather than prevent, cramp – dehydration is normally the cause of cramp (together possibly with a shortage of potassium)	High salt intakes may increase blood pressure, risk of stroke, fluid retention and upset the electrolyte balance of the body
May help to reduce blood pressure and encourage sodium excretion	Extra potassium is not known to enhance performance; may help to prevent cramp	Excess is excreted, therefore toxicity is very rare
Extra iron can improve the oxygen -carrying capacity of red blood cells, and therefore improve aerobic performance; can prevent or treat anaemia	Iron-deficiency anaemia can impair performance especially in aerobic activity; exercise destroys red blood cells and haemoglobin and increases loss of iron, therefore iron requirements of sportspeople may be slightly higher than that of sedentary people; iron is lost through menstruation, so supplements may be sensible for sports-women	High doses may cause constipation and stomach discomfort; they may also interact with zinc, reducing its absorption

Mineral	Function(s)	Sources	RNI and SUL*
Zinc	A component of many enzymes involved in the metabolism of proteins, carbohydrates and fats; helps to heal wounds; assists the immune system; needed for building cells	Meat, eggs, wholegrain cereals, milk and dairy products	Men: 9.5 mg/day Women: 7 mg/day SUL: 25 mg
Magnesium	Involved in the formation of new cells, in muscle contraction and nerve functions; assists with energy production; helps to regulate calcium metabolism; forms part of the mineral structure of bones	Cereals, vegetables, fruit, potatoes, milk	Men: 300 mg/day Women: 270 mg/day SUL: 400 mg
Phosphorus	Assists in bone and teeth formation; involved in tenergy metabolism as a component of ATP	Cereals, meat, fish, milk and dairy products, green vegetables	550 mg/day SUL: 250 mg from supplements

*RNI = Reference nutrient intake
USL = Upper safe levels are guides for self-supplementation. These are maximum levels which
   should not be exceeded unless advised by a qualified health professional.
**NV = no value published.

Sources:
Department of Health, 1991.
Food Standards Agency, 2003.

SUL = Safe Upper Limit recommended by the Expert Group on Vitamins and Minerals, an independent advisory committee to the Food Standards Agency.

Claim(s) of supplements	The evidence	Possible dangers of high doses
Suggest a possible role in high-intensity and strength exercises; may help to boost the immune system	Studies have failed to show that extra zinc is of any benefit to performance; sportspeople with a zinc deficiency may have an impaired immune system, so an adequate intake is important	High doses may cause nausea and vomiting; daily doses of more than 50 mg also interfere with the absorption of iron and other minerals, leading to iron-deficiency anaemia
Magnesium status may be related to aerobic capacity	Studies have failed to show that magnesium supplements are beneficial to performance	May cause diarrhoea
It has been claimed that phosphate loading enhances aerobic performance and delays fatigue	The consensus is that phosphate loading is of little benefit to performance	High intakes over a long period of time may lower blood calcium levels

List of Abbreviations

ACSM	American College of Sports Medicine	GI	glycaemic index
ADP	adenosine diphosphate	HDL	high density lipoprotein
ALA	alpha-linolenic acid	HMB	beta-hydroxy beta-methylbutyrate
ATP	adenosine triphosphate	IAA	indispensable amino acid
BCAA	branched-chain amino acids	IGF-I	insulin-like growth factor-I
BMI	Body Mass Index	IOC	International Olympic Committee
BMR	basal metabolic rate	LDL	low density lipoprotein
BV	Biological Value	MRP	Meal Replacement Product
DAA	dispensable amino acid	PC	phosphocreatine
DHA	docosahexanoic acid	RDA	Recommended Daily Amount
DHEA	dehydroepiandrosterone	RMR	resting metabolic rate
DoH	Department of Health	RNI	Reference Nutrient Intake
DRV	Dietary Reference Value	ST	slow-twitch (type I) muscle fibres
EFA	essential fatty acid	USL	upper safe level
EPA	eicosapentanoic acid	VO_2max	maximal aerobic capacit
FT	fast-twitch (type II) muscle fibres		

List of Weights and Measures

Symbols used:

g	gram
h	hour
kcal	kilocalorie
kJ	kilojoule
L	litre
m	metre
min	minute
mg	milligram (1000 g = 1 g)
ml	millilitre
mmol	millimole
mph	miles per hour
sec	seconds
tbsp	tablespoon
tsp	teaspoon
dl	decilitre (10 dl = 1 L)
µg	microgram (1000 µg = 1 mg)
<	less than
>	greater than
°C	degree Celsius

Conversions:

1 kcal	=	4.2 kJ		25 ml	=	1 fl oz
25 g	=	1 oz		600 ml	=	1 pint
450 g	=	1 lb		5 ml	=	1 tsp
1 kg	=	2.2 lb		15 ml	=	1 tbsp

REFERENCES

Aceto, C. (1997), *Everything You Need to Know about Fat Loss* (Adamsville TN: Fundco).

ACSM (1996), 'Position stand on exercise and fluid replacement', *Med. Sci. Sports and Ex.*, vol. 28, pp. i–vii.

ACSM/ADA/DC (2000), 'Position of the American Dietetic Association, Dietitians of Canada, and the American College of Sports Medicine: nutrition and athletic performance', Med. *Sci. Sports and Ex.*, vol. 32 (12), pp. 2130–45.

Ahlborg, B. *et al.* (1967), 'Human muscle glycogen content and capacity for prolonged exercise after different diets.' *Forsvarsmedicin*, vol. 3. pp. 85–99.

Albrink, M. J. (1978), 'Dietary fibre, plasma insulin and obesity', *Am. J. Clin. Nutr.*, vol. 31, S277–9.

American Dietetic Association (1993), 'Position of The American Dietetic Association and the Canadian Dietetic Association: nutrition for physical fitness and athletic performance for adults,' *J. Am. Diet. Assoc.*, vol. 93, pp. 691–6.

Anderson, M. *et al.* (2000), 'Improved 2000 rowing performance in competitive oars-women after caffeine ingestion', *Int. J. Sport Nutr.*, vol. 10, pp. 464–75.

Antonio, J. and Street, C. (1999), 'Glutamine: a potentially useful supplement for athletes', *Can. J. Appl. Physiol.*, vol. 24 (1): S69–S77.

Armstrong, L. E. (2002), 'Caffeine, body fluid-electrolyte balance and exercise performance', *Int. J. Sport Nutr.*, vol. 12, pp. 189–206.

Armstrong, L. E. *et al.* (1985), 'Influence of diuretic-induced dehydration on competitive running performance', *Med. Sci. Sports Ex.*, vol. 17, pp. 456–61.

– (1998), 'Urinary indices during dehydration, exercise and rehydration', *Int. J. Sport Nutr.*, vol. 8, pp. 345–55.

Ashenden, M. J. et al. (1998), 'Serum ferritin and anaemia in trained female athletes', *Int. J. Sport Nutr.*, vol. 8, pp. 223–9.

Barr S. I. and Costill D. L. (1989), 'Water. can the endurance athlete get too much of a good thing?' *J. Am. Diet. Assoc.* vol. 89, pp. 1629–32.

Barr, T. C. *et al.* (1995), 'Periodic carbohydrate replacement during 50 min. of high-intensity cycling improves subsequent spring performance', *Int. J. Sports Nutr.*, vol. 5, pp. 151–8.

Bazzare, T. L. *et al.* (1986), 'Incidence of poor nutritional status among triathletes, endurance athletes and controls', *Med. Sci. Sports Ex.*, vol. 18, p. 590.

Beals, K. A. & Manore, M. M. (1994), 'The prevalence and consequences of subclinical eating disorders in female athletes', *Int. J. Sport Nutr.*, vol. 4, pp. 157–95.

Bell, D. G. *et al.* (2001), 'Effect of caffeine and ephedrine ingestion on anaerobic exercise performance', *Med. Sci. Sport Exerc.*, vol. 33 (8), pp. 1399–1403.

Below, P. R. *et al.* (1994), 'Fluid and carbohydrate ingestion independently improve performance during one hour of intense exercise', *Med. Sci. Sports Ex.*, vol. 27, pp. 200–10.

Bergstrom, J. *et al.* (1976), 'Diet, muscle glycogen and physical performance', *Acta Physiol Scand.*, vol. 71. pp. 140–50.

Bishop, N. C. *et al.* (2002), 'Influence of carbohydrate supplementation on plasma cytokine and neutrophil degranulation responses to high intensity intermittent exercise', *Int. J. Sport Nutr.*, vol. 12, pp. 145–56.

Bledsoe, J. (1999), 'Can taking glutamine boost your immune system?', *Peak Performance*, vol. 116, pp. 1–4.

Bloomer, R. J. *et al.* (2000), 'Effects of meal form and composition on plasma testosterone, cortisol and insulin following resistance exercise', *Int. J. Sport Nutr.*, vol. 10, pp. 415–24.

Bosselaers, I. *et al.* (1994), 'Twenty-four-hour energy expenditure and substrate utilisation in bodybuilders', *Am. J. Clin. Nutr.*, vol. 59, pp. 10–12.

Bounous, G. & Gold, P. (1991), 'The biological activity of un-denatured whey proteins: role of glutathione', *Clin. Invest. Med.*, vol. 4, pp. 296–309.

Brilla, L. R. & Conte, V. (2000), 'Effects of a novel zinc-magnesium formulation on hormones and strength', J. *Exerc. Physiol. Online*, vol. 3 (4), pp. 1–15.

Broeder, C. E. *et al.* (2000), 'The Andro Project', *Arch. Intern. Med.*, vol. 160 (20), pp. 3093–104.

Brouns, F. *et al.* (1998), 'The effect of different rehydration drinks on post-exercise electrolyte excretion in trained athletes', *Int. J. Sports Med.*, vol. 19, pp. 56–60.

Brown, G. A. *et al.* (2000), 'Effects of anabolic precursors on serum testosterone concentrations and adaptations to resistance training in young men', *Int. J. Sport Nutr.*, vol. 10, pp. 340–59.

Brown, G. A. *et al.* (1999), 'Effect of oral DHEA on serum testosterone and adaptations to resistance training in young men', *J. A. P. Online*, vol. 87(6), pp. 2007–15,

Bryce-Smith, D. and Simpson, R. (1984), 'Anorexia, depression and zinc deficiency', *Lancet*, vol. 2, p. 1162.

Burke, D. G. *et al.* (2001a), 'The effect of alpha lipoic supplementation on resting creatine during acute creatine loading', (conference abstract). *FASEB Journal*, vol. 15 (5), pp. A814.

–(2001b), 'The effect of whey protein supplementation with and without creatine monohydrate combined with resistance training on lean tissue mass and muscle strength', *Int. J. Sport Nutr.*, vol. 11, pp. 349–64.

–(2000), 'The effect of continuous low dose creatine supplementation on force, power and total work', *Int. J. Sport Nutr.*, vol. 10, pp. 235–44.

–(1993), 'Muscle glycogen storage after prolonged exercise: effect of glycaemic index of carbohydrate feedings', *J. Appl. Physiol.*, vol. 75, pp. 1019–23.

–(1998), 'Glycaemic index – a new tool in sports nutrition', *Int. J. Sport Nutr.*, vol. 8, pp. 401–15.

Bussau, V. A. *et al.*, (2002), 'Carbohydrate loading in human muscle: an improved 1-day protocol.' *Eur J. Appl. Physiol.*, vol. 87, pp. 290–295.

Butterfield G. E. (1996), 'Ergogenic Aids: Evaluating sport nutrition products', *Int. Sport Nutr.* vol. 6, pp. 191-7.

Cahill, C. F. (1976), 'Starvation in Man', *J. Clin. Endocrinol. Metab.*, vol. 5, pp. 397–415.

Candow, D. G. *et al.* (2001), 'Effect of glutamine supplementation combined with resistance training in young adults', *Eur. J. Appl. Physiol.*, vol. 86 (2), pp. 142–9.

Cann, C. E. et al. (1984), 'Decreased spinal mineral content in amenhorreic women', *JAMA*, vol. 251, pp. 626–9.

Carbon, R. (2002), 'The Female athlete triad does not exist', *Sports Care News*, 26, pp. 3–5.

Castell, L. M. & Newsholme, E. A. (1997), 'The effects of oral glutamine supplementation on athletes after prolonged exhaustive exercise', *Nutrition*, vol. 13, pp. 738–42.

Catlin, D. H. et al. (2000), 'Trace contamination of over-the-counter androstenedione and positive urine tests for nandrolone metabolite', *J. Am. Med. Assoc.*, vol. 284, pp. 2618–21.

Chan, W. (2003), *Food & Diet Counter*, London: Hamlyn.

Cheuvront, S. N. (1999), 'The diet zone and athletic performance', *Sports Medicine*, vol. 27(4), pp. 213–28.

Christensen, E. H. & Hansen, O. (1939), 'Arbeitsfahigheit und Ernahrung', *Skand Arch Physiol*, vol. 81, pp. 160–71.

Chryssanthopoulos, C. *et al.* (2002), 'The effect of a high carbohydrate meal on endurance running capacity', *Int. J. Sport Nutr.*, vol. 12, pp. 157–71.

Clark, J. F. (1997), 'Creatine and phosphocreatine: a review', *J. Athletic Training*, vol. 32 (1), pp. 45–50.

Clark, N. (1995), 'Nutrition quackery: when claims are too good to be true', *Phys. Sports Med.*, vol. 23, pp. 7–8.

Coggan, A. R. & Coyle, E. F. (1991), 'Carbohydrate ingestion during prolonged exercise: effects on metabolism and performance', in J. Holloszy (ed.), *Exercise and Sports Science Reviews*, vol. 19 (Baltimore: Williams & Wilkins), pp. 1–40.

Igan, M. *et al.* (1991), 'Micronutrient status of endurance athletes affects haematology and performance', *J. Appl. Nutr.*, vol. 43(1), pp. 27–36.

CompEat 5 (Grantham: Nutrition Systems).

Cook, J. D. (1994), 'The effect of endurance training on iron metabolism', *Sem. Hemat.*, vol. 31, pp. 146–54.

Costill, D. L. & Hargreaves, M. (1992), 'Carbohydrate nutrition and fatigue', *Sports Med.*, vol. 13, pp. 86–92.

Costill, D. L. (1985), 'Carbohydrate nutrition before, during and after exercise', *Fed. Proc.*, vol. 44, pp. 364–368.

–(1986), *Inside Running: Basics of Sports Physiology* (Indianapolis: Benchmark Press), p. 189.

–(1988), 'Carbohydrates for exercise: dietary demands for optimal performance', *Int. J. Sports Med.*, vol. 9, pp. 1–18.

Costill, D. L. & Miller, J. (1980), 'Nutrition for endurance sport: carbohydrate and fluid balance', *Int. J. Sports Med.*, vol. 1, pp. 2–14.

Costill, D. L. *et al.* (1971), 'Muscle glycogen utilisation during prolonged exercise on successive days', *J. Appl. Physiol.*, vol. 31, pp. 834–8.

Cox, G. *et al.* (2002), 'Acute creatine supplementation and performance during a field test simulating match play in elite female soccer players', *Int. J. Sport Nutr.*, vol. 12, pp. 33–46.

Coyle, E. F. (1995), 'Substrate utilization during exercise in active people', *Am. J. Clin. Nutr.*, vol. 61 (suppl), pp. 968–79.

–(1991), 'Timing and method of increased carbohydrate intake to cope with heavy training, competition and recovery', *J. Sports Sci.*, vol. 9 (suppl.), pp. 29–52.

–(1988), 'Carbohydrates and athletic performance', *Sports Sci. Exch. Sports Nutr. Gatorade Sports Science Institute*, vol. 1.

Cupisti, A. *et al.* (2002), 'Nutrition knowledge and dietary composition in Italian female athletes and non-athletes', *Int. J. Sport Nutr.*, vol. 12, pp. 207–19.

Dangin, M. *et al.* (2000), 'The digestion rate of protein is an independent regulating factor of postprandial protein retention', *Am. Physiol. Soc. abstracts*, 7: 022E.

Davis, C. (1993), 'Body image, dieting behaviours and personality factors: a study of high-performance female athletes', *Int. J. Sport Psych.*, vol. 23, pp. 179–92.

Davis, J. M. *et al.* (1988), 'Carbohydrate-electrolyte drinks: effects on endurance cycling in the heat', *Am. J. Clin. Nutr.*, vol. 48, pp. 1023–30.

DeMarco, H. M. *et al.* (1999), *Med. Sci. Sports Ex.*, vol. 31(1), pp. 164–70.

Department of Health (1994), *Nutritional Food Guide* (Norwich: HMSO).

Dodd, S. L. *et al.* (1993), 'Caffeine and exercise performance', *Sports Med.*, vol. 15, pp. 14–23.

Dreon, D. M. *et al.* (1999), 'A very low-fat diet is not associated with improved lipoprotein profiles in men with a predominance of large low-density lipoproteins', *Am. J. Clin. Nutr.*, vol. 69, pp. 411-18.

Drinkwater, B. L. (1986), 'Bone mineral content after resumption of menses in amenorrheic athletes', *JAMA*, vol. 256, pp. 380-2.

–*et al.* (1984), 'Bone mineral content of amenorrheic and eumenorrheic athletes', *New England. J. Med.*, vol. 311, pp. 277–81.

Dulloo, A. G. *et al.* (1999), 'Efficacy of a green tea extract rich in catechins polyphenols and caffeine in increasing 24 hour energy expenditure and fat oxidation in humans', *Am. J. Clin. Nutr.*, vol. 70, pp. 1040–5.

Durnin, J. V. G. A. & Womersley, J. (1974), *Brit. J. Nutr.*, vol. 32, p. 77.

Dueck, C. A. et al. (1996), 'Role of energy balance in athletic menstrual dysfunction', *Int. J. Sport Nutr.*, vol. 6, pp. 165–90.

Edwards, J. R. *et al.* (1993), 'Energy balance in highly trained female endurance runners', *Med. Sci. Sports Ex.*, vol. 25(12), pp. 1398–1404.

Erasmus, U. (1996), *Fats that Heal: Fats that Kill* (Alive Books).

European Federation of Health Product Manufacturers and UK Council for Responsible Nutrition (1997), Report on upper safe levels for supplements.

Faff, J. (2001), 'Effects of antioxidant supplementation in athletes on the exercise-induced oxidative stress', *Biology of Sport*, vol. 18 (1), pp. 3–20.

Fairchild, T. J. *et al.* (2002), 'Rapid carbohydrate loading after a short bout of near maximal-intensity exercise.' *Med Sci Sports Exer.*, pp. 980–986.

Febbraio, M. A. & Stewart, K. L. (1996), 'CHO feeding before prolonged exercise: effect of glycaemic index on muscle glycogenolysis and exercise performance', *J. Appl. Phsyiol.*, vol. 81, pp. 1115–20.

Flatt, J. P. (1993), 'Dietary fat, carbohydrate balance and weight maintenance', *Ann NY Acad. Sci.*, vol. 683, pp. 122–40.

Fleck, S. J. & Reimers, K. J. (1994), 'The practice of making weight: does it affect performance?', *Strength and Cond.*, vol. 1, pp. 66–7.

Fogelholm, M. (1994), 'Effects of bodyweight reduction on sports performance', *Sports Med.*, vol. 18(14), pp. 249–67.

Food Standards Agency (2002), 'Consumer attitudes to Food Survey, 2001'.

Forsythe, W. (1995), 'Soy protein, thyroid regulation and cholesterol metabolism', *J. Nutr.*, vol. 125(3), pp. 619–23.

Fretsos, J. A. & Baer, J. T. (1997), 'Increased energy and nutrient intake during training and competition improves elite triathletes' endurance performance', *Int. J. Sport Nutr.*, vol. 7, pp. 61–71.

Galloway, S. D. R. & Maughan, R. (2000), 'The effects of substrate and fluid provision on thermoregulatory and metabolic responses to prolonged exercise in a hot environment', *J. Sports Sci.*, vol. 18 (5), pp. 339–51.

Garfinkel, P. E. & Garner, D. M. (1982), *Anorexia nervosa: a multidimensional perspective* (New York: Brunner/Mazel).

Gibala, M. J. (2000), 'Nutritional supplementation and resistance exercise: what is the evidence for enhanced skeletal muscle hypertrophy?', *Can. J. Appl. Physiol.*, vol. 25 (6), pp. 524–35

Gisolphi, C. V. et al. (1995), 'Effect of sodium concentration in a carbohydrate-electrolyte solution on intestinal absorption', *Med. Sci. Sports Ex.*, vol. 27(10), pp. 1414–20.

Goldfarb, A. H. (1999), 'Nutritional antioxidants as therapeutic and preventative modalities in exercise-induced muscle damage,' *Can. J. Appl. Physiol.*, vol. 24(3), pp. 249–66.

Gontzea, I. *et al.* (1975), 'The influence of adaptation to physical effort on nitrogen balance in man', *Nutr. Rep. Int.*, vol. 22, pp. 213–16.

Gonzalez-Alonzo, J. *et al.* (1992), 'Rehydration after exercise with common beverages and water', *Int. J. Sports Med.*, vol. 13, pp. 399–406.

Graham, T. E. & Spriet, L. L. (1991), 'Performance and metabolic responses to a high caffeine dose during prolonged exercise', *J. Appl. Physiol.*, 71(6): pp. 2292-8.

Grandjean, A. (2000), 'The effect of caffeinated, non-caffeinated, caloric and non-caloric beverages on hydration', *J. Am. Coll. Nutr.*, vol. 19, pp. 591–600.

Green, A. L. *et al.* (1996), 'Carbohydrate augments creatine accumulation during creatine supplementation in humans', *Am. J. Physiol.*, vol. 271, E821–6.

Greenhaff, P. L. (1997), 'Creatine supplementation and implications for exercise performance and guidelines for creatine supplementation', in A. Jeukendrup *et al.* (eds), *Advances in Training and Nutrition for Endurance Sports* (Maastrict: Novertis Nutrition Research Unit), pp. 8–11.

Halliwell, B. and Gutteridge, J. M. C. (1985), *Free Radicals in Biology and Medicine*, (Oxford: Clarendon Press), pp. 162–4.

Hargreaves, M. & Snow, R. (2001), 'Amino acids and endurance exercise', *Int. J. Sport Nutr.*, vol. 11, pp. 133–145.

Harris, R. C. (1998), 'Ergogenics 1', *Peak Performance*, vol. 112, pp. 2–6.

Harris, R. C. *et al.* (1992), 'Elevation of creatine in resting and exercised muscle of normal subjects by creatine supplementation', *Clin. Sci.*, vol. 82, pp. 367–74.

Haub, M. D. (1998), 'Acute l-glutamine ingestion does not improve maximal effort exercise', *J. Sport Med. Phys. Fitness*, vol. 38, pp. 240–4.

Haussinger, D. *et al.* (1996), 'The role of cellular hydration in the regulation of cell functioning', *Biochem. J.*, vol. 31, pp. 697–710.

Herman, P. and Polivy, J. (1991), 'Fat is a psychological issue', *New Scientist*, 16 Nov., pp. 41–5.

Hickey, H. S. *et al.* (1994), 'Drinking behaviour and exercise-thermal stress: role of drink carbonation', *Int. J. Sport Nutr.*, vol. 4, pp. 8–12.

Hitchins, S. *et al.* (1999), 'Glycerol hyperhydration improves cycle time trial performance in hot humid conditions', *Eur. J. Appl. Physiol. Occup. Physiol.*, vol. 80(5), pp. 494–501.

Holt, S. J. (1992), 'Relationship of satiety to postprandial glycaemic, insulin and cholecystokinin responses', *Appetite*, vol. 18, pp. 129–41.

Horton, T. J. *et al.* (1995), 'Fat and carbohydrate overfeeding in humans: different effects on energy storage', *Am. J. Clin. Nutr.*, vol. 62, pp. 19–29.

Houtkooper, L. B. (2000), 'Body composition', in Manore, M. M. & Thompson, J. L. *Sport Nutrition for Health and Performance*, Human Kinetics, pp. 199-219.

Hultman, E. *et al.* (1996), 'Muscle creatine loading in man', *J. Appl. Physiol.*, vol. 81, pp. 232–9.

Hunter, A. M. *et al.* (2002), 'Caffeine ingestion does not alter performance during a 100-km cycling time trial performance', *Int. J. Sport Nutr.*, vol. 12, pp. 438–52.

Hytten, F. E. & Leitch, I. (1971), *The Physiology of Human Pregnancy*, 2nd ed. (Oxford: Blackwell Scientific Publications).

Institute of Medicine (1990), *Nutrition during Pregnancy. Part 1: Weight Gain* (Washington DC: National Academy Press).

Ivy, J. L. *et al.* (1988a), 'Muscle glycogen synthesis after exercise: effect of time of carbohydrate ingestion', *J. Appl. Physiol.*, vol. 64, pp. 1480–5.

– (1988b), 'Muscle glycogen storage after different amounts of carbohydrate ingestion', *J. Appl. Physiol.*, vol. 65, pp. 2018–23.

Jacobs, K. A. & Sherman, W. M. (1999), 'The efficacy of carbohydrate supplementation and chronic high-carbohydrate diets for improving endurance performance', *Int. J. Sport Nutr.*, vol. 9, pp. 92–115.

Jenkins, D. J. *et al.* (1987), 'Metabolic effects of a low GI diet', *Am. J. Clin. Nutr.*, vol. 46, pp. 968–75.

Jowko, E. *et al.*, (2001) 'Creatine and HMB additively increase lean body mass and muscle strength during a weight training programme', *Nutrition*, vol. 17 (7), pp. 558–66.

Kamber, M. *et al.* (2001), 'Nutritional supplements as a source for positive doping cases?', *Int. J. Sports Nutr.*, vol. 11, pp. 258–63.

Kanter, M. M. & Eddy, D. M. (1992), 'Effect of antioxidant supplementation on serum markers of lipid peroxidation and skeletal damage following eccentric exercise', *Med. Sci. Sports Ex.*, vol. 24 (supp.), S17.

Kanter, M. M. *et al.* (1993), 'Effects of an antioxidant mixture on lipid peroxidation at rest and post-exercise', *J. Appl. Physiol.*, vol. 74, pp. 965–9.

Karlsson, J. & Saltin, B. (1971), 'Diet, muscle glycogen and endurance performance', *J. Appl. Physiol.*, vol. 31, pp. 201–6.

Keizer, H. A. et al. (1986), 'Influence of liquid or solid meals on muscle glycogen resynthesis, plasma fuel hormone response and maximal physical working capacity', *Int. J. Sports Med.*, vol. 8, pp. 99–104.

Kiens, B. *et al.* (1990), 'Benefit of simple carbohydrates on the early post-exercise muscle glycogen repletion in male athletes', *Med., Sci. Sports Ex.* (suppl.), S88.

King, D. S. *et al.* (1999), 'Effects of oral androstenedione on serum testosterone and adaptations to resistance training in young men', *J. Am. Med. Assoc.*, vol. 281(21), pp. 2020–8.

Kreider, R. B. *et al.* (2000), 'Effects of calcium-HMB supplementation during training on markers of catabolism, body composition, strength and sprint performance', *J. Exerc. Physiol.*, vol. 3 (4), pp. 48–59.

–(1996), 'Effects of ingesting supplements designed to promote lean tissue accretion on body composition during resistance training', *Int. J. Sport Nutr.*, vol. 63, pp. 234–46.

Krotkiewski, M. *et al.* (1994), 'Prevention of muscle soreness by pre-treatment with anti-oxidants', *Scand. J. Med. Sci. Sports*, vol. 4, pp. 191–9.

Krumbach, C. J. *et al.* (1999), 'A report of vitamin and mineral supplement use among University Athletes in a division I Institution', *Int. J. Sport Nutr.*, vol. 9, p. 416–25.

Lean, M. E. J. *et al.* (1995), 'Waist circumference as a measure for indicating need for weight management', *BMJ*, vol. 311, pp. 158–61.

Leeds, A., Brand Miller, J., Foster-Powell, K. & Colagiuri, S. (2000), *The Glucose Revolution* (London: Hodder & Stoughton), p. 29.

Lemon P. W. R. (1998), 'Effects of exercise on dietary protein requirements', *Int. J. Sport Nutr.*, vol. 8, pp. 426-47.

–(1992), 'Protein requirements and muscle mass/strength changes during intensive training in novice bodybuilders, *J. Appl. Physiol.*, vol. 73, pp. 767–75.

Lloyd, T. *et al.* (1986), 'Women athletes with menstrual irregularity have increased musculo-skeletal injuries', *Med. Sci. Sports Ex.*, vol. 18, pp. 3427–9.

Lohman T. G. (1992), Basic concepts in body composition assessment, in *Advances in Body Composition Assessment*, Human Kinetics, pp. 109-118.

Loucks, A. B. *et al.* (1989), 'Alterations in the hypothalamic-pituitary-ovarian and the hypothalamic-pituitary axes in athletic women', *J. Clinical Endocrinol. Metab.*, vol. 68, pp. 402–22.

McConnell, G.K., Burge, C. M, Skinner, S.L. & Hargreaves, M. (1997), 'Influence of ingested fluid volume on physiological responses during prolonged exercise', *Acta Phys. Scan.*, vol. 160, pp. 149-56.

Macintosh, B.R. *et al.* (1995), 'Caffeine ingestion and performance of a 1500-metre swim',. *Can. J. Appl. Physiol.*, 20(2): p. 168-77.

McLean, D. A. *et al.* (1994), 'Branch-chain amino acids augment ammonia metabolism while attenuating protein breakdown during exercise', *Am. J. Physiol.*, vol. 267, E1010–22.

McNaughton, L. R. *et al.* (1998), 'The effects of creatine supplementation on high intensity exercise performance in elite performers', *Eur. J. Appl. Physiol.*, vol. 78, pp. 236–40.

Madsen, K. *et al.* (1996), 'Effects of glucose and glucose plus branched chain amino acids or placebo on bike performance over 100 km', *J. Appl. Physiol.*, vol. 81, pp. 2644–50.

MAFF/RSC (1991), *McCance and Widdowson's The Composition of Foods*, 5th ed. (Cambridge: MAFF/RSC).

Maffucci, D. M. & McMurray, R. G. (2000), 'Towards optimising the timing of the pre-exercise meal', *Int. J Sport Nutr.*, vol. 10, pp. 103–13.

Maughan, R. J. *et al.* (1996), 'Rehydration and recovery after exercise', *Sports Sci. Ex.*, vol. 9(62), pp. 1–5.

Mason, W. L. *et al.* (1993), 'Carbohydrate ingestion during exercise: liquid vs solid feedings', *Med. Sci. Sports Ex.*, vol. 25, pp. 966–9.

Mayhew, D. L. *et al.* (2002), 'Effects of long term creatine supplementation on liver and kidney function in American Football players', *Int. J. Sport Nutr.*, vol. 12, pp. 453–60.

Melby, C. *et al.* (1993), 'Effect of acute resistance exercise on resting metabolic rate', *J. Appl. Physiol.*, vol. 75, pp. 1847–53.

Mihic, S. *et al.* (2000), 'Acute creatine loading increases fat free mass but does not affect blood pressure, plasma creatinine or CK activity in men and women', *Med. Sci. Sport. Exerc.*, vol. 32, pp. 291–6.

Miller, S. L. *et al.* (2002), 'Metabolic responses to provision of mixed protein-carbohydrate supplementation during endurance exercise attenuate the increases in cortisol', *Int. J. Sport Nutr.*, vol. 12, pp. 384–97.

Minehan, M. R. *et al.* (2002), 'Effect of flavour and awareness of kilojoule content of drinks on preference and fluid balance in team sports', *Int. J. Sport Nutr.*, vol. 12, pp. 81–92.

Mountain, S. J. & Coyle, E. F. (1992), 'The influence of graded dehydration on hyper-thermia and cardiovascular drift during exercise', *J. Appl. Physiol.*, vol. 73, pp. 1340–50.

Mujika, I. *et al.* (1996), 'Creatine supplementation does not improve sprint performance in competitive swimmers', *Med. Sci. Sports. Exerc.*, vol. 28, pp. 1435–41.

Mullins, V. A. *et al.* (2001), 'Nutritional status of US elite female heptathletes during training', *Int. J. Sport Nutr.*, vol. 11, pp. 299–314.

National Institutes of Health (1994), 'Weight cycling', *J. Am. Med. Assoc.*, vol. 272(15), pp. 1196–1202.

Nelson, A. *et al.* (1997), 'Creatine supplementation raises anaerobic threshold', *FASEB J.*, vol. 11, A586 (abstract).

Nelson, M. E. *et al.* (1986), 'Diet and bone status in amenorrheic runners', *Am. J. Clin. Nutr.*, vol. 43, pp. 910–16.

Nissan, S. *et al.* (1996), 'Effect of leucine meta-bolite HMB on muscle metabolism during resistance exercise training', *J. Appl. Physiol.*, vol. 81, pp. 2095–2104.

– (1997), 'Effect of feeding HMB on body composition and strength in woman', *FASEB J.*, vol. 11, A150 (abstract).

Noakes, T. D. (1993), 'Fluid replacement during exercise', *Exerc. Sport Sci. Rev.*, vol. 21, pp. 297-330.

Paddon-Jones, D. *et al.* (2001), 'Short term HMB supplementation does not reduce symptoms of eccentric muscle damage', *Int. J. Sport Nutr.*, vol. 11, pp. 442–50.

Pannomans, D. L. *et al.* (1997), 'Calcium excretion, apparent calcium absorption and calcium balance in young and elderly subjects: influence of protein intake', *Brit. J. Nutr.*, Vol. 77(5), pp. 721–9.

Parry-Billings *et al.* (1992), 'Plasma amino acid concentrations in over-training syndrome: possible effects on the immune system', *Med. Sci. Sport Ex.*, vol. 24, pp. 1353–8.

Peters, E. M. *et al.* (2001), 'Vitamin C supplementation attenuates the increases in circulating cortisol, adrenaline and anti-inflammatory polypeptides following ultra-marathon running', *Int. J. Sports Med.*, vol. 22 (7), pp. 537–43.

–(1993), 'Vitamin C supplementation reduces the incidence of post-race symptoms of upper-respiratory-tract infection in ultra-marathon runners', *Am. J. Clin. Nutr.*, vol. 57, pp. 170–4.

Petrie, T. A. (1993), 'Disordered eating in female collegiate gymnasts', *J. Sport Ex. Psych.*, vol. 15, pp. 434–36.

Pollock, M. L. & Jackson, A. S. (1984), 'Research progress invalidation of clinical methods of assessing body composition', *Med. Sci. Sport Ex.*, vol. 16, pp. 606–13.

Poortmans, J. R. & Francaux, M. (1999), 'Long-term oral creatine supplementation does not impair renal function in healthy athletes', *Med. Sci. Sports Ex.*, vol. 31(8), pp. 1103–10.

Powers, M. E. (2002), 'The safety and efficacy of anabolic steroid precursors: What is the scientific evidence?', *J. Athol. Training*, vol. 37 (3), pp. 300–5.

Prentice, A. M. *et al.* (1989), 'Metabolism or appetite: questions of energy balance with particular reference to obesity', *J. Hum. Nutr. Diet.*, vol. 2, pp. 95–104.

Ready, S. L. *et al.* (1999), 'The effect of two sports drink formulations on muscle stress and performance', *Med. Sci. Sports Exerc.*, vol. 31(5), pp. S119

Robertson, J. *et al.* (1991), 'Increased blood antioxidant systems of runners in response to training load', *Clin. Sci.*, vol. 80, pp. 611–18.

Robinson. T. M. *et al.* (2000), 'Dietary creatine supplementation does not affect some haematological indices, or indices of muscle damage and hepatic and renal function', *Brit. J. Sports Med.*, vol. 34, pp. 284–8.

Rokitzki, L. *et al.* (1994), 'α-tocopherol supplementation in racing cyclists during extreme endurance training', *Int. J. Sports Nutr.*, vol. 4, pp. 235–64.

Rolls, B. J. & Shide, D. J. (1992), 'The influence of fat on food intake and body weight', *Nutr. Revs*, vol. 50(10), pp. 283–90.

Rosen, L. W. *et al.* (1986), *Physician Sports Med.*, vol. 14, pp. 79–86.

Rowbottom, D. G. *et al.* (1996), 'The energizing role of glutamine as an indicator of exercise stress and overtraining', *Sports Med.*, vol. 21 (2), pp. 80–97.

Samaha, F. F. *et al.* (2003) 'A low-carbohydrate as compared with a low-fat diet in severe obesity', *New England J. Med*, vol. 348, pp. 2074–2081.

Schokman, C. P. *et al.* (1999), 'Pre- and post game macronutrient intake of a group of elite Australian Football Player', *Int. J. Sport Nutr.*, vol. 9, pp. 60–9.

Sen, C. K. (2001) 'Antioxidants in exercise nutrition', *Sports Med.*, vol. 31(13), pp. 891-908.

Sherman, W. M. *et al.* (1981), 'Effect of exercise-diet manipulation on muscle glycogen and its subsequent utilisation during performance', *Int. J. Sports Med.*, vol. 2, pp. 114–18.

Shirreffs, S. M., *et al.* (1996), 'Post-exercise rehydration in man: effects of volume consumed and drink sodium content', *Med. Sci. Sports Ex.*, vol. 28, pp. 1260–71.

Short, S. H. & Short, W. R. (1983), 'Four-year study of university athletes' dietary intake', *J. Am. Diet. Assoc.*, vol. 82, pp. 632.

Sinning W. E. (1998), 'Body composition in athletes', in *Human Body Composition*, Roche A. F., Heymsfield S. B. & Lohman T. G., eds. Human Kinetics, pp. 257-73.

Slater, G. *et al.* (2001), 'HMB supplementation does not affect changes in strength or body composition during resistance training in trained men', *Int. J. Sport Nutr.*, vol. 11, pp. 383–96.

Sohlstrom, A. *et al.* (1992), 'Evaluation of simple methods to estimate total body fat in healthy women', *Scand. J. Sci. Med. Sport*, 2(4), pp. 207–11.

Speedy D. B., Noakes, T. D., Rogers, I. R., Thompson, J. M. D., Campbell, R. G. D., Kuttner, J. A., Boswel,l D. B., Wright, S. & Hamlin. M., (1999), 'Hyponatremia in ultradistance triathletes', *Med. Sci. Sports Exerc.*, 31: 809-15.

Spriet, L. (1995), 'Caffeine and performance', *Int. J. Sport Nutr.*, vol. 5 pp. S84–S99.

Steen, S. N. & McKinney, S. (1986), 'Nutrition assessment of college wrestlers', *Physician and Sports Med.*, vol. 14, pp. 100–106.

Steenge, G. R. *et al.* (1998), 'The stimulatory effect of insulin on creatine accummulation in human skeletal muscle', *Am. J. Physiol.*, vol. 275, pp. E974–9.

Stunkard, A. J. *et al.* (1986), 'An adoption study of human obesity', *New England J. Med.*, vol. 314, pp. 193–8.

– (1990), 'The body mass index of twins who have been reared apart', *New England J. Med.*, vol. 322, pp. 1483–7.

Subudhi, A. W. *et al.* (2001), 'Antioxidant status and oxidative stress in elite Alpine ski racers', *Int. J. Sport Nutr.*, vol. 11, pp. 32–41.

Sundgort-Borgon, J. (1994a), 'Eating disorders in female athletes', *Sports Med.*, vol. 17(3), pp. 176–88.

– (1994b), 'Risk and trigger factors for the development of eating disorders in female elite athletes', *Med. Sci. Sports Ex.*, vol. 26, pp. 414–19.

– and Larsen, S. (1993), 'Nutrient intake and eating behaviour in elite female athletes suffering from anorexia nervosa, anorexia athletica and bulimia nervosa', *Int. J. Sport Nutr.*, vol. 3, pp. 431–42.

Swaminathan, R. *et al.* (1980), 'Thermic effect of feeding carbohydrate, fat, protein and mixed meal in lean and obese subjects', *Am. J. Clin. Nutr.*, vol. 42, pp. 177–81.

Tarnopolsky, M. & MacLennan, D. P. (2000), 'Creatine monohydrate supplementation enhances high-intensity exercise performance in males and females', *Int. J. Sport Nutr.*, vol. 10, pp. 452–63.

–(1997), 'Post exercise protein-carbohydrate and carbohydrate supplements increase muscle glycogen in males and females'. *J. Appl. Physiol., Abstracts*, vol. 4, p. 332A

–(1992), 'Evaluation of protein requirements for trained strength athletes', *J. Appl. Physiol*, vol. 73, pp. 1986–95.

–(1988), 'Influence of protein intake and training status in nitrogen balance and lean body mass', *J. Appl. Physiol*, vol. 64, pp. 187–93.

Thomas, D. E. *et al.* (1991), 'Carbohydrate feeding before exercise: effect of glycaemic index', *Int. J. Sports Med.*, vol. 12, pp. 180–6.

– (1994), 'Plasma glucose levels after prolonged strenuous exercise correlate inversely with glycaemic response to food consumed before exercise', *Int. J Sports Nutr.*, vol. 4, pp. 261–73.

Thompson, D. *et al.* (2001), 'Prolonged vitamin C supplementation and recovery from demanding exercise', *Int. J. of Sport Nutr.*, vol. 11 (4), pp. 466–81.

Thomson, J. L. *et al.* (1996), 'Effects of diet and diet-plus-exercise programs on resting metabolic rate: a meta analysis', *Int. J. Sport Nutr.*, vol. 6, pp. 41–61.

Tiptan, C. M. (1987), *Physician and Sports Med.*, vol. 15, p. 160.

Tsintzas, O. K. *et al.* (1995), 'Influence of carbohydrate electrolyte drinks on marathon running performance', *Eur. J. Appl. Physiol.*, vol. 70, pp. 154–60.

Vahedi, K. (2000), 'Ischaemic stroke in a sportsman who consumed mahuang extract and creatine monohydrate for bodybuilding', *J. Neur., Neurosurgery and Psych.*, vol. 68, pp. 112–13.

Volek, J. S. (1997), 'Response of testosterone and cortisol concentrations to high-intensity resistance training following creatine supplementation', *J. Strength Cond. Res.*, vol. 11, pp. 182–7.

Volek, J. S. *et al.* (1999), 'Performance and muscle fibre adaptations to creatine supplementation and heavy resistance training', *Med. Sci. Sports Ex.*, vol. 31(8), pp. 1147–56.

– and Kraemer, W. J. (1996), 'Creatine supplementation: its effects on human muscular performance and body composition', *J. Strength Cond. Res.*, vol. 10(3), pp. 200–10.

Volek, J. S. *et al.* (1996), 'Creatine supplementation enhances muscular performance during high intensity resistance exercise', *J. Am. Diet Assoc.*, vol. 97, pp. 765–70.

Wagenmakers, A. J. M. *et al.* (1996), 'Carbohydrate feedings improve one-hour time-trial cycling performance', *Med. Sci. Sports Ex.*, vol. 28, supp. 37.

Walberg-Rankin, J. (20000, 'Forfeit the fat, leave the lean: optimising weight loss for athletes', *Gatorade Sports Science Exchange*, vol. 13 (1).

Welbourne, T. (1995), 'Increased plasma bicarbonate and growth hormone after an oral glutamine load', *Am. J. Clin. Nutr.*, vol. 61, pp. 1058–61.

Wemple, R. D. *et al.* (1997) 'Caffeine vs. Caffeine-free sports drinks: effects on urine production at rest and during prolonged exercise', *Int. J. Sports Med.* 18(1): pp. 40-6.

Wilk, B. & Bar-Or, O. (1996), 'Effect of drink flavour and sodium chloride on voluntary drinking and hydration in boys exercising in the heat', *J. Appl. Physiol.*, vol. 80, pp. 1112–17.

Williams, C. & Devlin, J. T. (eds) (1992), *Foods, Nutrition and Performance: An International Scientific Consensus* (London: Chapman & Hall).

Williams, M. H. (1992), *Nutrition for Fitness and Sport* (Dubuque, IO: William C. Brown).

– (1998), *The Ergogenics Edge* (Illinois: Human Kinetics).

– (1999), *Nutrition for Health, Fitness and Sport*, 5th ed. (New York: McGraw-Hill).

Williams, M. H. *et al.* (1999), *Creatine: The Power Supplement* (Illinois: Human Kinetics).

Wilmore, J. H. (1983), 'Body composition in sport and exercise', *Med. Sci. Sports Ex.*, vol. 15, pp. 21–31.

Zawadzki, K. M. *et al.* (1992), 'Carbohydrate-protein complex increases the rate of muscle glycogen storage after exercise', *J. Appl Physiol.*, vol. 72, pp. 1854–9.

Ziegenfuss, T. *et al.* (1997), 'Acute creatine ingestion: effects on muscle volume, anaerobic power, fluid volumes and protein turnover', *Med. Sci. Sports Ex.*, vol. 29, supp. 127.

Ziegler, P. J. *et al.* (1999), Nutritional and physiological status of US National Figure Skaters', *Int. J. Sport Nutr.*, vol. 9, pp. 345–60.

FURTHER READING

Aceto, Chris (1997), *Everything You Need to Know about Fat Loss* (Adamsville, TN: Fundco Printers).

Applegate, L. (2001) *Eat Smart Play Hard*, Rodale.

Bean, A. (2001) *The Complete Guide to Strength Training* 2nd ed, A & C Black.

Bean, A. (2002) *Food For Fitness* 2nd ed, A & C Black.

Bean, A. (2002) *Kids' Food For Fitness*, A & C Black.

Benardot, D. (2000), *Nutrition for Serious Athletes* (Illinois: Human Kinetics).

Brouns, Fred (1993), *Nutritional Needs of Athletes* (Chichester: J. Wiley).

Clark, Nancy (1997), *Nancy Clark's Sports Nutrition Guidebook*, 2nd ed. (Illinois: Human Kinetics).

Dorfman, Lisa (2000), *The Vegetarian Sports Nutrition Guide* (New York: J. Wiley).

Food Standards Agency (2002) *McCance & Widdowson's The Composition of Foods*, 6th summary ed, Royal Society of Chemistry.

Gastelu, Daniel and Hatfield, Fred (1997), *Dynamic Nutrition for Maximum Performance* (New York: Avery Publishing Group).

Girard Eberle, S. (2000) *Endurance Sports Nutrition*, Human Kinetics.

Hawley, John and Burke, Louise (1998), *Peak Performance* (St Leonards, NSW, Australia: Allen & Unwin).

Kleiner S. M. (2001), *Power Eating* 2nd ed., Human Kinetics.

Leeds, A., Brand-Miller, J., Foster-Powell, K. & Colagiuri, S. (1998), *The Glucose Revolution*, Hodder & Stoughton.

Reader's Digest Guide to Vitamins, Minerals and Supplements (2000) (London: Reader's Digest Association Ltd).

Thompson, R. A. and Sherman, R. T. (1993), *Helping Athletes with Eating Disorders* (Illinois: Human Kinetics).

Williams, C. and Devlin, J. T. (eds) (1992), *Foods, Nutrition and Performance: An International Scientific Consensus* (London: Chapman and Hall).

Williams, M. H. (1998). *The Ergogenics Edge* (Illinois: Human Kinetics).

Williams, M. H., Kreider, R. B. and Branch, J. D. (1999), *Creatine: The Power Supplement* (Illinois: Human Kinetics).

Wilmore, J. and Costill, D. (1994), *Physiology of Sport and Exercise* (Illinois: Human Kinetics).

USEFUL ADDRESSES

British Dietetic Association
5th floor, Charles House
148–9 Great Charles Street
Queensway
Birmingham   B3 3HT
www.bda.uk.com

British Nutrition Foundation
High Holborn House
52–54 High Holborn
London   WC1V 6RQ
www.nutrition.org.uk

Dietitians in Sport and Exercise Nutrition
PO Box 22360
London   W13 9FL

Eating Disorders Association
1st floor, Wensum House
103 Prince of Wales Road
Norwich   NR1 1DW
www.edauk.com

Food Standards Agency
Room 621, Hannibal House
PO Box 30080
London   SE1 6YA
www.foodstandards.gov.uk

**National Sports Medicine Institute
   of the UK**
32 Devonshire Street
London   W1G 6PX
www.nsmi.org.uk

The Nutrition Society
10 Cambridge Court
210 Shepherds Bush Road
London   W6 7NJ
www.nutsoc.org

Vegetarian Society
Parkdale
Dunham Road
Altrincham
Cheshire   WA14 4QG
www.vegsoc.org

ON-LINE RESOURCES

www.eatright.org, the website of the American Dietetic Association, gives nutrition news, tips and resources.

www.sdasolutions.com details nutrition and fitness software, including the dietary analysis software, Nutrition Publisher.

www.nutrition.org.uk The website of the British Nutrition Foundation provides nutrition fact sheets, information, and educational resources.

www.USDA.gov The website of the US Department of Agriculture contains useful and authoritative nutritional information.

www.intelihealth.com Daily news, health features, interactive quizzes, 'Ask the Expert,' and access to the USDA database for nutrient analysis can all be found here.

www.hsis.org provides good information on vitamins, minerals and supplements.

www.phys.com This website helps you work out your ideal weight, body fat percentage and calorie, fat, protein and carbohydrate needs.

www.mayohealth.org This US site offers good nutrition information in a fun, user-friendly format.

www.nsmi.org.uk has the largest sports medicine library in Europe, including up-to-date summaries of sports nutrition research.

www.edauk.com The website of the Eating Disorders Association where you will find information and help on all aspects of eating disorders

www.foodstandards.gov.uk The website of the government's Food Standards Agency has news of nutrition surveys, nutrition and health information.

www.vegsoc.org The Vegetarian Society's website provides information on general nutrition as well as hundreds of vegetarian recipes.

www.nutrio.com A US website that provides nutrition news, diet and fitness plans, menus and recipes.

www.webmd.com This comprehensive US website has a directory of food topics and advice on many aspects of nutrition and fitness.

INDEX